ISCHAEMIC HEART DISEASE AND EXERCISE

Ischaemic Heart Disease and Exercise

ROY J. SHEPHARD, M.D. (London), Ph.D.
Director, School of Physical & Health Education
and
Professor of Applied Physiology, Faculty of Medicine,
University of Toronto

A CROOM HELM BOOK

Distributed by
YEAR BOOK MEDICAL PUBLISHERS, INC.
35 East Wacker Drive, Chicago

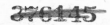

Distributed in Continental North, South and Central America, Hawaii, Puerto Rico and The Philippines by
Year Book Medical Publishers, Inc.
(ISBN 0-8151-7649-X)

by Arrangement with Croom Helm Ltd Publishers

CONTENTS

PREFACE

Exercise in the prevention and treatment of ischaemic heart disease remains a controversial issue. Exercise enthusiasts insist blindly that vigorous physical activity will both prevent and cure cardiac disease. If they commit their ideas to writing, it is usually in popular format, a lurid jacket spelling out a concept such as 'exercise and your heart'. At the other extreme are conservative physicians who know little of exercise, but argue with an aura of great dignity that statistical proof of the value of physical activity is lacking. If they choose to write, it is in sombre medical prose, a dark-blue spine carrying the gold-leaf lettering that spells the end of a patient's productive life — 'ischaemic heart disease' — period.

The present title — 'ischaemic heart disease *and* exercise' — reflects the author's personal philosophy. The book navigates carefully the treacherous strait that separates the Scylla-like temptations of euphoric popular commendation of exercise from the Charybdic whirlpool of cold statistical disdain. The voyage is charted from the perspective of varied and multidisciplinary ventures. After a period as cardiac research fellow at Guy's Hospital under the legendary Maurice Campbell, founder of the *British Heart Journal*, I gained broad experience in applied physiology, working in England, the US and Canada. More recently, I have served as professor to the Department of Preventive Medicine and Biostatistics at the University of Toronto. Now I find myself with a larger office, a carpet and the title of Director of the School of Physical and Health Education. The 'stress' of this somewhat chequered career has probably shortened my personal lifespan by several years, but at least it has provided insight into the respective viewpoints of exercise enthusiasts and agnostics. As in most arguments, the truth lies somewhere between the opposing factions. The present short volume sets on record the views I have formed in mediating many heated discussions. It attempts a careful, balanced and up-to-date review of both the advantages and the dangers of physical activity in cardiac disease.

A natural starting point is found in a brief description of the underlying pathology of cardiac disease. This is discussed in simple terms for the benefit of those who lack an extensive medical background. Attention is then focused on factors responsible for the waxing and waning of the 'cardiac epidemic', and the question is posed as to whether changing patterns of daily activity have contributed to this intriguing phenomenon of twentieth-century medicine. A critical look is then taken at the hazards of exercise, particular attention being directed to the possibility that physical activity will precipitate myocardial infarction and sudden death. Evidence that physical activity has therapeutic value is next discussed in the context of the primary, secondary and tertiary prevention of ischaemic heart disease. Possible beneficial effects of exercise are reviewed, and details of current therapeutic trials are carefully examined. Normal and pathological reactions of the heart to exercise are considered in the light of modern non-invasive diagnostic procedures — the electrocardiogram, echocardiography and the use of radionuclides. Practical principles of exercise prescription are related to the needs of hospital, outpatient and home phases of treatment. Mediators of the exercise response are discussed, and some important contraindications to exercise are noted. Drugs commonly taken by the cardiac patient are examined with particular reference to their impact upon stress testing and training patterns. Psycho-social variables are reviewed, including the influence of mood upon two key measures of successful treatment — return to normal employment and full sexual activity after myocardial infarction. Special problems of patients with angina, by-pass operations and peripheral vascular disease are covered, and comment is made upon particular features of cardiac disease in the female patient. A final chapter examines the topical issue of cost-benefit analyses from the standpoint of the patient, the physician and the community.

Such a broadly ranging book is intended to attract a broad readership, spanning the spectrum of medical and paramedical workers with an interest in the prevention and treatment of ischaemic heart disease. The text is written with a minimum of technical jargon, to accommodate a multidisciplinary audience. Nevertheless, all propositions are founded on sound medical, scientific and (where necessary) statistical discussion. Further research is facilitated by a bibliography of more than 1,300 recent references selected from the world literature.

As in previous writing, I must acknowledge with warm thanks my profound debt to many teachers, colleagues and students who have helped in shaping my present views. I still remember the crowded outpatient department of the early 1950s, with Dr Maurice Campbell vividly demonstrating simple clinical methods of distinguishing angina from benign chest pain. More recently, it has been a great pleasure to work closely with my good friend Dr Terence Kavanagh as physiological consultant to the Toronto Rehabilitation Centre. I have rejoiced in the practical triumphs of his innovative pattern of treatment, as new hope has come to some 2,000 'post-coronary' patients. I have shared Dr Kavanagh's excitement, as some of the patients from the Centre have completed marathon events in a little over three hours. Above all, I have had the total cooperation of Centre and patients in realising the tremendous research potential afforded by this programme. Such material is identified in this monograph as Toronto Rehabilitation Centre data. The past decade has also seen a most fruitful collaboration with Dr Peter Rechnitzer of the University of Western Ontario, and a distinguished group of investigators involved in the Southern Ontario multicentre exercise-heart trial. The team has included Drs G. Andrew, C. Buck, D. Cunningham, N. Jones, T. Kavanagh, N. Oldridge, J.C. Parker, P. Rechnitzer (director), S. Sangal and M. Yuhasz. Where not specifically attributed to one or more of these authors, such material is identified as Southern Ontario multicentre data. Again, this has brought budget, research material and above all a tremendous cross-fertilization of ideas. Several trained graduate students — Veena Pandit, Ken Sidney, Veli Niinimaa, Don Paterson, Mike Cox and Tony Verde — have greatly helped forward the departmental programme of cardiac research. Three decades of reading and scientific meetings have also played their part in the writing of this book. Where possible, I have acknowledged the sources of my information; however, material is sometimes absorbed almost subconsciously and, if a debt has been overlooked, I trust the donor will accept my apology.

The book poses a very practical question. Should we recommend that the coronary-prone and the cardiac patient become involved in vigorous exercise? The reader must judge how far an answer is given. Possibly, as he reads the final page a larger question mark will be forming in his brain. However, this is preferable to a facile and intellectually dissatisfying endorsement of exercise. At least the unanswered problems about physical activity will have been brought into focus. If confusion remains, it is a clearer confusion! This is the first step on the road towards definitive answers. If the book has done no more than facilitate the search for knowledge, I shall feel well rewarded as an author.

Roy J. Shephard
October 1980

1 PATHOLOGY OF ISCHAEMIC HEART DISEASE

I am in anguish! I writhe with pain!
Walls of my heart!
My heart is throbbing!

(Jeremiah 4[19], Jerusalem translation)

Ancient literature contains many passages that could be interpreted as describing manifestations of coronary vascular disease. Thus it is conceivable that the prophet Jeremiah personally experienced the anguish of anginal pain, and translations such as the Jerusalem Bible interpret his warning of a northern invasion of Israel in the tragic poetry of a cardiac analogy. The Ebers Papyrus from ancient Egypt likewise gives a clear account of cardiac failure: 'When the heart is diseased, its work is performed imperfectly; the vessels proceeding from the heart become inactive, so that you cannot feel them' (J.B. Hurry, 1926); however, there is no direct indication that coronary disease was responsible for the pathology thus described.

Hippocrates reported the pain of angina (strangling) as 'extending from the collar-bone', 'like a weight in the forearm'. 'It causes very great pain and orthopnoea; it may suffocate the patient even on the first day' (A.M. Katz & Katz, 1962). Other descriptions in the Hippocratic literature are less characteristic of angina pectoris, and we must conclude that Greek physicians had not fully differentiated this condition from such diseases of the throat as acute tonsillitis and diphtheria. Nevertheless, suggestive evidence that ischaemic heart disease led to occasional fatalities is provided by the messenger Pheidippides, who died suddenly after running 40.0 kilometres to bring the news of victory from Marathon to Athens; the modern Marathon race covers a distance of 42.2 km.

Many more recent authors have shared in the confusion of terminology as they have discussed problems of cardiac oxygen lack (ischaemia). In particular, they have failed to differentiate the primary effects of anoxia (angina, myocardial infarction and sudden death), the immediate reaction to tissue destruction (myocardial fibrosis) and later consequences of such scarring and chronic hypoxia (persistent dysrhythmia, abnormal motion of the cardiac wall and pump failure). To avoid this problem, we will start our review of ischaemic heart disease and exercise with a brief discussion of terminology and the underlying pathology.

Atherosclerosis and Ischaemic Heart Disease

Atherosclerosis

Atherosclerosis is a general condition of the arteries in which the lumina are partially blocked by an accumulation of fat, complex carbohydrates, blood and blood products, fibrous tissue and calcium deposits in their walls, with associated medial changes (World Health Organization, 1958).

The build-up of lipids in arterial lesions has been recognised since R. Virchow (1856). The earliest changes probably occur in the arterial endothelium (M.D. Haust, 1970). One hypothesis is that injurious 'factors' from within the lumen of the blood vessels, either blood-borne chemicals or haemodynamic stresses (M. Texon, 1971), increase the permeability of the endothelium. This allows an 'insudation' of blood constituents into the intimal tissue of affected vessels, disturbing the metabolism of both cells and fibres. Alternatively, the injurious 'factors' may pass through the endothelium without causing initial harm, but resultant changes in the metabolism of the intimal cells lead to secondary effects upon the permeability of the endothelium, with resultant insudation. In either event, there is an increase in the muco-polysaccharide content of the tissue and an extracellular deposition of lipid, particularly cholesterol; accumulation of the latter substance probably reflects both more ready penetration of the intima and an increased retention due to changes in intimal metabolism (E.P. Smith, 1977). As the fatty plaques develop, they bulge into the arterial lumen and become enlarged by inflammation, haemorrhage and thrombus formation.

The first manifestation of coronary atherosclerosis is a fatty streaking of the major vessels; this can be detected in quite young children dying of inter-current disease (G.R. Osborn, 1963; D. Jaffé & Manning, 1971). Studies of young men killed in battle, air crashes and automobile accidents often reveal substantial (although clinically silent) atheroma (W.F. Enos *et al.*, 1953; J.C. Geer & McGill, 1967; H.H. Clarke, 1979). In one study of 20-year-old subjects, 40 per cent of the sample showed atherosclerosis, and in 15 per cent there was more than 75 per cent blockage of a main coronary artery (R. Gorlin, 1976). The disease process advances progressively with age (E.B. Smith *et al.*, 1967), and in many subjects eventually gives rise to symptoms.

Atherosclerotic changes within the coronary arteries predispose to such manifestations of ischaemic heart disease as angina, myocardial infarction and electrical failure of the heart.

Arteriosclerosis

Arteriosclerosis may co-exist with atherosclerosis, but should be distinguished from it (T.R. Harrison & Reeves, 1968). The arteriosclerotic blood vessel shows a progressive loss of elasticity and a hardening of its walls, often with radiologically visible calcification. Many older people are affected to some degree by arteriosclerosis. If severe, it can cause a substantial increase of systolic blood pressure, a narrowing or incompetence of the cardiac valves and ultimately a weakness of the vessel walls.

Plainly, such changes can contribute to and complicate the picture of ischaemic heart disease. The coronary vessels become narrow and rigid, with little potential for dilatation during exercise, while the valvular changes increase the work-load of the heart. However, many older authors have attributed almost every case of cardiac failure occurring in a man over the age of 50 years to arteriosclerotic heart disease, with the result that the term now lacks scientific precision.

Ischaemic heart disease

Ischaemic heart disease is a composite term referring to the several possible manifestations of relative oxygen lack in the myocardium (T.R. Harrison & Reeves, 1968). It is currently preferred to its apparent rival atherosclerotic heart disease.

Although the latter term is sometimes used as a synonym for ischaemic heart disease, the two rubrics do not encompass identical pathologies. Atherosclerosis may be present for many years without the development of clinically recognisable ischaemic heart disease. Clinical manifestations await a second, triggering factor. This may be haemorrhage into a plaque, lodgment of a thrombus at a point of vascular narrowing, coronary vascular spasm (R.C. Schlant, 1974), an unusual myocardial oxygen demand or some metabolic abnormality of the myocardium (T.W. Anderson, 1978a). Furthermore, if the immediate cause of death is ventricular fibrillation or myocardial infarction due to increased cardiac work rather than a specific blockage of the coronary vessels, post-mortem evidence of atherosclerosis may be rather slight. Finally, there are a number of non-atheromatous causes of ischaemic heart disease. These are uncommon, but nevertheless are well documented, including congenital abnormalities of the coronary vessels (H.A. Blake *et al.*, 1964), obstruction of the coronary ostium by syphilitic aortitis or a dissecting aneurysm (T.R. Harrison & Reeves,

1968), various types of aortic arteritis, vascular obstruction by non-atheromatous emboli (air, fat or tumour fragments) and pathological increases in the work-load of the left or right ventricle (for example, aortic stenosis or pulmonary hypertension; J.D. Woods, 1961). This substantial conglomerate of cardiac disorders is conveniently encompassed by the term ischaemic heart disease.

Angina

The classical clinical description of angina was furnished by W. Heberden (1772). He noted the sense of strangling, 'a painful and most disagreeable sensation in the breast, which seems as if it would extinguish life, if it were to continue'; it developed while the patient was 'walking (more especially if it be uphill and soon after eating) . . . but the moment they stand still, all this uneasiness vanishes.' It was plainly a harbinger of sudden death — if 'the disease go on to its height, the patients all suddenly fall down and perish almost immediately.' It also responded in some measure to regular exercise — 'I knew one who set himself a task of sawing wood for half an hour every day and was nearly cured.'

Despite this clear description of the clinical features, Heberden and his contemporaries were unaware of the pathological basis for the disorder. John Hunter drew attention to a bony hardening of the coronary arteries when conducting an autopsy of a patient with angina, but this contribution was ignored by nineteenth-century cardiologists. Laennec considered angina as a type of neuralgia, while William Osler listed angina among the cardiac neuroses. C.S. Keefer & Resnick (1928) seem the first authors to have recognised clearly that angina was due to a *relative* oxygen lack in the myocardium; this could reflect coronary narrowing, an increase of cardiac work-rate or a combination of these two factors.

The oxygen lack of an anginal attack is usually of insufficient duration to cause death of the myocardial tissue (A. Kattus & MacAlpin, 1969), but metabolic changes during the period of anoxia ('accumulation of a P substance'; R.C. Schlant, 1974) can sometimes be acutely painful. In earlier stages of the disease, there may be no more than a mild sense of oppression in the chest or a tightness of the throat which is difficult to diagnose. As the syndrome advances, its features become more characteristic. The patient is gripped by a severe, vice-like pain the midline of the chest, often radiating upwards into the root of the neck, or extending along the inner aspect of the left arm. There is usually a clear precipitating cause — anxiety, or a walk uphill (particularly in cold weather, when cutaneous vasoconstriction is maximal and nerve endings within the airway are stimulated by cold, dry air). Symptoms last no longer than two minutes, and do not cause general collapse; rest and medication such as glyceryl trinitrate help in providing rapid relief.

Myocardial Infarction and Fibrosis

Myocardial infarction

This is the usual cause of the 'coronary attack' of popular parlance. For one of the various reasons discussed when dealing with ischaemic heart disease (see above), an area of heart wall becomes starved of blood for sufficient time (five to ten minutes) to cause irreversible tissue damage. If the affected segment of the myocardium is large, the immediate or early demise of the patient is likely. Death results from an abnormality of cardiac rhythm (the irregular and ineffective pattern of ventricular contraction known as ventricular fibrillation), asystole (a complete cessation of cardiac contractions) or the onset of cardiac failure. Overall, 30–40 per cent of patients die before medical attention is received, and a further 30–35 per cent succumb while in hospital (W.B. Kannel *et al.*, 1971a, b; Council on Rehabilitation, 1973). Nevertheless, a proportion of patients, particularly younger individuals, those with less severe disease (C.K. Friedberg & Unger, 1967; H.I. Russek & Zohman, 1971; D.G. Julian, 1973) and those receiving early first-aid treatment (L. Cobb *et al.*, 1975; D.A. Chamberlain, 1978a; P. Siltanen, 1978) survive the immediate insult. In such cases the infarcted area (infarcted means literally 'stuffed with blood') is replaced by dense scar tissue over a period of some three months. The prognosis for conservatively treated patients is summarised in Table 1.1. The five-year death rate is at least ten times that indicated by standard life-assurance tables. Nevertheless, the normal function of the heart can be restored partially or completely by an extended programme of physical rehabilitation.

Papers describing the importance of the coronary circulation to the nutrition of the heart were published by Marshall Hall, Adam Hammer and George Dock among others, but J.B. Herrick (1912) gave the first detailed account of four possible clinical presentations:

Table 1.1: Five-year Mortality Following Recovery from Acute
Myocardial Infarction

Year of study	Sample size	Five-year mortality (%)	Authors
1920–30	162	51	Richards *et al.* (1956)
1932–41	285	33	Cole *et al.* (1954)
1934–6	—	29	Metropolitan Life (1953)
1935–52	224	45	Juergens *et al.* (1960)
1935–54	389	34	Biorck *et al.* (1957)
1940–9	286	42	Helander & Levander (1959)
1940–55	202	17	Dimond (1961)
1950–2	503	31	Beard *et al.* (1960)
1950–4	348	39	Honey & Truelove (1957)
1952–9	120	21	Little *et al.* (1965)
1956–61	932	26	Pell & D'Alonzo (1964)
1961–8	407	22*	Weinblatt *et al.* (1968)
1966–74	2,789	21	Coronary Drug Project (1975)

*   4½ years.

Source: Based on data collected by C.K. Friedberg & Unger (1967); P. Rechnitzer *et al.* (1971); T. Kavanagh & Shephard (1973b); and D.H. Paterson (1977). See original papers for details.

(i)   sudden and unanticipated death;

(ii)   severe pain, with profound shock and death in a few minutes;

(iii)   anginal pain without a precipitating cause, usually lasting longer than two minutes; and

(iv)   pictures intermediate between (ii) and (iii).

Diagnosis became more certain with the development of precordial electrocardiographic leads by F.N. Wilson (1944), and the demonstration of increases in certain serum enzymes such as glutamic oxaloacetic transaminase (SGOT), lactic dehydrogenase (LDH) and creatine phosphokinase (CPK) (J.S. La Due *et al.*, 1954; L. Cohen, 1967). The electrocardiographic changes include displacement of the ST segment and abnormal Q and T waves, these signs evolving in the first few hours following symptoms. The elevation of serum enzyme concentrations begins some twelve hours after infarction, peaks in two to three days, and persists for 14-21 days.

Anatomical features influencing the extent of a myocardial infarct and the likelihood that the patient will recover include the volume of tissue to which the normal arterial pathway has been interrupted, and the extent of anastomotic connections between the two main coronary vessels (collateral circulation).

Myocardial fibrosis

If an infarct is small, the clinical symptoms may be mistaken for indigestion or even overlooked. Nevertheless, a segment of the heart wall dies and is replaced by scar tissue. Thus a series of such 'silent' infarcts can lead to a progressive fibrosis of the myocardium, with a deterioration in pump function.

Sudden Death

Ischaemic heart disease is the commonest cause of sudden death in a middle-aged or older individual (G.E. Burch & De Pasquale, 1965; L. Kuller, 1966; V. Manninen & Halonen, 1978). In 80-90 per cent of cases where death occurs within an hour of the onset of symptoms, the problem is of cardiovascular origin, but if the definition of 'sudden' death is extended to include all fatalities occurring within 24 hours of the primary complaint, the proportion of cases attributable to cardiovascular disease drops to 50-60 per cent. Some 90 per cent of cardiovascular deaths are in turn attributable to coronary atherosclerosis, although there are other possible pathologies, including acute left-ventricular failure due to aortic stenosis, aortic insufficiency or coarctation of the aorta, right-ventricular failure due to pulmonary hypertension, a dysrhythmia precipitated by a viral myocarditis and rupture of a dissecting aneurysm of the aorta or a berry aneurysm in the circle of Willis at the base of the skull. In one series of 1,348 deaths due to coronary atherosclerosis, 26 per cent had known coronary disease, 33 per cent had undiagnosed symptoms and in 41 per cent the condition had remained silent until immediately before death (R.J. Myerburg & Davies, 1964).

The immediate reason for death in the patient with ischaemic heart disease is thought to be ventricular fibrillation or asystole. However, few electrocardiograms are available except from severely ill patients dying in intensive care units. M.W. Stroud & Feil (1948) noted that, of 16 such cases, seven showed ventricular fibrillation and nine ventricular standstill. J.S. Robinson *et al.* (1965) found 24 examples of ventricular fibrillation and 14 episodes of ventricular asystole. Both reports noted that 'instantaneous' deaths tended to be associated with ventricular fibrillation, while a more prolonged period of shock and poor myocardial function led to ventricular standstill.

The explanation for the early episodes of ventricular fibrillation lies in the pathology of this condition. The abnormal rhythm is often provoked and usually maintained by a unidirectional blockage in transmission of the electrical impulse through an ischaemic portion of the myocardium. This situation allows re-entry of the impulse into a region of the myocardium that is capable of re-excitation, and a vicious cycle of abnormal electrical pathways is established (Figure 1.1; Y. Watanabe & Dreifus, 1972). Within 15–20 minutes of the development of coronary occlusion, the majority of the ischaemic cells have become totally unresponsive, and can no longer participate in re-entrant circuits (D. Durrer *et al.*, 1978).

Figure 1.1: To illustrate how an ischaemic, unidirectional block in transmission of the cardiac impulse can allow an abnormal ('re-entrant') impulse to re-excite an area of the myocardium (Y. Watanabe & Dreifus, 1972)

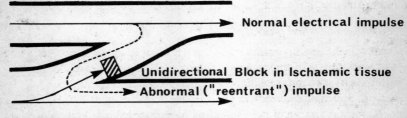

Normal electrical impulse

Unidirectional Block in Ischaemic tissue

Abnormal ("reentrant") impulse

Later Complications

Cardiac failure

A non-fatal episode of myocardial infarction is usually followed by an acute failure of the cardiac pump (D.E. Harken, 1972; H.O. Hirzel *et al.*, 1973). About a third of patients show shock within six hours, a half within 24 hours and two thirds by 36 hours (S. Scheidt *et al.*, 1970). The minimum recorded systemic blood pressure gives an indication of the severity of this reaction.

After the formation of scar tissue, the effectiveness of the cardiac pump may still be handicapped by various types of abnormal motion in the affected portion of the ventricular wall. M.V. Herman *et al.* (1967) distinguish *akinesis* (a total lack of movement in a part of the heart wall), *asyneresis* (diminished motion), *dyskinesis* (paradoxical expansion of the wall) and *asynchrony* (a disturbed temporal sequence of contraction).

Occasionally, there may be rupture of a bulging (aneurysmal) area of the heart wall (R.A. Van Tassel & Edwards, 1972). However, an aneurysm is in itself rather uncommon among patients referred for exercise rehabilitation (14 of 610 cases in the series of R.J. Shephard *et al.*, 1980), and rupture is an even rarer event.

Ventricular fibrillation

The risk of ventricular fibrillation is greatest in the first 24 hours after infarction. Nevertheless, even after many months of apparently successful rehabilitation, the person who has sustained an infarct remains at an increased risk of death from dysrhythmia relative to an age-matched control. There is sometimes a premonitory phase, an increase in the frequency of multifocal premature ventricular contractions occurring during the 'vulnerable' part of the cardiac cycle (the R wave of the premature beat being superimposed on the preceding T wave of the electrocardiogram), but in 25-50 per cent of cases ventricular fibrillation develops without warning (M.G. Wyman & Hammersmith, 1974; K.I. Lie *et al.*, 1975; D.G. Julian *et al.*, 1978).

Extension of disease process

Development of a myocardial infarction is commonly a warning of advanced disease of the coronary vasculature and, unless the clinical episode serves to induce a dramatic change in the lifestyle of the patient, a further extension of the atherosclerotic process is likely.

Recurrent attacks of ischaemia lead to a progressive deterioration of myocardial function. A stage may be reached where exercise induces a decrease of stroke volume and a fall rather than a rise of systemic blood pressure, such phenomena being harbingers of recurrence of the infarction and of death (R.J. Shephard, 1979a). In such patients there is a real danger that exercise may provoke acute cardiac failure with a fatal waterlogging of the lungs, and for this reason exercise rehabilitation may be unwise for the individual with severe exercise-induced angina (J.O. Parker *et al.*, 1966).

International Classification of Diseases

It will be useful in concluding this chapter to relate the various
conditions discussed to the International Classification of Disease
(World Health Organisation, 1968). Unfortunately, the scheme of
classification has undergone several changes over the years, as
diagnoses have become more precise; for example, the 1968 revision
increased the apparent incidence of coronary deaths by a factor of
1.146 (W.J. Walker, 1977).

The rubrics cited here refer to the eighth (1971) revision of the
classification.

Acute ischaemic heart disease: angina pectoris, sudden death,
coronary thrombosis and acute myocardial infarction (410,
411, 413).
Chronic ischaemic heart disease: fatty heart, myocardial degeneration
(412).
Heart failure, cause unspecified (427-9).
Valvular heart disease (390-8, 421, 424).

2 THE CURRENT EPIDEMIC OF ISCHAEMIC HEART DISEASE

A stimulating popular book entitled *The Medical Runaround* (A. Malleson, 1973) exposes many medical fallacies. One trend for which British physicians had claimed great credit was the drop of suicides in the United Kingdom, from a peak of 5,600 per year in the early 1960s to just over 4,000 per year in 1970. Unfortunately for this piece of self-congratulation, careful analysis of the statistics disclosed that the overall decrease in suicides was the result of two opposing trends — a decrease in deaths from domestic coal-gas poisoning (as the Gas Council replaced coal gas by natural gas), and an increase in suicides by the use of medicaments over which the physicans supposedly had complete control.

The epidemic of ischaemic heart disease has given rise to much similar loose speculation. We will therefore scrutinise closely not only the extent of the epidemic, but also its origins and likely course.

Extent of the Epidemic

Incidence and prevalence

At first inspection, it might seem a simple matter to calculate the incidence and prevalence of ischaemic heart disease in a given community. Thus:

$$\text{Incidence rate} = \frac{\text{number of new cases of disease}}{\text{population at risk}}$$

over a specified period of time such as one year, while

$$\text{Prevalence rate} = \frac{\text{number of existing cases of disease}}{\text{total population}}$$

at any given time.

In practice, there are a number of complications to the derivation of such statistics.

Criterion of disease

It is first necessary to decide upon a criterion of disease. This could be the onset of cardiac symptoms such as anginal pain, the appearance

of an abnormal electrocardiogram, the development of a frank
'coronary' attack or a 'cardiac' death. Each of these various approaches
has its own inherent uncertainties.

Anginal pain. The patient may confuse anginal pain with indigestion or
the discomfort of an arthritic shoulder. Further, the threshold for the
reporting of the symptom varies greatly with the personality of the
patient and the level of physical activity that he habitually undertakes.
One reason why angina pectoris is more frequent in London bus
conductors than in the drivers (J.N. Morris *et al.*, 1953) is that the
former are more likely to undertake a sufficient rate of physical work
to reveal an impairment of their coronary blood supply.

Ischaemic exercise electrocardiogram. The exercise electrocardiogram
shows much day-to-day variation. In the Saskatoon experiment
(D.A. Bailey *et al.*, 1974), a randomly selected sample of adults were
cleared for exercise by a medically supervised sub-maximal stepping
test; nevertheless, when the same physician carried out a sub-maximal
cycle-ergometer test on these subjects a few days later, he found it
necessary to halt the test in four per cent of individuals because of
electrocardiographic abnormalities. The exercise electrocardiogram is
also liable to substantial inter-observer differences of interpretation.
H. Blackburn (1968) commented that the frequency of 'positive'
diagnoses in a set of exercise electrocardiograms varied from five to 55
per cent when interpretations were made by 14 different 'experts'!
Interestingly, technical personnel were more consistent and as accurate
as cardiologists in classifying ischaemic abnormalities of the electrocardiogram. Lastly, there are numerous physiological reasons for the
development of a falsely positive ischaemic appearance in the exercise
electrocardiogram (A.M. Katz, 1977; Table 7.4).

Clinical diagnosis. A severe 'coronary' attack is usually diagnosed fairly
readily, but minor infarcts are difficult to distinguish from other
medical problems, even if there is assistance from objective data such
as serial electrocardiograms and serum enzyme determinations
(Chapter 1).

It might be thought that the diagnosis of sudden death would leave
little room for uncertainty. However, in practice it is often difficult to
find reliable witnesses who can describe the time of onset of discomfort
or the exact minute of death.

The completion of death certificates provides an apparent wealth of information, but unfortunately the details given are notoriously imprecise, with much scope for both temporal and regional fashions when recording the principal cause of death. Interpretation of death rates is further complicated by successive changes in the International Classification of Diseases (Chapter 1).

Survey methods

Having decided upon the criterion of disease, it is then necessary to determine its incidence or prevalence. It is plainly impractical to wait for the patient himself to make a complaint. K.L. White & Ibrahim (1963) estimated that 150 of each 1,000 people in the United States had diagnosable cardiac disease, but that only 60 of the 150 would report their illness. Possible approaches are to conduct household, laboratory or community surveys.

Household surveys. In the usual form of household survey, a suitably trained nurse or health visitor visits randomly selected homes, questioning those encountered about cardiac disease or carrying out a simple exercise test (J. Murphy, 1980; R.J. Shephard, 1980a). If but one call is made to each home, the selected householder may be absent, and there is a danger that the sample will become unduly weighted by those who are confined to their homes. Particular care must be taken to include an appropriate proportion of individuals who live permanently in institutions (old people's homes, hospitals, prisons and the armed services), along with those who are frequent travellers (transport workers, business men and commercial representatives) or shift workers. Cooperation may be refused, questions may be misunderstood and, if an exercise test is performed a lack of habituation to the observer and the test procedure may give a high pulse rate, a high blood pressure and an unusually large secretion of catecholamines (R.J. Shephard, 1969).

Laboratory surveys. If randomly selected subjects are invited to attend a laboratory for a diagnostic procedure, attrition of the intended test population is even more dramatic than with a household survey. D.A. Bailey *et al.* (1974) carried out a fitness survey in the city of Saskatoon by taking names at random from the telephone directory. This approach immediately excluded those with unlisted telephone numbers, the poor who could not afford a telephone and the majority of those living in institutions. Of respondents (Table 2.1), about a third were frankly unwilling to attend the laboratory, and a further third made

Table 2.1: To Illustrate Sample Attrition When Subjects for a 'Fitness Test' are Selected Randomly from the Telephone Directory

Initial exclusions:		Institutionalised subjects
		No telephone
		Unlisted number
Initial sample:	2648	telephone responses
	118	judged as unsuitable for testing
	982	refused test
	649	stated test time inconvenient or similar excuse
	49	failed to report for testing
	72	excluded by screening physician
	778	undertook fitness test

Source: Based on data of D.A. Bailey *et al.* (1974).

some excuse or failed to appear for testing at the appointed time. The group finally examined was thus a slender 32 per cent of the original telephone sample.

Community surveys. A final possibility is a community survey. In a small town, one may attempt to examine the entire population, while in a medium-sized city attention is directed to all citizens of a specific age group (such as all men born in 1913). Such approaches have been adopted with considerable success in Tecumseh, Michigan (H. Montoye, 1975), Framingham, Mass. (W.B. Kannel *et al.*, 1971a,b), Göteburg (L. Wilhelmsen *et al.*, 1972) and Malmö (N.H. Sternby, 1977). Close personal contacts with the population allow a much higher response rate in a small-town setting; for example, Montoye and his associates were able to examine 88 per cent of the 9,500 people living in Tecumseh in 1959-60, and to repeat examinations on 82 per cent of the population between 1961 and 1965.

The main disadvantage of a small-town survey is uncertainty concerning the relevance of the results to the modern metropoli in which most people currently live.

National differences

Keeping in mind these limitations of household, laboratory and community surveys, it is interesting to compare figures for the incidence of

Table 2.2: Age-standardised Average Yearly Incidence of Ischaemic Heart Disease Manifestations in Seven Countries, Expressed as Annual Incidence Rates per 10,000 Men Aged 40–59 Years, Free of Disease at Beginning of Study and Followed up for Five Years

Nation	Deaths	Myocardial infarctions	Angina	Other manifestations of ischaemic heart disease
Japan	9		between 15 and 20*	
Greece	8	8	1	15
Yugoslavia	11	8	18	16
Italy	12	18	30	40
Netherlands	27	33	23	56
US railways	37	28	67	45
Finland	26	31	71	70

* Documentation of non-fatal episodes for Japan is imprecise.

Source: A. Keys (1970).

ischaemic heart disease in different parts of the world (Table 2.2). In almost all nations, ischaemic heart disease is a major cause of disability and death, although there is a several-fold gradient in the occurrence rate for new events between countries such as Japan and Greece (where the incidence is relatively low) and Finland and the United States (where the incidence is particularly high). Some authors (for example, A. Keys, 1970) have attempted to correlate these differences with the average level of such risk factors as the percentage of energy taken in the form of saturated (animal) fat among the populations concerned.

Economic implications

The World Health Organisation (1976) noted that in 29 technologically advanced countries in 1967, cardiovascular disease accounted for 39 per cent of deaths among men aged 25 to 64 years, some three quarters of this total being due to ischaemic heart disease. In the US, cardio-vascular disease accounts for 53 per cent of all deaths in men and women, 'coronary' attacks being responsible for 65 per cent of this total (R.A. Bruce, 1974).

The Canadian Government has assessed the economic impact of various health problems in terms of 'lost productive years.' The calculation is made noting deaths that occur after the age of one but

Table 2.3: Annual Loss of Productive Years in Canada through Deaths Occurring between the Ages of One and 70 Years, Based on Data for 1971

Cause of death	Annual loss of productive years	
	Men	Women
Ischaemic heart disease	157,000	36,000
Motor-vehicle accidents	154,000	59,000
Other accidents	136,000	43,000
Respiratory diseases	90,000	50,000
Suicide	51,000	18,000

Source: Lalonde (1974).

before the age of 70 years, each death being multiplied by the number of years that would have elapsed if the individual in question had lived to the age of 70 years (M. Lalonde, 1974; Table 2.3). On this criterion, ischaemic heart disease is the main health problem of Canadian men, and is an important consideration in women also.

Source of the Epidemic

Antiquity of the disease

Many people have viewed ischaemic heart disease as purely a twentieth-century epidemic, associated in some way with the 'evils' of modern civilisation. This concept has been supported by superficial comparisons of the incidence of the disease between the 'developed' and less-developed nations of our day.

Possibly in previous generations the problem was confined to an over-fed and pampered upper class of society. However, the writings of classical and neo-classical physicians (Chapter 1) leave little doubt that, since ancient times, a proportion of the human race has suffered from such manifestations of ischaemic heart disease as angina and sudden death. What has emerged over the past half-century has been a recognition by physicians of the symptoms and signs associated with acute myocardial infarction.

Twentieth-century trends

Although the disease process is not new in itself, vital statistics have shown a dramatic increase in most manifestations of ischaemic heart

Figure 2.1: Annual death rate for age-specific groups of the English and Welsh populations, based upon an analysis of the Registrar-General's statistics for 1931–48. Line (a) shows deaths from acute ischaemic heart disease (coronary arterial disease plus angina, including coronary atheroma — or atherosclerosis — and coronary, ischaemic — or arteriosclerotic — heart disease, particularly the syndrome of thrombosis, occlusion, and infarction and its variants). Line (b) shows chronic myocardial diseases (including late deaths from myocardial infarction). Line (c) is the sum of (a) and (b).

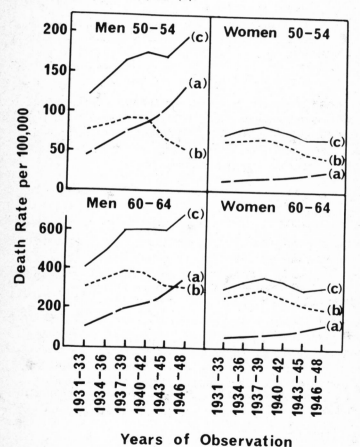

Source: J.N. Morris (1951).

disease over the first half of the present century. J.N. Morris (1951) examined figures for England and Wales, taken from the Registrar General and covering the period 1931-48. Data for men aged 50-4 years and 60-4 years showed a progressive increase in deaths attributed to ischaemic heart disease, this trend being attributable to acute rather than to chronic manifestations of the disorder (Figure 2.1). Among women of comparable age, deaths due to coronary vascular disease were less frequent, but nevertheless they also showed an increase of 'acute' deaths. Subsequent analyses from the United States and Canada revealed similar trends.

It could be argued that part, if not all, of the increase in deaths from ischaemic heart disease is an artefact, reflecting changes in fashions of diagnosis and the completion of death certificates. Some authors have alleged that previous generations of physicians were wont to ascribe sudden and unexpected deaths to vague, non-specific causes such as 'acute indigestion', 'apoplexy' and 'chronic myocardial degeneration'. T.W. Anderson and his colleagues thus devoted considerable effort to establishing that the epidemic was a real phenomenon. An examination of vital statistics for the Province of Ontario showed them an increase in certification of deaths from ischaemic heart disease similar to that described for Britain (Figure 2.2; T.W. Anderson & Le Riche, 1970). They next studied figures for sudden deaths, the majority of which are attributable to ischaemic heart disease (Chapter 1); again they observed a progressive upward trend. Lastly, they re-examined the original death certificates, re-interpreting the information where this seemed appropriate. Contrary to previous suggestions, they found no deaths from 'acute indigestion', and few deaths attributed to 'apoplexy'. The revised statistics thus confirmed that there was a large increase in the death rate due to ischaemic heart disease, particularly between 1931 and 1961.

As a further check upon the reality of the epidemic, death rates were compared for men and for women (T.W. Anderson, 1976; T.W. Anderson & Halliday, 1979; M. Halliday & Anderson, 1979). It was reasoned that if there had been a change of diagnostic fashion, statistics for men and women would have been affected by approximately the same extent. However, in practice the sex ratios for heart disease (all types) remained close to unity until the mid-1920s, when there was a dramatic increase of disease in the men, similar in timing and in magnitude for Canada, the United States and England and Wales (Figure 2.3). Furthermore, there was no decrease in the sex ratio for other conditions that might have been confused with cardiac disease

Figure 2.2: Deaths from ischaemic heart disease in the Province of Ontario. The figure illustrates official mortality data for ischaemic heart disease — angina pectoris, coronary thrombosis, myocardial infarction and arteriosclerotic heart disease — in men aged 45–64 years, the probable incidence of ischaemic heart disease deaths (based upon the authors' reinterpretation of the death certificates; probable ischaemic heart disease includes ischaemic heart disease and non-specific heart disease — heart failure, cardiac dropsy, organic heart disease, myocarditis, etc.), and the incidence of sudden death (adjusted to allow for certificates with no information on duration of illness). Note that, in contrast to the graphs of J.N. Morris (Figure 2.1), a logarithmic scale has been used upon the ordinate.

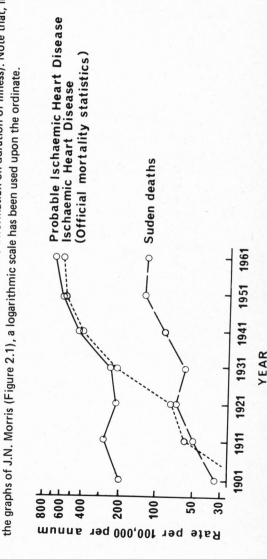

Source: Based on an analysis of T.W. Anderson and Le Riche (1970).

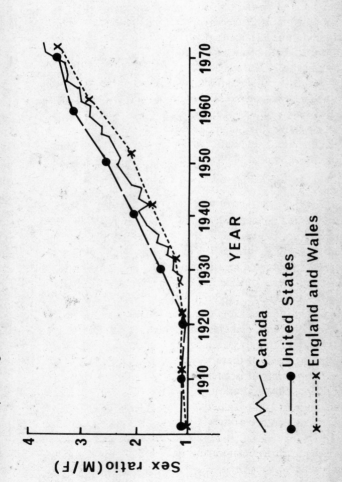

Figure 2.3: The sex ratio (male/female) for all forms of heart disease in subjects aged 45 to 64 years. Data for Canada, United States, and England and Wales.

Source: T.W. Anderson (1976).

(other diseases of the circulation, nephritis, indigestion, asthma and diabetes mellitus). There must therefore have been a true increase of ischaemic heart disease deaths among the men, or (much less likely) a decrease among the women, over the period of inquiry.

Calculation of the sex ratios revealed two other interesting facets of the cardiac epidemic. Firstly, although one might consider coronary atherosclerosis as but one manifestation of a general vascular disorder, there was no evidence of a time-related change in the sex ratio for other vascular conditions such as cerebral vascular accidents; T.W. Anderson (1976) thus suggested that some local factor had increased the vulnerability of the myocardium over the period of observation. Secondly, there had been a progressive change in the social characteristics of those affected by ischaemic heart disease (M. Halliday & Anderson, 1979). In the 1920s, ischaemic heart disease was a problem of the gentry, the rise of sex ratio occurring largely in British social class one (the professional workers). More recently, the disease has extended progressively to blue-collar groups, with a rapid rise in the sex ratio for social class five (the manual labourers).

Factors associated with the current waning of the epidemic are dicussed in the next section of this chapter.

Risk factors and diseases

A number of 'risk factors' (Table 2.4) increase an individual's chances of developing ischaemic heart disease (J. Truett *et al.*, 1967; W.B. Kannel *et al.*, 1971a, b; G.F. Fletcher & Cantwell, 1971, 1974; R.A. Bruce, 1974; J.P. Strong, 1977). Some of these variables, such as age, sex, race, geographic location and the mineral content of the drinking water, are largely outside of personal control, but other factors are strongly related to lifestyle. In the latter context, we may note specifically hypertension, cigarette smoking, physical inactivity, a high serum cholesterol, diabetes and obesity.

It is interesting to search for a parallel between changes to the population levels of these various risk factors and the onset of the current epidemic of ischaemic heart disease, although in so doing we are handicapped by limitations in the data available and uncertainties concerning the time lag between the development of a given risk factor and the appearance of overt disease.

Hypertension. There are many causes of high blood pressure, including some factors over which the hypertensive individual has no control. Nevertheless, population levels of systemic blood pressure are affected

Table 2.4: Risk Factors Predisposing to Ischaemic Heart Disease*

Cigarette smoking/impaired pulmonary function/carboxyhaemoglobin

Hypertension

Blood lipid abnormalities/hereditary hypercholesterolaemia

Physical inactivity/high resting heart rate

Excess body mass

Heredity/family history of 'heart attacks'/blood group other than O

Personality and behaviour patterns/socio-economic status/'stress'

Abnormal ECG

Carbohydrate intolerance/diabetes

Increased serum uric acid/gout

Softness of drinking water

Disorders of blood coagulation

Hypothyroidism

Diet (excess animal fat/sucrose/heavy meals)

Male sex (especially before menopause)

Age

---

*   Note that: (1) many of these factors are inter-related (American Heart Association, 1972; R. Paffenbarger, 1977; W.B. Kannel, 1979); (2) a given risk factor has more predictive value in some populations than in others (A. Keys, 1975); and (3) it is by no means proven that the risk of developing clinical disease can be changed by modifying these factors (Council on Rehabilitation, 1973; Hickey *et al.*, 1975).

by lifestyle, particularly the dietary intake of table salt, and the extent of exposure to 'stress'.

Historic details of salt consumption are limited. In some parts of Africa and Asia where salt is still in short supply, the incidence of hypertension is much lower than in Europe and North America (I. Maddocks, 1964). It might be thought that the western use of salt was greater before the general availability of fresh foods and refrigeration. H. Kaunitz (1956) noted that wars were fought over sources of salt, and for centuries its trade was more important than that of any other material. However, B. Friend *et al.* (1979) estimated that in the US an increased consumption of processed food increased the average daily sodium intake by 14 per cent from 1909-13 to 1976.

The 'stress' associated with the life of the modern city dweller is still keenly debated (R.S. Eliot, 1974). H.I. Russek & Russek (1977) reported that one in twenty of US workers had two jobs, and some had three; further, among coronary victims 25 per cent had been holding

Table 2.5: Prevalence of Coronary Disease by Age and Arbitrary Assessment of Occupational Stress

Occupational stress	Prevalence of disease (%)		
	Age 40–9 years	Age 50–9 years	Age 60–9 years
Low: Dermatologists, orthodontists, patent lawyers, periodontists	0.70	5.42	7.38
Moderate: Oral surgeons, other lawyers, pathologists, security analysts, trial lawyers	2.09	6.42	13.46
High: Anaesthesiologists, general practice dentists, general practice lawyers, general practice physicians, security traders	4.20	11.40	19.43

Source: Based on data of H.I. Russek & Russek (1977).

down two jobs, and a further 46 per cent had been working 60 or more hours per week prior to the onset of symptoms. Likewise, T. Kavanagh & Shephard (1973a) noted that in the year prior to a coronary attack business problems had been increased in 71 per cent of their patients, were normal in 27 per cent and decreased in only two per cent, a very different pattern of response from that reported by control subjects from the same occupations. H.I. Russek & Russek (1977) further observed a gradient in the occurrence of ischaemic heart disease that was correlated with the pre-judged stressfulness of 20 different occupations (Table 2.5).

Such views are by no means novel. William Osler (1896) noted that the typical case of angina pectoris was a 'keen and ambitious man, the indicator of whose engines is always set "full speed ahead" ', and others have repeatedly reiterated this assessment (for example, J.A. Arlow, 1945; C. Kemple, 1945). There is clearly some association between the time-oriented, competitive ('Type A') personality and an increased risk of hypertension and ischaemic heart disease (M. Friedman & Rosenman, 1974), although many coronary victims do not show the classical 'Type A' picture of excessively rapid movement, tense musculature, explosive conversation, excessive gesturing and a general air of impatience (H.I. Russek & Zohman, 1958).

It is possible that present-day society encourages the development of 'Type A' characteristics in the 'successful' executive. Several authors have pointed to an association between urban living and hypertension (for example, J. Stamler *et al.*, 1967). However, other investigators have emphasized that not everyone reacts to modern city living in the same manner. Thus L.E. Hinckle & Wolff (1962) found more hypertension in young business executives with only a high-school education than in those who were university graduates; they concluded that business was stressful only for those who were upwardly mobile. Likewise, C. Hames (1975) observed a correlation between the prevalence of coronary disease and the recent acquisition of status symbols such as education and ownership of property. The two points of view may be reconcilable, since it can be argued that the 'Type A' person is the most aggressive in climbing the ladder of success.

Sceptics have claimed that the main stresses faced by many business men are over-large lunches, too frequent cocktails and a lack of physical activity! Certainly, there is no strong evidence that the pressures of daily life have increased over the last 50 years. Furthermore, Japan has had a very high incidence of hypertension over this period, but it has only recently begun to experience the cardiac epidemic (C.P. Wen & Gershoff, 1973). It thus seems unlikely that a salt- or stress-induced outbreak of hypertension is the prime cause of the increase is ischaemic heart disease over the present century.

Cigarette smoking

Cigarette smoking is a much stronger candidate habit for explanation of the cardiac epidemic. It is thought to have a long-term influence upon the course of atherogenesis (N. Wald *et al.*, 1973), hypoxia of the blood vessel walls associated with carboxyhaemoglobin formation and a shift of the oxygen dissociation curve both favouring the formation of atherosclerotic plaques (P. Åstrup *et al.*, 1966; P. Åstrup, 1977; H.C. McGill, 1977). Smoking also has more immediate effects upon myocardial irritability and the dimensions of the coronary vasculature, increasing the frequency of premature ventricular contractions (H.J.L. Marriott & Myerburg, 1974) and speeding the development of exercise-induced angina (W.S. Aronow *et al.*, 1968).

The first cigarette-rolling machines appeared about 1870, and the habit rapidly gained ground in the early 1900s, becoming epidemic among the generation of young men serving in the first world war (Figure 2.4). There is thus a fairly close temporal relationship between

Figure 2.4: Percentage of US men currently smoking cigarettes. Data for 1955, 1966 and 1970, shown in relation to age at time of survey and birth cohort. Note that cigarette smoking first becomes epidemic in the cohort reaching manhood during the first world war.

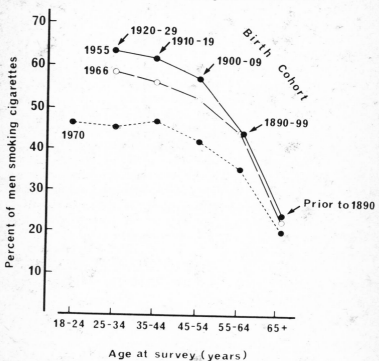

Source: Based on data in *The Health Consequences of Smoking, 1974* (US Dept. of Health, Education and Welfare, Washington, DC).

the development of cigarette consumption in the western world and the appearance of an increased number of male cardiovascular deaths.

In women, smoking first became widespread during the second world war, and over the period 1921 to 1971 the increase in incidence of ischaemic heart disease among women remained relatively small (T.W. Anderson & Halliday, 1979): if we are to accept the hypothesis that cigarette consumption contributed to the male epidemic, we must therefore postulate that other factors have intervened to protect women from the consequences of a similar lifestyle.

Habitual physical inactivity

Daily activity fell progressively over the first half of the present century. One significant change was in the amount of energy used for personal transportation. This can be documented in terms of motor vehicle registrations. In the US, the number of cars rose from a very small number in 1900 to a peak about 1928, this being surpassed only in the 1950s. Since 1950, the main increase has been in the number of families owning two or more cars (Table 2.6), with about a sixth of the population (the poor, the disabled and the elderly) still not owning a car.

Until the recent renaissance of recreational cycling, rising sales of cars were linked with corresponding mass closures of factories manufacturing bicycles.

The ever-increasing industrial and domestic power consumption suggests that automation has also reduced the energy demands of occupational and domestic pursuits over the present century, although O.G. Edholm (1970) has advanced the provocative hypothesis that new technology has increased the output of goods per worker, leaving the energy cost of his daily activity unchanged.

The overall food consumption of the US population showed a per capita decline of some 1.25 Megajoules (MJ) per day from 1930 to 1960 (Table 2.7); although there has been some recovery of energy usage in the 1970s, if account is taken of the greater height and mass of the present-day population, energy consumption would need to have increased by about 0.6 MJ per day in order to sustain the level of daily activity seen in the 1930s. Part of the observed decrease in energy usage could be attributed to such factors as ageing of the population (basal

Table 2.6: Car Ownership in the United States (per family)

Year	No car (%)	One car (%)	Two or more cars (%)
1950	41	52	7
1955	30	60	10
1960	23	62	15
1965	21	55	24
1970	21	50	29
1974	18*	49	33

* But two per cent have some form of light truck, leaving only 16 per cent without personal transportation.

Table 2.7: Daily per Capita Food Consumption in the United States

Year	Total energy value (MJ)	Carbohydrate (g)	Fat (g)	Protein (g)
1930	14.4	474	134	93
1940	14.0	429	143	93
1950	13.6	402	145	94
1960	13.1	375	143	95
1965	13.1	372	144	96
1970	13.8	380	157	100
1975	13.6	377	152	99
1977	14.1	391	159	103

metabolism decreases with age) and an increased use of processed food (with a decrease of kitchen wastage). However, casual observation suggests that the wastage of food has increased rather than decreased as the population has become more affluent. The data therefore strongly suggest that there has been a decrease of physical activity, particularly between 1930 and 1960.

Nevertheless, the contribution of physical inactivity to the cardiac epidemic is probably rather small. In terms of motor-car usage, relatively few citizens of the United Kingdom owned vehicles before world war II, and during the war most civilians were unable to obtain petrol for the operation of personal transportation. However, the cardiac epidemic was well established in 1946-8 (Figure 2.1), and indeed the male/female ratio increased with only slight retardation relative to US statistics (Figure 2.3). Automation is also unlikely to have been a major factor, since in the Britain of J.N. Morris's study there had been little attempt to modernise industry or to reduce the physical demands upon the worker. Even patterns of leisure activity had shown little change in Britain by 1948; although public television broadcasting was introduced in 1936, the majority of the population did not purchase television sets until the mid-1950s.

We must conclude that, while habitual activity has undoubtedly undergone changes over the present century, the pace of change has shown quite large differences between North America and western Europe, without parallel differences in the time course of the cardiac epidemic.

Serum cholesterol

Much of the serum cholesterol is normally manufactured in the liver (H.S. Sodhi *et al.*, 1977). Nevertheless, there is some evidence that the level of serum cholesterol is influenced by the balance between habitual activity and the dietary intake of animal fat. J.J. Groen *et al.* (1959) noted low cholesterol levels in Trappist monks who did not eat fish, meat, eggs or butter. Likewise, Somali camel-herders (V. Lapiccirella *et al.*, 1962) and the East African Masai (G.V. Mann *et al.*, 1965) seem relatively free of ischaemic heart disease despite a diet rich in dairy fat, presumably because they counter their adverse diet by a much higher level of physical activity than is usual in western man.

Many western peoples have increased their fat consumption over the present century, but this is due more to an increase in the consumption of salad oil, cooking oil and margarine than to an increased intake of other forms of fat (Table 2.8). If the present intake of animal fat is undesirably high, it would seem that this situation was already established in the early part of the present century, at least in the United States.

An interesting contrast is provided by data for occupied Europe during world war II. Between 1942 and 1946, the diet dropped to a total energy input of 3.4–4.2 MJ per day, with some 5–10 g in the form of fat. The mean body mass was 10–15 kg below normal, and the serum cholesterol fell from a pre-war average of around 200 mg·dl^{-1} to about 140 mg·dl^{-1}. Given this drastic modification of national diets, atherosclerotic deaths due to conditions such as myocardial infarction

Table 2.8: Patterns of Fat Consumption in the United States, 1909–13 to 1976

Year	Total fat consumed (g)	Salad oil, cooking oil and margarine (g)	Other fat (g)
1909–13	125	3.4	121.6
1935–9	132	10.9	121.1
1947–9	140	14.7	125.3
1957–9	143	22.5	120.5
1965	144	27.5	116.5
1970	156	33.6	122.4
1976	157	38.5	118.5

Source: Based on data of B. Friend *et al.* (1979).

were substantially reduced relative to pre-war statistics (Malmros, 1950; G. Schettler, 1977).

Refined carbohydrate and diabetes

A second major historical change of diet has involved a progressive increase in the consumption of sucrose and other refined carbohydrates. Early statistics suggest that there was an annual per capita usage of 5 lb (2.3 kg) of sucrose in 1750 and 25 lb (11.4 kg) in 1850. More recent US data (B. Friend *et al.*, 1979) show a further rise from 75 lb (34 kg) in 1909–13 to a peak of 104 lb (47 kg) at the time of prohibition. Subsequent consumption has hovered just under 100 lb per year, with a peak of 102 lb (46 kg) in 1973 (probably due to the ban on the sale of cyclamates), and a decrease in 1974 (probably related to a substantial rise in world sugar prices).

The increased sugar intake could influence cardiovascular health at least indirectly. Diabetes is a well-recognised risk factor for ischaemic heart disease, and the likelihood of maturity-onset diabetes is influenced by the balance between habitual activity and the dietary intake of sucrose. However, the chain of events is somewhat tenuous, and again the increase of sugar consumption began long before the onset of the cardiac epidemic.

Obesity

The epidemiological significance of obesity is still a matter of some controversy. A Keys *et al.* (1972) claimed that an excessive body weight was not a risk factor for ischaemic heart disease if prior allowance was made for the associated risks of high systemic blood pressure and a high serum cholesterol level. Such computer analyses are interesting, but unfortunately they cannot prove whether hypertension or obesity is the primary disorder. There is certainly an association between gross obesity and death from cardiovascular disease (Society of Actuaries, 1959). In men aged 15–69 years, the mortality due to diseases of the heart and circulation is 131 per cent of standard for those 24 kg above the ideal mass, rising to 155 per cent with 33 kg excess mass, and 185 per cent with 42 kg of excess mass. Furthermore, there is good evidence that a reduction of excess mass will reduce both hypertension and cholesterol (F.W. Ashley & Kannel, 1974). Thus in a practical sense, if there has been an increase in the proportion of obese individuals in a country, this could have contributed to the appearance of a cardiac epidemic.

Historical information on obesity is limited, and inter-survey comparisons are complicated by (i) the secular trend to an increase of standing height, and (ii) uncertainties concerning the adjustments that investigators have made for the mass of clothing and the height of shoes when reporting their data. Portrait galleries from previous centuries suggest that many of the wealthy were quite obese. In contrast, in poor and underdeveloped societies, a low incidence of ischaemic heart disease today remains coupled with extremely low skinfold readings, and a body mass that is often 10–15 kg below the actuarial ideal value (R.J. Shephard, 1974a, 1978a).

Many Europeans are currently much heavier than their counterparts were during world war II. Thus the Birmingham workers of 1960 studied by T. Khosla & Lowe (1967) were 6–7 kg heavier than the men of wartime Britain (W.F.F. Kemsley, 1951–3), even when the two sets of data were standardised to a common height of 175 cm. Nevertheless, such increases of body mass do not parallel the time course of the cardiac epidemic in England and Wales (Figure 2.1).

Conclusion

The cause or causes of the cardiac epidemic have yet to be identified with certainty. Cigarette smoking is one major aspect of lifestyle that does appear to have changed in parallel with the epidemic, but its influence is not strong enough to account for the entire phenomenon. Heavy smoking approximately doubles the risk of a fatal coronary attack (R. Paffenbarger, 1977) and, since some 50 per cent of men developed a heavy cigarette habit over the period in question, smoking could have increased the attack rate by about 50 per cent. In fact, there was at least a three- to four-fold increase of mortality between the early 1900s and 1960 (Figures 2.1–2.3). We must thus presume that smoking interacted with other risk factors yet to be delineated. On the statistics of R. Paffenbarger (1977), the entire increase might be explained by a combination of smoking, low energy output and hypertension secondary to obesity.

Recent Course of Epidemic

The downturn

Epidemiologists in the United States and Canada have been fascinated to note that over the past 15 years the trend to an increase of ischaemic heart disease deaths has been reversed (T.W. Anderson, 1978b; Figure 2.5). In Britain, mortality only began to decrease in 1974 (Du V.C. Florey *et al.*, 1978), but the North American epidemic apparently

Figure 2.5: Course of ischaemic heart disease epidemic 1950–76. Data for Canadian and US 'white' subjects aged 55–64 years, adjusted to allow for the change in classification of ischaemic heart disease (1968, USA; 1969, Canada).

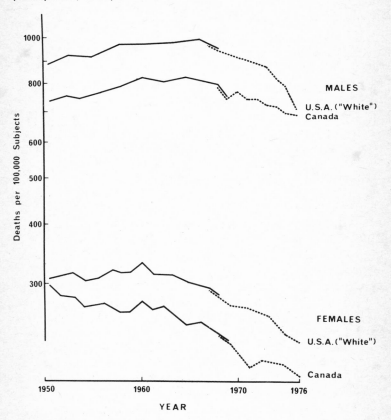

Source: T.W. Anderson (1978b).

peaked about 1967, and 'cardiac deaths' among middle-aged adults have subsequently fallen by about 25 per cent (Table 2.9). The decrease has occurred equally in 'white' and 'non-white' groups, but it has been some four per cent larger in those with recorded hypertension than in those without this sign, while the improvement of prognosis for acute myocardial infarction (the first eight weeks after the attack) has been almost twice as large as for those dying of chronic ischaemic heart

Table 2.9: Decrease in Age-specific Coronary Mortality of US Citizens, 1963-75, Adjusted for Changes in Eighth Revision of International Classification of Disease

Age (years)	Decline of age-specific coronary mortality (%)
35–44	27.2
45–54	27.4
55–64	23.5
65–74	25.3
75–84	12.8
Over 85	19.3

Source: W.D. Walker (1977).

disease. It has been less clearly established that the incidence of non-fatal attacks has changed.

Naturally, many groups, ranging from exercise enthusiasts to cardiac surgeons, have been eager to claim responsibility for this favourable trend of vital statistics.

Improved treatment

A part of the reduction in 'coronary' deaths is probably due to recent advances in the medical and surgical treatment of ischaemic heart disease. In particular, it could be argued that fewer young and middle-aged patients who sustain 'heart attacks' are dying of their disease.

In the past, a large number of cardiac fatalities occurred before the patient could reach hospital, and it might thus be inferred that the improved prognosis was related to the widespread instruction of ambulance crews and of the general public in techniques of cardiac resuscitation (L. Cobb *et al.*, 1975; D.A. Chamberlain, 1978a; J.R. Hampton & Nicholas, 1978; A.F. MacKintosh *et al.*, 1978; P. Siltanen, 1978). Over a third of the Seattle population, for example, is now qualified to undertake such emergency treatment. While gains are to be anticipated from such training, in fact they have yet to be realised. P. Siltanen (1978) found that the specially trained ambulance crews reached about a half of the cases of cardiac arrest where medical aid was summoned before death had occurred, but they were able to treat less than five per cent of all cases of unexpected cardiac arrest. Perhaps because of fears generated by arrival of the special 'cardiac' ambulance, the early mortality for mobile coronary care units has also equalled or slightly exceeded that for patients transported by normal ambulance (J.R. Hampton & Nicholas, 1978; P. Siltanen, 1978).

It might be anticipated that a large reduction of 'coronary' mortality would have resulted from the introduction of expensively equipped intensive-care wards. However, again possibly because of fears aroused by the special treatment, controlled trials have shown that the acute coronary care unit offers little advantage of prognosis relative to treatment in the patient's own home (J.D. Hill *et al.*, 1978).

Early trials of β-adrenoceptor antagonists had disappointingly little influence upon mortality following myocardial infarction (R. Balcon *et al.*, 1966; J. Clausen *et al.*, 1966; Multicentre Trial, 1966; R.M. Norris *et al.*, 1968), but it has been suggested that the dose of propranolol used was too small. D.A. Chamberlain (1978b) has now presented evidence that large doses of cardio-selective β-blocking drugs such as practolol and alprenolol reduce the number of cardiac deaths in the period one month to one year post-infarction, although the effect observed (a halving of events) would reduce the overall mortality from ischaemic heart disease by about two per cent rather than 25 per cent.

By-pass surgery may also improve prognosis in selected cases (Table 2.10), particularly patients with multiple-vessel disease (A.V.G. Bruschke, 1977) or left-main-stem coronary-artery disease (M.H. Frick *et al.*, 1978). Frick *et al.* comment that 'in no report has the surgical treatment been inferior to medical management' but that 'data analyzed do not strongly favor surgical therapy as a means of reducing the rate of sudden death nor death in general for that matter.'

We must thus conclude that the overall contribution of improved treatment to the decline in mortality has been relatively small, and certainly much less than 25 per cent.

Increased physical activity

Voluntary leisure-time physical activity has undoubtedly increased in popularity among North Americans over the past 15 years. In one survey of Harvard alumnae, R. Paffenbarger *et al.* (1978) observed that the proportion of physically active individuals had increased from 35 per cent to 70–80 per cent over the course of a longitudinal study. Sales of recreational bicycles, cross-country skis and other equipment for endurance activity have increased vastly since the early 1960s. Nevertheless in North America, as in Scandinavia (S. Stensassen, 1978), this

Table 2.10: Influence of Surgical Treatment on Survival Following Myocardial Infarction

Type of disease	Period of follow-up (years)	Medical treatment (%)	Surgical treatment (%)
Single-vessel disease	5	89.0	94.6
Two-vessel disease	5	70.0	94.1
Three-vessel disease	4	65.0	92.7
Aneurysm	4	59.0	84.1
Diffuse myocardial impairment	3	23.9	33.0

Source: Based on data of A.V.G. Bruschke (1977).

change of attitude is predominantly a middle-class phenomenon, and the great mass of lower-class Americans have yet to turn from their sedentary lifestyle.

Among the telephone sample of the Saskatoon population (D.A. Bailey *et al.*, 1974), 60 per cent of men and 64 per cent of women were still taking only one session or less of endurance activity per week. On the limiting assumptions that (i) a half of the remaining 38 per cent were new converts to exercise, and (ii) that such exercise halved the chances of a fatal heart attack (R. Paffenbarger, 1977; R. Paffenbarger *et al.*, 1978), the maximum reduction in mortality from this cause would be ten per cent.

Cigarette smoking

The proportion of male cigarette smokers in the coronary-prone age categories has dropped steadily over the period of inquiry. The US sample reached a peak of about 63 per cent smokers in 1955 (Figure 2.4), dropping to about 46 per cent in 1970. Figures for Canada are similar, with 44 per cent of continuing smokers in 1973 (*Smoking in Canada*, 1973).

On the basis that smoking doubles the risk of sudden death (Framingham Heart Study, 1966), this change of behaviour would in itself account for a twelve per cent decrease in deaths from ischaemic heart disease. Many of the fatalities in continuing smokers are sudden deaths due to the onset of ventricular fibrillation. The contribution of reduced smoking to the waning of the epidemic is thus supported by the greater relative reduction of acute than of chronic deaths.

Table 2.11: Change in Per Capita Consumption of Tobacco and Fat (US Citizens, 1963 to 1975)

Product	Change in per capita consumption (%)
Tobacco (all forms)	−22.4
Animal fat and oils	−56.7
Vegetable fat and oils	+44.1
Butter	−31.9
Milk and cream	−19.2
Eggs	−12.6

Source: Based on an analysis by W.D. Walker (1977).

Intake of animal fat

North Americans have shown a substantial increase in the intake of supposedly unsaturated fat over the present century (Tables 2.8 and 2.11). However, the trend was initiated at a time when the incidence of ischaemic heart disease was still rising steeply. A long lag period between fat intake and disease must thus be postulated if the recent decline in mortality is to be attributed to the dietary change. Such is indeed possible. A reduced intake of animal fat probably does little to reverse established atherosclerotic lesions, but it may well prevent the formation of the initial fatty plaques in younger individuals who as yet have healthy arteries.

Conclusion

Much of the decrease in deaths from ischaemic heart disease over the past fifteen years can apparently be attributed to favourable changes in the lifestyle of the average North American (Table 2.11). There is *prima facie* evidence that a combination of reduced cigarette smoking and enhanced physical activity account for over 20 per cent of the observed change, with the remaining five per cent possibly due to long-term changes in eating habits and improved patterns of treatment for established disease.

This conclusion is particularly encouraging for those concerned with preventive medicine. Until recently, cynics have insisted that human behaviour cannot be changed. They have pointed out that gains from health education seem few and short-lived. For example, the massive report of the US surgeon-general on *Smoking and Health*

(1964) apparently produced no more than a five per cent decrease of US cigarette consumption, which disappeared over the next one to two years. Nevertheless, graphs such as Figure 2.4 show that in a more long-term sense the efforts of the health educators are modifying human behaviour, and this in turn is now having a positive influence upon the health of the North American population.

3 ISCHAEMIC HEART DISEASE AND THE RISKS OF EXERCISE

Newspapers frequently publicise fatalities involving well-known athletes, particularly if death has occurred during physical activity. R. Medved *et al.* (1973) describe a 29-year-old member of the Yugoslavian national soccer team who died suddenly, soon after competition, with narrowing of the aorta as a possible contributory cause. K.S. Zakopoulos (1973) collected histories of seven such episodes in Greek soccer players over the course of twenty years; one 24-year-old man died of cardiac arrest, and another man aged 29 died of acute myocardial infarction. Personal experience of this type of incident includes an apparently healthy 23-year-old university student who died after hanging for several minutes from the parallel bars in the gymnasium, and a middle-aged janitor who died while rushing up several flights of stairs to attend to a broken water-main. The latter individual had completed a multistage stress test some weeks previously; the laboratory exercise had been symptomless, but the electrocardiogram had shown marked ST segmental depression and multiple abnormalities of cardiac rhythm as maximum effort was approached (see Chapter 8).

Before proceeding to consider the possible therapeutic value of exercise, it is thus necessary to examine the alternative hypothesis that physical activity increases the immediate mortality of seemingly normal adults, of the 'coronary-prone' and of patients with established clinical ischaemic heart disease. After noting the basic risk of a coronary attack in the average adult, we shall look at the patho-physiology of those dying during exercise, epidemiological data and the experience gained through exercise testing and prescription. The issues of more general injury and infection attributable to exercise will be discussed briefly in Chapter 9.

The Basic Risk of Myocardial Infarction and Sudden Death

Even if physical activity was not a precipitating factor, a certain number of 'coronary' events would be anticipated in exercising subjects as a matter of chance. The likely statistics can be calculated from the incidence of ischaemic heart disease (Chapter 2). In an older man of working age, for example, the risk of developing a heart attack in any given year is about one chance in three hundred, and only about a third of these cases will die during the acute episode.

Given that the average bout of voluntary exercise lasts about 30 minutes, the chances that the attack will occur during this specific session are about two in ten million, with the risk of a fatality about six in 100 million. Figures for women are only about a third as large. Statistics can be further improved if training programmes educate the general public in the techniques of cardiac resuscitation (Chapter 2).

On the other hand, if exercise is repeated 150 times per year, there is a corresponding increase in the *a priori* likelihood that an attack will occur while the individual is physically active.

Patho-physiology of Sudden Death during Exercise

Possible mechanisms

E. Jokl (1958) and more recently E. Jokl & McClellan (1971) have maintained that exercise never causes the death of a normal heart, at least in a temperate climate. Likewise L.E. Hinckle *et al.* (1969) suggested that, if abnormalities of cardiac rhythm were provoked by ordinary physical activity, there was usually some underlying cardiac disease. While such views are probably correct, they are not particularly helpful in elucidating the dangers of exercise, for as we have already noted there is evidence of atherosclerosis in the hearts of most North Americans from a relatively early age (W.F. Ebos *et al.*, 1955; D. Jaffé & Manning, 1971).

Sudden death has many patho-physiological connotations, particularly if statistics are extended to include all patients dying within 24 hours of the onset of symptoms. However, if interest is restricted to the first one or two hours, ventricular fibrillation or asystole is largely responsible (Chapter 1; H.K. Hellerstein & Turrell, 1964; H. Grendahl, 1967; T.N. James, 1972). There are several possible mechanisms whereby an increase of physical activity could enhance myocardial irritability and thus provoke fibrillation or asystole.

The cardiac work-rate may be augmented four- or five-fold by increases in: (i) heart rate; (ii) systolic pressure; and (iii) myocardial contractility (Chapter 8). A combination of shortened diastole and increase of systolic pressure restricts perfusion of left-ventricular muscle, increasing the chances that a relative oxygen lack will develop. The sub-endocardial tissue is particularly vulnerable, and hypoxia may persist in this region during the recovery period. At this stage, a catastrophic fall of blood pressure and thus coronary perfusion may arise from passive standing in a humid changing room or use of an excessively hot shower (R.A. Bruce *et al.*, 1968), while slowing of the heart rate enhances the danger of re-entry of the electrical impulse (Chapter 1). The excitability of the myocardium is further disturbed by alterations of the balance between sodium and potassium ions across the cell membranes of the myocardium, as potassium ions leak from skeletal and cardiac muscle (R.J. Shephard & Kavanagh, 1975) and fluids with an excessive content of potassium ions are administered (T. Kavanagh & Shephard, 1978). If the patient becomes anxious, hyperventilation and an increased liberation of catecholamines add to the irritability of the heart.

Ventricular premature contractions are generally held to be of two types (G. Bourne, 1927; R.H. Mann & Burchell, 1952). One is present at rest and becomes less frequent during exercise. This form of dysrhythmia is quite common (for example, R.G. Hiss & Lamb, 1962, found a prevalence of 0.8 per cent among 122,000 asymptomatic Air Force personnel aged 16 to 50 years). It appears to be relatively benign (J.M. Clarke *et al.*, 1976; M. Brodsky *et al.*, 1977). The other type of premature ventricular contractions is aggravated by exercise or appears for the first time during exercise (B. Lown *et al.*, 1969; H. Blackburn *et al.*, 1973; J.M. Atkins *et al.*, 1976), and becomes even more apparent in the recovery period. This second type of dysrhythmia is an accompaniment of otherwise symptomless atheroma in the middle-aged person and, particularly if of multifocal origin, it is associated with both ischaemic depression of the ST segment of the electrocardiogram and progression to sudden death from ventricular fibrillation or asystole (B. Chiang *et al.*, 1969; L.E. Hinckle *et al.*, 1969; J.A. Vedin *et al.*, 1972).

Exercise may also contribute to the development of a frank myocardial infarct. This could arise from a relative ischaemia of the myocardium, due to the various factors discussed above. Alternatively, an exercise-induced increase of coronary blood flow or an enhanced movement of the ventricular wall could precipitate haemorrhage into a pre-existing atheromatous plaque (A.C. Burton, 1965) or lead to the breaking away of an embolic fragment of plaque and overlying clot which becomes impacted in a more distal branch of the coronary arterial tree. There are thus good patho-physiological grounds for suggesting that exercise can sometimes precipitate death through dysrhythmia, asystole or myocardial infarction.

Post-mortem findings

E. Jokl (1958) collected post-mortem reports on 76 cases of sudden death during exercise. The majority date from the period prior to world war II, but nevertheless the material is of some interest in indicating the commonest pathological findings.

Coronary insufficiency or occlusion was noted in 34 cases. Rupture of the heart or a major blood vessel occurred in 22 instances, although two of these episodes associated with advanced tuberculosis and one related to tertiary syphilis would be unlikely in a more recent series; 4 of the lesions developed in the heart wall, eleven in the aorta, five in cerebral blood vessels and two in the pulmonary vessels. Cardiac rupture is often associated with an unsuspected myocardial infarction. The diagnosis is sometimes missed because of a psychosis (W.W. Jetter & White, 1944), but even in psychiatrically normal individuals up to 25 per cent of infarctions pass unrecognised under such guises as a self-medicated 'attack of indigestion' (W.B. Kannel *et al.*, 1970). Cardiac failure was blamed in 17 of the 76 deaths discussed by E. Jokl, eight being examples of chronic infection or degenerative conditions and five acute viral or bacterial infections. We have noted the decrease in popularity of chronic myocardial degeneration as a descriptor of the cause of death (Chapter 2). Nevertheless, degeneration can develop with repeated small infarcts, or as a consequence of malnutrition (for example, in alcoholics and in many of the patients from under-developed countries). Acute infections may sometimes account for the general malaise that is a frequent precursor of myocardial infarction. Congenital lesions (four cases) were a relatively infrequent diagnosis, while in three of the 76 reports the cause of death was not clearly established.

About a third of the 76 cases presented a history of sustained isometric effort before death. Examples included 'weight-lifting', 'carrying heavy luggage', 'cranking a motor-car', 'lifting a heavy couch' and 'killing animals with a 25 pound hammer'. However, some deaths had been preceded by more moderate activities such as walking, and the remaining third had been associated with sustained rhythmic activities such as long-distance running, cycling, games of football, tennis and swimming.

Several other pathological reports point to similar conclusions. L. Schmid & Hornof (1973) described 76 deaths in Czechoslovak athletes. The average age was 31.2 years, and (probably as a consequence of relative participation rates) 94.7 per cent of the sample were men. In 30 of the 76, coronary disease was implicated, and in 20

Table 3.1: Activities Undertaken by 174 Athletes Sustaining
Cardiovascular Deaths while Exercising

Baseball	1	Quoits	1
Basketball	17	Riding	1
Bowls	2	Running	57
Boxing	2	Shot-put	4
Climbing	2	Skiing — downhill & Nordic	13
Cricket	2	Skipping	1
Curling	4	Softball	1
Cycling	4	Squash	1
Dancing	4	Swimming	8
Football (rugby, soccer & US)	25	Wrestling	3
Golf	4	Weight lifting	1
Gymnastics	3	Yachting	2
Hockey	1		
Judo	3		
Pentathlon	1		

Source: Data compiled from the reports specified in the text.

of the remainder other cardiac disorders were held to be responsible.
N.D. Graievskaia & Markov (1973) reported on the deaths of five
Russian athletes; they thought it significant that all of the fatalities
occurred in individuals who were training irregularly (although it is
arguable that this may have been an effect rather than the cause of
their problem). I. Vuori (1975) examined details of deaths during
20–90-km cross-country skiing events; unfortunately, autopsy reports
were available for only seven of ten fatalities, three of the seven being
acute myocardial infarctions. J. Moncur (1973) obtained reports of
63 deaths in Scottish sportsmen; 43 were due to environmental
exposure or trauma, but twelve of the remaining 20 were attributed
to coronary occlusion. In West Germany, a Documentation Centre has
recorded 110 sports deaths over ten years (H. Munscheck, 1980); 40
of 85 organic disorders were coronary atherosclerosis, and a further ten
were instances of myocarditis. One somewhat divergent report was
from the US Armed Forces Institute of Pathology (B.J. Maron, 1980);
among 19 competitive atheletes who died suddenly, the commonest
anatomic lesion (six cases) was said to be hypertrophy. Nevertheless,
severe coronary atherosclerosis was seen in three cases, and congenital

coronary arterial anomalies in a further three cases.

Information on the nature of the sport being undertaken is available from a total of 174 reports (E. Jokl, 1958; T.N. James *et al.*, 1971; T. Izeki, 1973; R. Medved *et al.*, 1973; K.S. Zakopoulos, 1973; R.J. Shephard, 1974b; I. Vuori, 1975; B.J. Maron, 1980). Interpretation is hampered by the specific interests of many of the investigators, and by differences in the average ages of competitors in different sports. Nevertheless, almost no type of sporting activity seems immune from such attacks (Table 3.1).

Epidemiological Data

General considerations

If physical activity contributes significantly to myocardial infarction and sudden death, as the above data suggest, one should find a differing incidence of 'coronary' episodes during the parts of the day devoted to sleep, employment (usually sedentary or light physical activity) and leisure (when most of the intense and unusual expenditures of energy are undertaken).

Unfortunately, a simple epidemiological analysis of this sort is rarely possible. Published reports commonly suffer from a dilution of the data. Information on attacks in the middle-aged and relatively healthy wage-earner is often confounded with data for very elderly patients (for example, R. Kala *et al.*, 1978) and, as W.M. Yater *et al.* (1971) have noted, the proportion of coronary victims dying at rest increases with their age. Even among the middle-aged, the consequences of physical activity could well be masked by statistics for that 70–90 per cent of the population who take little physical activity either at work or in their leisure hours (R.J. Shephard, 1976a; R.J. Shephard *et al.*, 1968c; D.A. Bailey *et al.*, 1974). Any activity that is undertaken is usually of brief duration, and the allowable latent period between exercise and death is uncertain. In one of the cases cited by E. Jokl (1958), twelve weeks had elapsed between the supposedly unusual exercise and death! A maximum of six hours should probably be allowed, and the evidence is most convincing if death occurs during or within 15 minutes of the completion of exercise. R. Kala *et al.* (1978) found that strenuous activity was more than twice as common during or immediately before an attack as on the preceding day.

A further problem is that data are usually collected retrospectively, and there is then a risk that relatives will have searched vigorously for a 'cause' of death, attaching excessive importance to some trivial incident. Death is usually ascribed to a 'coronary attack' or 'ischaemic heart disease', without distinguishing the several possible pathologies (ventricular fibrillation, relative ischaemia, haemorrhage into an atheromatous plaque, lodgement of an embolus or cardiac failure following progressive thrombosis of a major coronary vessel). Whereas the first four of these conditions could be precipitated by exercise, the last seems more likely to arise while the coronary blood flow is sluggish (for example, during sleep). R. Kala *et al.* (1978) noted that physical activity was 2.4 times more common in subjects dying instantaneously than in their total sample of 'coronary' deaths.

A final difficulty is that the classification of activity may be inadequate if not misleading. Bed rest, for example, may be a modest description which hides a substantial number of attacks brought about by sexual activity.

Previous investigations

C.K. Friedberg (1966) has summarised much of the older literature on this topic. C. Phipps (1936) assembled a series of 437 cases. Deliberate physical exercise was noted in 13 per cent, and moderate or unusual exertion in a further 18 per cent, while only eight per cent of subjects were sleeping at the time of attack. A.M. Master (1946) apparently set out to disprove the association between disease and exertion, and claimed to have substantiated his argument when only two per cent of 1,108 cases gave a history of unusual exertion. However, a surprising 16 per cent were walking, and another nine per cent were engaged in moderate activity, bringing the total who were exercising to 27 per cent of his series. G. Fitzhugh & Hamilton (1933) found 24 per cent of their population had been involved in violent exertion, and 33 per cent in moderate activity. Other of the older authors repeat this story. Unusual exertion was noted in 17 per cent (W.B. Cooksey, 1939), 33 per cent (A.J. French & Dock, 1944) or even 60 per cent of patients (C. Smith *et al.*, 1942). W.M. Yater *et al* (1971) looked at 'coronary attacks' in young soldiers, and commented that during physical effort the incidence was twice the anticipated figure for resting conditions. G. Fitzhugh & Hamilton (1933) observed that the critical episode was often associated with fatigue, inadequate sleep and emotional strain. This point is well illustrated by Werkmeister's patient, who died while walking to college on his examination day (E. Jokl, 1958). A.J. French & Dock (1944) provided examples of the type of daily activity associated with myocardial infarction — cranking a car in cold weather, lifting a heavy trunk, pushing a stalled car and long walks uphill. They emphasised that many of the individuals concerned had either not attempted these tasks previously, or at least had not carried them out for many years.

A.R. Moritz & Zamcheck (1946) looked at the antecedents of sudden and unexpected death in soldiers. Their subjects were presumably younger and in better physical condition than the average coronary victim, yet the number of sudden deaths occurring during vigorous activity was about twice the anticipated figure. L. Adelson (1961) found that 55 per cent of his sample were engaged in light activity, five per cent in strenuous activity and only 21 per cent were asleep at the time of attack. However, his population was atypical, consisting largely of 'alcoholics and vagabonds'. D.M. Spain & Bradess (1960a) examined episodes of sudden 'coronary' death in Westchester County, New York; they reported that 14 per cent of those with atherosclerotic lesions and 16 per cent of those with thrombotic lesions had been involved in unusual activity at the moment of attack. A. Armstrong *et al.* (1972) noted that, of 226 medically unattended sudden deaths, a surprisingly large proportion (19 per cent) occurred 'on the street'. B. Wikland (1971) scrutinised all medically unattended fatal cases of ischaemic heart disease in a defined population; he observed that 27 per cent of the men and 25 per cent of the women were walking at the time of attack. Only four per cent of the men and six per cent of the women in his sample were asleep, but a relatively large percentage (52 per cent of the men and 56 per cent of the women) were said to be resting.

Against this long list of reports stressing the association between physical activity and attack, S. Pell & D'Alonzo (1964) stated that 60 per cent of ischaemic heart disease in wage-earning men occurred during sleep or rest, while L. Kuller *et al.* (1967) found no relationship of sudden death to time of day, season, place, occupation or activity. As already noted, some of the discrepancy in conclusions is related to the suddenness of death (R. Kala *et al.*, 1978). M. Friedman *et al.* (1973) distinguished sudden death (within 24 hours of the onset of symptoms) from instantaneous death (within 30 seconds of the onset of symptoms). The latter type of fatality was almost always due to a dysrhythmia, and in more than a half of cases it developed during or immediately after physical exertion.

E. Simonson & Berman (1972) have summarised the experience of Russian investigators. Findings seem much as in the west. Myocardial infarction is by no means a rarity in young Russians. The male/female ratio is much higher for young than for older patients, and excessive physical effort — vigorous bouts of running, skiing, athletic games and the lifting of heavy loads — seems the commonest cause of attack in the young.

The antecedents of coronary attacks in women have received relatively little study. C. Bengtsson (1973) reported that two per cent of women were under mental stress, and 15 per cent were physically active at the time of attack. M. Romo (1972) compared the activity patterns of men and women dying suddenly from ischaemic heart disease. Some six per cent of the men were actually engaged in strenuous physical activity, and a further nine per cent presented such a history immediately prior to attack (items cited included formal sports, snow-shovelling and the carrying of heavy loads). However, perhaps because such activities were infrequent among the women of Helsinki in 1972, only one per cent of the females had been engaged in vigorous work at the time of attack. As in most other studies, both sexes showed a small deficit of cases between midnight and 6 a.m.

To summarise previous epidemiological data, most authors have found some relationship between physical activity and sudden death, at least in men. On the other hand, the strength of the association has varied widely from one study to another, being greater for near-instantaneous deaths than for episodes where some hours had elapsed between the onset of symptoms and death.

The Toronto study

T. Kavanagh & Shephard (1973a) made a further study of the antecedents of myocardial infarction in relatively young coronary victims (average age 45 years) who had survived the acute episode and were attending an exercise-centred rehabilitation programme.

Events were reviewed for one year, one week and one day prior to attack. By way of control, the same questionnaire was administered to healthy colleagues of the 'post-coronary' sample. Data were available from 203 primary and 30 recurrent non-fatal attacks. In the year preceding the primary episode, 79 of the 203 men noted an increase in body mass, and only 16 a decrease; however, 28 of 57 controls also reported a gain in body mass. Physical activity was regarded as 'normal' by most of the coronary group, but 130 of the 203 reported an increase of business problems, and only three men a decrease ($P < 0.001$); 61 also noted increased social and domestic problems, and only two a decrease ($P < 0.001$).

One week before attack, there was still no change in physical activity, but business problems (increased in 106/203, decreased in 8/203) and social or domestic problems (increased in 42/203, decreased in 4/203) were again perceived as important. Only nine of the 203 patients identified a clear-cut fever or upper respiratory infection, but 73 felt vaguely 'unwell' in the week preceding the attack (compared with eleven who noted an improvement of health; $P <$ 0.001). In about two thirds of the group, the complaints could perhaps be interpreted as incipient myocardial oxygen lack, but the remainder merely complained of tiredness, nervous tension or depression. In some instances, an accumulation of business worries may have led to excessive smoking, an abnormally large intake of coffee, loss of physical condition or an increase in body mass. In other cases, acute infection or a disturbance of electrolyte balance may have had a more direct impact upon myocardial irritability.

On the day prior to attack, information was incomplete for two individuals, 85 of 201 felt unwell, vigorous physical activity was noted by 51/201 and heavy lifting by 47/202. In contrast, unusual annoyance (41/203), business problems (40/203) and social or domestic problems (25/203) were less common than in the entire year preceding the attack. Humid heat was reported by 35/203; the association between heat stress and cardiac deaths is well recognised in the United States (G.S. Berenson & Burch, 1952). Fresh, wet snow was reported by 25/202, cold or very cold weather by 87/203, and snow-shovelling by 9/203. Despite frequent newspaper headlines in northern cities, snow-shovelling is a relatively infrequent antecedent of heart attacks. This is partly because the total number of minutes devoted to shovelling is relatively few in any given year, and partly because the cardiac work-load varies widely with such variables as the depth and wetness of the snow, the chill factor and the possible physiological and psychological strains of rapid shovelling immediately after breakfast.

Among the control sample, complaints of increased business worries were made by only 16 of 57 subjects at one year, 14 of 57 at one week, and four of 57 at one day prior to completion of the questionnaire. Likewise, social and domestic problems were increased in only 14 of 57 at one week, and two of 57 on the day prior to questioning. Only eight of the 57 noted annoyance on the preceding day, and only four of 57 a deterioration of health in the preceding week. It would thus appear that business and social problems along with a general malaise are common features of the period before a frank coronary attack. Nevertheless, it remains arguable that the perception of such problems has been heightened by the critical experience of the acute episode.

Perhaps the most intriguing comparison is between the activities actually reported at the time of attack and the anticipated daily activity pattern of the average Toronto business man. We expected, for example, about 7.7 hours of sleep per day, which would have yielded 81 sleep-related attacks among our total sample of 233 primary and recurrent episodes; however, in fact there were only 48 such attacks. Likewise, at least 70 attacks should have occurred at the place of employment, but there were only 30 such incidents. In contrast, odd jobs and sports should not have accounted for more than five cases apiece, yet the totals were 21 and 30 cases, respectively. Walking also accounted for 13 rather than the anticipated three cases. Other significant concentrations were for running (eight cases), various sports (13 cases, including one in the shower area), snow-shovelling (nine cases), various other heavy domestic chores (15 cases) and sexual intercourse (two cases). In a number of instances, the physical activity closely followed a heavy meal, or was associated with emotional stress (for instance, defending a curling championship). Other episodes were related to the patient's aggressive 'Type A' behaviour, for example determination to beat an opponent at tennis after some years away from the courts, and reluctance to admit exhaustion (well illustrated by a politician entered in a long-distance charity run). A number of histories referred to unusual isometric activity, such as a professor who had spent a whole day moving 25 kg cartons of mineral specimens after a sabbatical leave, and a 'cottager' who had carried his canoe for almost 1 km when closing his summer home for the season.

Several incidents occurred while attending a hospital or a doctor's office, apparently for treatment of an unrelated condition. It is possible that the premonitory malaise of a coronary attack had contributed to the decision to undergo medical examination, but it is also arguable that anxiety associated with the examination precipitated the attack. The latter viewpoint has two practical corollaries — effort should be given to making medical examinations a less frightening experience, and over-zealous medical supervision may on occasion provoke the calamity it is trying to avoid.

Because of the location of the Toronto Rehabilitation Centre, the majority of our patients are 'white-collar' workers. It is thus possible that more employment-related episodes might be encountered in other communities where physical labour was the norm. In Brisbane, the State Compensation Board accepts some 500 cases per year (about a third of the total coronary victims among employed males in Queensland) as being caused or aggravated by daily work. Usually, the work accepted for purposes of compensation is of a physical nature, although occasional episodes have been attributed successfully to unusual mental stresses that have arisen in the course of employment.

Both the Toronto and the Brisbane statistics support the view that exercise increases the immediate risk of myocardial infarction. Adverse features include activity that is unusual for the patient, is excessive relative to his level of physical fitness, and is accompanied by emotional stress.

Experience during Exercise Testing and Prescription

Another possible tactic is to review the experience of exercise test facilities and gymnasia. The problem with such an approach is that we are dealing with an infrequent occurrence. Even a very busy laboratory hardly accumulates enough data to yield accurate statistics. If the test facility is in a hospital, the population examined is usually biased in the direction of the middle-aged and the coronary-prone, and performance of the test involves not only vigorous exercise, but also anxiety concerning the test result.

Exercise testing

J.R. McDonough & Bruce (1969) set the hazard of clinical exercise testing at one attack of ventricular fibrillation for every 3,000 maximum-effort tests, and one attack for every 15,000 sub-maximum tests. Many of their cases of ventricular fibrillation were successfully resuscitated, partly because the coronary vasculature of those tested was adequate for rest if not for maximum effort, and partly because a well-trained emergency team was always close at hand.

P. Rochmis & Blackburn (1971) found 16 fatal incidents in pooled data from 72 North American laboratories. It was estimated that the investigators concerned had carried out a total of about 170,000 maximum or sub-maximum tests. Thirteen of the fatal episodes began within one hour of exercise, an attack rate of one in 13,000; all were patients with known cardiac disease, but unfortunately there were no means of determining how many of the 170,000 individuals who were tested also fell into this 'high-risk' category.

Other researchers have had a somewhat similar experience. L. Brock (1967) encountered three fatal episodes in a series of 17,000 work evaluation tests. M. Ellestad *et al.* (1969) had no deaths in 4,000 symptom-limited maximum tests, but about 0.9 per cent of his patients developed ventricular tachycardia. A. Kattus & McAlpin

(1968) reported two attacks of ventricular fibrillation (one fatal) in 500 treadmill tests, while B. Phibbs *et al.* (1968) noted 'three major complications including a massive current of injury and ventricular flutter' in 787 tests.

There is some evidence that the Master two-step exercise is less hazardous than maximum exercise; three series (A.J. Brody, 1959; L.E. Lamb & Hiss, 1962; G.P. Robb & Marks, 1964) observed no significant dysrhythmias other than one evanescent tachycardia in a total of 4,266 cases.

The attack rate of P. Rochmis & Blackburn is equivalent to 674 attacks per 1,000 man-years, even neglecting the effect of the three subjects who died in the period between one and 24 hours after testing. If we assume that the base population was mainly male, half being average middle-aged adults with a coronary risk of 3.5 attacks per 1,000 man-years, and half 'coronary' patients with a recurrence rate of 25 attacks per 1,000 man years, the observed frequency of attacks during exercise would be 47 times the anticipated figure. Conclusions of a similar order can be drawn from the other reports concerning maximum and sub-maximum exercise tests.

Operation of gymnasia

Anecdotal reports suggest that vigorous physical activity can have appreciable risk for middle-aged adults. Thus S. Fox (personal communication) noted that, over a one-year period, eight deaths of men wearing jogging clothes occurred in Orange County, California.

The mass ski contests of Scandinavia provide sufficient man-hours of exercise to allow risk calculations. P.O. Åstrand (personal communication) comments that two large cross-country events in Sweden have attracted about 10,000 entrants for each of 50 years, with only two fatalities, both in 1971. The Finnish experience is similar. I. Vuori (1975) found ten fatalities in twelve million man-hours of cross-country skiing. Between a half and three quarters of the villagers participated in the events that he examined, and he estimated that the death rate was about four times that of a comparable population under resting conditions. Uncertainties include the impact of conditioning and competition, but this is probably a minimum estimate of the danger of sustained exercise, since the unhealthy members of a community would tend to avoid the ski races. A further imponderable is the relationship between brief and extended activity. Many of the harmful effects of exercise, such as the rise in systemic blood pressure and the secretion of catecholamines, are cumulative phenomena, so that the hazard of a six-hour ski race might be much greater than a 30-minute 'work-out' in a gymnasium; on the other hand, there are specific risks associated with the warm-up (R.J. Barnard *et al.*, 1973) and the warm-down (J.R. McDonough & Bruce, 1969), and in this sense a number of short bouts of activity create more danger than one long race.

Almost a quarter of the patients attending the Toronto Rehabilitation Centre perceived their 'coronary' attacks as occurring during exercise (T. Kavanagh & Shephard, 1973a). It is unlikely that the average member of this group was spending more than 30–60 minutes per day in such physical activity prior to infarction, and on this basis we would estimate that the risk of a non-fatal coronary incident was increased between six- and twelve-fold during exercise. The patients studied were of course a high-risk group, heavy smokers, with a high serum cholesterol, 'Type A' personalities and other disadvantages of the 'coronary-prone' person.

A few years ago, calculations based on reports reaching Toronto newspapers suggested that the attack rate in unsupervised gymnastic programmes for the coronary-prone middle-aged male might be as high as one in 2,500 man-hours (Shephard, 1971). Subsequent to publication of this pessimistic statistic, admission criteria were greatly tightened in Ontario and elsewhere, and the frequency of such episodes decreased dramatically. More recent figures refer to patients with known ischaemic heart disease. H.R. Pyfer *et al.* (1975) have experienced one episode of cardiac arrest for every 7,000 man-hours of supervised training, all patients being successfully resuscitated. W.L. Haskell (1978) collected data on 949,568 man-hours of exercise from 86 exercise programmes. Considering all available information, the risk of cardiac arrest was one in 29,674 man-hours, but in recent years a more cautious approach to operation of the clubs had apparently reduced the risk to one in 268,922 man-hours. Ten years' experience in Toronto has yielded similar statistics. T. Kavanagh and I have now accumulated 242,420 hours of supervised and 700,840 hours of unsupervised activity, with a total of eight incidents (four of which were successfully resuscitated); our attack rate is thus one in 117,907 man-hours of exercise. This is low, but is nevertheless equivalent to an annual rate of 7.43 per cent, more than four times the overall coronary recurrence rate for our particular sample of patients.

The Southern Ontario multicentre exercise-heart trial has followed 750 post-coronary patients prospectively for a total of four years. About a quarter of the recurrent infarctions in this group were associated with exercise (R.J. Shephard, 1979a). Even taking account of substantial exercise prescriptions, the attack rate during physical activity was at least six times as large as expected.

Conclusions

Available data suggest that in normal subjects, coronary-prone individuals and post-coronary patients exercise increases the immediate risk of a 'coronary attack' by a factor of between four and twelve. Statistics of this order show the need for individualised exercise prescription, with avoidance of excessive competition and unusual activity for which a person is ill prepared; in patients, there must also be a careful monitoring of the training response, with a graded progression and avoidance of isometric effort.

Some reports indicate a risk of group exercise that is between 10- and twenty-fold greater than the currently accepted North American figure. It is not clear how far this can be explained simply by factors of patient selection. One adverse factor may be emotional stress, whether due to the task itself (for example, a crucial competition), the outcome of the exercise (a stress test) or some unrelated circumstance of business or domestic life.

Paradoxically, such figures are not an argument against advising people to exercise. Although exercise may precipitate a 'coronary' attack, it is serving mainly to reveal the presence of a badly damaged coronary arterial tree. The affected individual is likely to succumb to ischaemic heart disease over the next few months, and it is preferable for the critical incident to develop in a gymnasium where help is at hand, rather than in some remote area of the countryside. Furthermore, our analysis has to this point merely focussed on the brief period of the day when the victim has been active, and a complete examination of prognosis must consider whether the chances of a critical event are reduced in the intervals between exercise bouts. A four-fold worsening of prognosis during one hour of activity could well be counteracted by a 13 per cent improvement of prognosis for the remaining 23 hours of the day!

Avoiding Exercise-induced Catastrophes

There are unfortunately few specific clues to the individual who will develop cardiac arrest, fibrillation or infarction while he is exercising. An analysis of 230 episodes in patients referred to the Toronto Rehabilitation Centre (R.J. Shephard & Kavanagh, 1978a) noted that those individuals who were active at the time of attack were less likely to have detected an abnormal cardiac rhythm or a general malaise than those who were inactive, but were more likely to have been aware of nervous tension or depression. It also seems likely that they approached exercise in a more competitive spirit, since their subsequent training response was marked by a larger gain of aerobic power (21 per cent, compared with 13.5 per cent), and a small decrease (0.5 kg) as compared with a small gain (0.6 kg) in body mass. After the attack, the blood pressure of the two groups showed no difference, either at rest or during graded exercise; however, it is probable that blood pressures were modified by the acute episode, and in any event there are considerable differences between a laboratory stress test and participation in competitive sports.

In the Southern Ontario multicentre exercise-heart trial, the main features that distinguished patients who developed a recurrence of their infarction while exercising (Table 3.2) were persistent resting ECG abnormalities, a poor exercise compliance and an ST segmental depression of more than 0.2 mV during exercise stress testing (R.J. Shephard, 1980b). Sequential testing further established that immediately prior to reinfarction a number of patients showed an impaired cardiac response to exercise, with a low stroke volume and cardiac output, plus a compensatory broadening of the arterio-venous oxygen difference (R.J. Shephard, 1979a).

Despite this limited information, certain general suggestions can be made to increase the safety of both exercise testing and subsequent exercise prescription. Within the doctor's office or laboatory, care must be taken to allay anxiety. Unnecessary apparatus should be removed from the room, and staff should cultivate a relaxed, non-authoritarian manner. It is often helpful to carry out a brief preliminary practice of the test, deferring formal assessment to a second visit. The safety of the test is increased by a careful preliminary medical examination (K.H. Cooper, 1970; K.L. Andersen *et al.*, 1971), the continuous monitoring of blood pressure and electrocardiograms during the tests with rigid criteria for halting an investigation and the presence of an efficient, well-trained and well-equipped resuscitation team.

If a significant dysrhythmia or ST segmental depression develops during the laboratory test, the heart rate corresponding to this occurrence should be noted, and the prescribed activity so arranged that the intensity of effort falls just below this danger level. Particularly when dealing with the post-coronary patient, close adherence to the exercise prescription should be stressed. Individual class members should be taught to count their pulse rate and to recognise such

Table 3.2: A Comparison of Patients Sustaining a Recurrence of Myocardial Infarction during Exercise with Those Sustaining Attack at Other Times

Variable	Recurrence during exercise (%)	Recurrence at other times (%)	P
Exercise compliance (average attendance at sessions over previous 3 months)	38.4	62.4	$0.2 > P > 0.1$
Current smoking	60.0	64.5	n.s.
Angina	60.0	58.1	n.s.
Systemic hypertension (resting pressure > 150/100 mm Hg)	0	11.1	n.s.
Serum cholesterol (> 270 mg/100 ml)	0	9.1	n.s.
Persistent resting ECG abnormalities	83.3	53.3	$0.2 > P > 0.1$
Exercise ST segmental depression > 0.2 mV	50.0	22.6	$0.1 > P > 0.05$
Ventricular premature beats	0	4.9	n.s.

Source: Based on preliminary data from Southern Ontario multicentre exercise-heart trial (R.J. Shephard, 1979a).

symptoms as angina and premature ventricular contractions. They should be advised to train regularly, avoiding both peaks of unusual activity and intense competition. Further, they should be warned to reduce their prescription temporarily in any unfavourable situation, be it climatic (very hot or very cold weather), medical (the sensing of ischaemic prodromata) or psychological (mental tension or depression).

Despite such precautions, some risks will remain. This may seem a negative conclusion to the committed exercise enthusiast. However, it is important to credibility that exercise scientists admit this hazard. And to set the matter in perspective, I would finally endorse the view (P.O. Åstrand & Rodahl, 1977) that, while physical activity carries some small risks, there is evidence (Chapter 4) that a careful medical examination is even more necessary for the person who plans to take no further exercise!

4 EXERCISE AND THE PRIMARY PREVENTION OF ISCHAEMIC HEART DISEASE

Textbooks of epidemiology distinguish the primary, secondary and tertiary prevention of disease (J.S. Mausner & Bahn, 1974). Primary prevention will be the main focus of this chapter. It is applied in the phase of susceptibility, and operates through a change of exposure to disease-causing agents or a reduction in the susceptibility of the individual. Since the initial changes of atherosclerosis develop at an early age (Chapter 1), exercise can have no role in primary prevention if it is not applied from childhood. Certain principles of secondary prevention will also be introduced, to be discussed more fully in Chapter 5. Secondary prevention involves the early detection and treatment of disease, usually while it is in the pre-clinical stage. In the context of ischaemic heart disease, we face the typical situation of the middle-aged adult who becomes involved in an exercise programme. Tertiary prevention, discussed in Chapter 6, is concerned with the restoration of effective function after clinical manifestations of disease have appeared. A typical example is the patient who has sustained a non-fatal myocardial infarction, and subsequently joins an exercise rehabilitation programme with a view to speeding his return to normal life and minimising his chances of a second infarction.

A comprehensive scheme of primary prevention involves both general measures of health promotion and specific action to protect the individual. Relevant techniques for the encouragement of physical activity in the community and the individual will be covered in Chapter 9. The present chapter will review normal reactions to regular endurance training, will consider the possible relevance of such changes to the prevention of ischaemic heart disease and will finally examine the fate of animals encouraged to exercise for long periods of their lives.

Normal Responses to Endurance Training

General considerations

The pattern of exercise most widely suggested as a means of preventing ischaemic heart disease is endurance training. Definitions vary somewhat from one investigator to another, but the usual implication is activity at 60–70 per cent of the individual's maximum oxygen intake, carried out in bouts of 30 minutes' duration or longer three or more times per week (R.J. Shephard, 1977a). In the context of primary prevention, the training must begin in childhood, and continue throughout the lifetime of the subject.

Physiological responses to endurance training were at one time inferred from cross-sectional comparisons between endurance athletes and the general public. This approach has the advantage that the activity considered has been intense and followed for a number of years. However, conclusions are hampered by the fact that top athletes represent a highly selected population sample; probably between a half and two thirds of their unusual ability is due to genetic endowment rather than endurance training (R.J. Shephard, 1978a, 1980c). Much current data is thus drawn from longitudinal studies. Often exercise is initiated as a young adult rather than as a child, and the period of observation is short in the context of chronic disease prevention; nevertheless, a number of interesting physiological changes can be demonstrated over a typical two-to-three month study. Appropriate control groups are an important precaution, since the exercise response can also be altered by habituation to the test environment (R.J. Shephard, 1969), learning of the test procedure (R.J. Shephard *et al.*, 1968a; R.J. Shephard & Lavallée, 1977), seasonal changes in fitness levels (R.J. Shephard *et al.*, 1978b), and long-term trends in the lifestyle of a community (for example, the acculturation of primitive societies to western patterns of diet and inactivity; R.J. Shephard, 1978a).

Recent reports have emphasised the specificity of training. While there is little dispute that the effects of 'weight' training are not the same as those induced by regular distance running, there are also differences in response to different types of endurance exercise, particularly if the total mass of muscle involved in the activity is fairly small. Gains of performance developed on the treadmill are largely transferable to cycle-ergometer exercise, but the reverse is not necessarily true. J.P. Clausen *et al.* (1973) found that some 50 per cent of the response to regular cycle-ergometer training was transferred to an arm-ergometer task, but that arm-ergometer training did little to improve the response to leg ergometry. Likewise, I. Holmér & Åstrand (1972) reported that a trained swimmer showed a larger difference of maximum oxygen intake from her twin sister when swimming than when exercising on an arm ergometer.

Many body systems are modified by regular endurance training

(A. Steinhaus, 1933; P.O. Åstrand & Rodahl, 1977; R.J. Shephard, 1980c). We will consider specifically changes in the heart and cardio-vascular system, the respiratory system, metabolism and body composition (Table 4.1), along with one convenient overall index of endurance fitness, the maximum oxygen intake (R.J. Shephard, 1977a). The average gain of maximum oxygen intake when a sedentary adult undergoes endurance training is about 20 per cent (R.J. Shephard, 1965a, 1977a), but the increase can be much larger if the exercise programme is both heavy and sustained (B. Saltin *et al.*, 1968; R.J. Shephard, 1979b); Dr T. Kavanagh and I have observed one middle-aged man develop from a value of 27 ml·kg^{-1}·min^{-1} immediately after myocardial infarction to about 65 ml·kg^{-1}·min^{-1} five years later (R.J. Shephard, 1979b). Individual responsiveness is modified by many variables, particularly initial fitness and the intensity of training (R.J. Shephard, 1968a, 1975a; M.L. Pollock, 1973). Gains are further augmented if the subject has been 'deconditioned' by a preliminary period of two to three weeks' bed rest (H.L. Taylor *et al.*, 1949; B. Saltin *et al.*, 1968; T. Fried & Shephard, 1969). Suggestions that older subjects train less readily than children or young adults (for example, B. Saltin, 1969) seem a fallacy, caused by judging initial fitness levels in terms of maximum oxygen intake without adjusting this variable for normal age-related changes. If the increase in maximum oxygen intake with training is expressed as a percentage of the initial value, the response of a sedentary 65-year-old adult is at least as large as that observed in his 25-year-old counterpart (K.H. Sidney & Shephard, 1978; R.J. Shephard, 1978b).

The deconditioning experiments illustrate the truth that fitness cannot be stored; indeed, much of the advantage of the endurance athlete is dissipated by a few weeks of inactivity (P.S. Fardy, 1969; M. Katila & Frick, 1970; W. Siegel *et al.*, 1970; Z.B. Kendrick *et al.*, 1971; Å. Kilböm, 1971; M.H. Williams & Edwards, 1971; B. Drinkwater & Horvath, 1972).

Cardiovascular changes

The most obvious cardiovascular response to endurance training is a decrease of heart rate at rest and during sub-maximum exercise (R.J. Barnard, 1975). Whereas the resting heart rate of a sedentary person is 70–80 beats·min^{-1}, that of a superbly conditioned athlete can be 30 beats·min^{-1} or less. The maximum heart rate is reached at a higher oxygen intake after training, and the peak heart rate may show a small (5–10 beats·min^{-1}) decrease (C.T.M. Davies, 1967; R.J. Shephard, 1980c).

Table 4.1: A Comparison of Physiological Variables between a Sedentary Normal Individual, a Trained Normal Individual and a World-class Endurance Athlete

Variable	Sedentary normal		Trained normal		Endurance athlete	
	Rest	Maximum	Rest	Maximum	Rest	Maximum
Cardiovascular						
Heart rate (beats•min^{-1})	71	185	59	183	36	174
Stroke volume (ml)	65	120	80	140	125	200
Cardiac output (l•min^{-1})	4.6	22.2	4.7	25.6	4.5	34.8
Blood pressure:						
systolic (mm Hg)	135	210	130	205	120	210
diastolic (mm Hg)	78	82	76	80	65	65
Heart volume (ml)	750		820		1,200	
Blood volume (l)	4.7		5.1		6.0	
Respiratory						
Resp. min. volume (l•min^{-1} BTPS)	7	110	6	135	6	195
Frequency of respiration (breaths•min^{-1})	14	40	12	45	12	55
Tidal volume (l)	0.5	2.75	0.5	3.0	0.5	3.5
Vital capacity (l)	5.8		6.0		6.2	
Residual volume (l)	1.4		1.2		1.2	
Metabolic						
Oxygen intake (ml•kg^{-1}•min^{-1})	3.5	40.5	3.7	49.8	4.0	76.7
Blood lactate (mg•dl^{-1})	10	110	10	125	10	185
Arterio-venous oxygen difference (ml•dl^{-1})	6.0	14.5	6.0	15.0	6.0	16.0
Body composition						
Body mass (kg)	79.5		77.3		68.2	
Fat mass (kg)	12.7		9.7		5.1	
Lean mass (kg)	66.8		67.6		63.1	
Relative fat (%)	16.0		12.5		7.5	

Source: J.H. Wilmore & Norton (1974).

There is also an increase in the stroke volume of the heart at rest and in sub-maximal exercise (B. Saltin *et al*., 1968; R. Simmons & Shephard, 1971a), while output per beat is better maintained in maximum effort (V. Niinimaa & Shephard, 1978). Consequently, the maximum output of the heart is increased roughly in proportion to the gain of maximum oxygen intake (B. Ekblom *et al*., 1968; R. Simmons & Shephard, 1971a).

Oxygen delivery is further facilitated by a widening of the maximum arterio-venous oxygen difference (B. Saltin *et al.*, 1968; R. Simmons & Shephard, 1971a; H. Roskamm, 1973a). Each litre of blood that is pumped by the heart may yield 160 rather than 140 ml of oxygen to the tissues. This reflects a redistribution of blood flow away from the regions of limited oxygen extraction such as the skin (R. Simmons & Shephard, 1971a) and the viscera (L.B. Rowell, 1974), with a possible increase of oxygen extraction in the working muscles. During sub-maximum exercise, muscle perfusion may be reduced (F.G.V. Douglas & Becklake, 1968; F. Treumann & Schroeder, 1968; J.P. Clausen *et al.*, 1973), but in maximum effort the flow to the muscles is increased (R.H. Rochelle *et al.*, 1971; H. de Marées & Barbey, 1973). The latter change may reflect in a part a strengthening of the working muscles, so that they contract at a small fraction of their maximum force during vigorous effort; this in turn reduces the impedance to their perfusion (C. Kay & Shephard, 1969).

As training proceeds, the drive to the heart from the sympathetic nervous system diminishes both at rest and during exercise. This affects not only the heart rate, but also the myocardial contractility (J. Crews & Aldinger, 1967; S. Penpargkul & Scheuer, 1970). At rest, such indices of myocardial contractility as the maximum rate of rise of intraventricular pressure are the same in sedentary and in trained individuals, but in maximum effort the rate of pressure rise is decreased by training (B.D. Franks & Cureton, 1969; J.F. Wiley, 1971; H. Roskamm, 1973a, b).

Most (L.H. Hartley *et al.*, 1969; Å. Kilböm *et al.*, 1969; J. Chrastek & Adimirova, 1970; H.A. de Vries, 1970; J.S. Hanson & Nedde, 1970; E. Jokl *et al.*, 1970; G. Choquette & Ferguson, 1973) but not all (M.H. Frick *et al.*, 1963; B.S. Tabakin *et al.*, 1965; B. Ekblom *et al.*, 1968) reports have indicated that regular physical exercise lowers the resting systemic blood pressure, both in hypertensive individuals and in those with 'normal' pressures. Blood-pressure readings may also be reduced at a given sub-maximal rate of working. On the other hand, the maximum attained blood pressure may be increased, particularly in hearts where there was difficulty in sustaining stroke output at high work rates prior to training (R.J. Shephard, 1978b).

Hypertrophy of the rat heart is more readily induced in young than in older animals (A.S. Leon & Bloor, 1970; R.J. Tomanek, 1970). In the dog, both the mass and the thickness of the ventricular wall can be increased by as little as twelve weeks of endurance training (H.L. Wyatt & Mitchell, 1974). Cardiac hypertrophy can also occur in human hearts (for example, children with congenital valvular abnormalities), and endurance athletes typically have large hearts (H. Reindell *et al.*, 1966); however, attempts to induce hypertrophy by the moderate endurance training of adolescents and young adults have had far from uniform success (H. Roskamm & Reindell, 1972; J. Cermak, 1973; H. Roskamm, 1973a; R.A. Bruce *et al.*, 1975).

The cardiac work-load comprises effort expended against friction and turbulence in the blood stream, internal work needed to develop and maintain tension in the ventricular walls and smaller energy losses associated with the basal metabolism of the heart muscle, activation of the myocardial fibres and internal friction as the fibres shorten (G. Blomqvist, 1974; E.F. Blick & Stein, 1977; C.R. Jorgensen *et al.*, 1977). Considering only the two main components, the rate of working $\dot{W}$ of each ventricle is approximated by the equation:

$$\dot{W} = (\int_{V_d}^{V_s} P_v \, \delta V + \alpha \int_0^t T \delta t) f_h$$

where P_v is the ventricular pressure, integrated between diastolic and systolic volumes; δV is the instantaneous change of ventricular volume; T is the tension in the ventricular wall integrated over the systolic phase of the cardiac cycle; δt is the instant of time at which a specific value of T is recorded; α is a constant to convert the tension integral to units of work; and f_h is the heart rate. The first term of the equation corresponds to frictional and turbulent work, and the second to tension work. Common non-invasive indices of cardiac work rate are: (i) the heart rate; (ii) the product of systolic pressure and heart rate, sometimes called the double product or the tension-time index; and (iii) the triple product (systolic pressure × heart rate × duration of systole). Heart rate (Y. Wang, 1972; C.R. Jorgensen *et al.*, 1977) is proportional to cardiac work rate only if ventricular pressure, stroke volume and cardiac contraction time all remain constant. The tension-time index depends on the constancy of stroke volume and contraction time. During exercise, the second variable changes less than the first and, fortunately for the index, the tension item is by far the largest component of cardiac work; perhaps for this reason the tension-time index is said to correlate well with direct measurements of myocardial oxygen consumption (C.R. Jorgensen *et al.*, 1977). The triple product is theoretically more precise, but in practice its use is limited by the difficulty in making non-invasive measurements of cardiac contraction times.

Training modifies several components of the cardiac work load.

There may be a small fall in systemic pressure, particularly at rest and in sub-maximum exercise. At the same time, the trained heart tends to empty more completely than the untrained heart, so that the radii of the heart tend to decrease. The relationship between ventricular pressure P_v and tension T is approximated most simply by the law of Laplace for a thin-walled structure:

$$T = (R_1 + R_2)P_v$$

where R_1 and R_2 are the principal radii of the heart; plainly, a decrease of mean dimensions leads to a drop in wall tension. With more sustained conditioning, the cardiac dimensions may be increased by hypertrophy; while this increases the overall tension, the thickening of the ventricular wall further lessens the force exerted by unit cross section of muscle. Heart rate is decreased mainly by a lengthening of the diastolic phase; the term relating to frictional and turbulent work is affected relatively little, since stroke volume per beat is increased, but the slow heart rate greatly diminishes the work performed against intra-mural tension. Finally, the work rate is modified by any changes of myocardial contractility that develop with training.

In the context of ischaemic-heart-disease prevention and treatment, much importance attaches to the delicate balance between the rate of working of the heart and the myocardial blood flow. Oxygen extraction from the coronary blood is relatively complete even at rest, so that the oxygen needs of exercise demand an increase of flow. The left ventricle is more vulnerable to ischaemia than is the right, as it has a heavier work rate and the coronary vessels are exposed to much greater external forces from the myocardium. Flow to the left side of the heart wall occurs mainly during diastole (D.E. Gregg & Fisher, 1963), and the training-induced lengthening of the diastolic phase of the cardiac cycle aids myocardial perfusion. The diastolic pressure may be reduced some-what by training, but this is offset by a reduction of intramural vascular compression, since wall tension is reduced by a decrease of cardiac size and a thickening of the ventricular wall. Substantial anastomoses occur between the two main coronary arteries, particularly at the apex of the heart. Such collaterals are important in reducing the area of heart muscle subject to infarction if flow through the normal pathway fails to satisfy metabolic demand. Some authors have postulated that regular exercise provides a 'hypoxic' stimulus that encourages the opening up of potential anastomotic pathways. Experiments in dogs exercised after surgically induced narrowing of the coronary vessels have sometimes shown such an effect (R.W. Eckstein, 1957; V.F. Froehlicher, 1972; but not F.R. Cobb *et al.*, 1968). The coronary arterial tree is also enlarged (J. Tepperman & Pearlman, 1961; J.A.F. Stevenson, 1967), and the capillary/muscle-fibre ratio is increased at least in experimental animals (R.J. Tomanek, 1970; R.L. Rasmussen *et al.*, 1978). On the other hand, primary prevention (exercise prior to occlusion) does not seem to protect animals against subsequent blockage of their coronary vessels (J.J. Burt & Jackson, 1965; E. Kaplinsky *et al.*, 1968; T.M. Sanders *et al.*, 1978). Observations in man have been limited to tertiary exercise therapy for anginal and 'post-coronary' patients. In general, no collateral formation has been observed (A. Kattus & Grollman, 1972; R.J. Ferguson *et al.*, 1974; M.H. Ellestad, 1975; H.K. Hellerstein, 1977; T. Semple, 1977; N.K. Wenger, 1977). However, it could be objected that: (i) the technique used in man (coronary angiography) only detects vessels larger than 100 μ; and (ii) caution of the patients or their physician leads to exercise of insufficient intensity to stimulate collateral formation.

Respiratory system

The respiratory system has only a modest influence upon the oxygen transport of a healthy adult (R.J. Shephard, 1977a, 1978a). Nevertheless, endurance training modifies a number of respiratory variables. The respiratory minute volume is reduced both at rest and during sub-maximum effort, and the ventilatory equivalent (the ventilatory volume in litres BTPS per litre SPTD of oxygen intake) diminishes towards a limiting value of 25 litres per litre. This reflects partly the adoption of a slower and deeper pattern of breathing, and partly an increase of the threshold work-rate for anaerobic effort (with its associated disproportionate hyperventilation; J. Karlsson *et al.*, 1972). The ventilation attained during maximum effort is increased with training. This is due in part to a strengthening of the respiratory muscles, and in part to an increase in pulmonary blood flow; the latter change augments the critical respiratory minute volume at which the oxygen cost of breathing exceeds the added oxygen intake derived from a further increase in ventilation (A.B. Otis, 1964; R.J. Shephard, 1966a).

Vital capacity shows a moderate correlation with athletic performance (T. Ishiko, 1967), even after allowance for body size (K. Sidney & Shephard, 1973) or body mass (T. Ishiko, 1967). This is attributable partly to selection, and partly to a strengthening of the chest muscles by exercise (L. Delhez *et al.*, 1967–8); modest gains of vital capacity can sometimes be observed after training (Table 3.1).

In the context of ischaemic heart disease, W.B. Kannel (1967) reported an association between a low vital capacity and both attacks of angina and coronary heart disease deaths:

	Anginal attacks (% expected)	Coronary heart disease deaths (% expected)
Low vital capacity	116	171
Normal vital capacity	95	82

Kannel interpreted vital capacity as one indicator of habitual activity, although it is possible that the coronary deaths and the low vital capacity also had a mutual association with cigarette smoking.

Recent research (V. Niinimaa *et al.*, 1980) has established that most subjects augment nose breathing by the oral inhalation of air when the respiratory minute volume exceeds 35 $l \cdot min^{-1}$ BTPS. This leads to a significant deterioration in the 'conditioning' of inspired air. The impingement of cold, dry air on the tracheal mucosa not only tends to provoke bronchospasm, but may also lead to an increase in systemic blood pressure and a reflex reduction in coronary blood flow (Bezold-Jarisch reflex). If training reduces the ventilatory cost of a given activity below the oral augmentation point, this may thus lead to an appreciable improvement in the balance between the cardiac work rate and the oxygen supplied via the coronary vessels.

Metabolism

Much effort has been directed to exploring the metabolic conse-quences of habitual activity. If the exercise is of sufficient vigour, there is an increase in the mitochondrial fraction of skeletal muscle (K.H. Kiessling *et al.*, 1973). On the other hand, myocardial enzyme activity usually remains unchanged (L. Oscai *et al.*, 1971), and some authors have observed mitochondrial degeneration in the heart muscle of the rat following strenuous exercise (J.C. Arcos *et al.*, 1968; E.E. Aldinger & Sohal, 1970; E.W. Banister *et al.*, 1971).

Animal experiments and human biopsies of skeletal muscle both show augmented activity of enzymes concerned in glycogen synthesis and breakdown, glucose breakdown, pyruvate oxidation and the coupling of chemical energy to muscle proteins (B. Saltin, 1973; J.O. Holloszy, 1973; A.W. Taylor, 1975). While there are also 'central' (cardiovascular and nervous) responses in the child and young adult, it has been argued that much of the training response in middle-aged adults and 'post-coronary' patients is of the peripheral type (J.P. Clausen *et al.*, 1971). Evidence advanced to support this view includes: (i) an apparent correlation between gains of maximum oxygen intake and measures of mitochondrial function such as increased enzyme activity; and (ii) a supposed increase in peripheral oxygen extraction as indicated by a widening of the arterio-venous oxygen difference.

The increase in enzyme activity is not in fact a strong argument, since much larger changes of enzyme activity are induced by isometric or anaerobic than by endurance training (P. Gollnick & Hermansen, 1973). Furthermore, the increase in enzyme activity usually develops more rapidly than the gain in maximum oxygen intake. It is also difficult to envisage any great increase in oxygen extraction in the active muscles as a result of increased enzyme activity; L.H. Hartley & Saltin (1969), for example, found that the normal oxygen content of femoral venous blood was only 6 ml of oxygen per litre, while E. Doll *et al.* (1968) noted no difference in femoral-venous oxygen tension between athletes and sedentary subjects. An alternative explanation of the widened arterio-venous oxygen difference is that a trained person directs a larger proportion of his total cardiac output to the working tissues (R. Simmons & Shephard, 1971a); this reflects: (i) an increase in maximum cardiac output; (ii) a reduction in cutaneous blood flow associated with earlier sweating and a loss of subcutaneous fat; and (iii) a possible further reduction in visceral blood flow.

What then is the reason for the doubling of enzyme activity that accompanies endurance training? It can hardly be regarded as a compensation for muscle hypertrophy, for although there are sometimes increases of muscle-fibre dimensions with training, these are roughly matched by an increase in the capillary bed of the muscles (R.E. Carrow *et al.*, 1967; R.J. Tomanek, 1970; L. Hermansen & Wachtlová, 1971; K. Rakusan *et al.*, 1971). One advantage of the increased enzyme concentrations is that the body does not need to go so far into oxygen debt to 'switch on' mechanisms of oxygen transport at the beginning of a bout of vigorous work (B. Saltin & Karlsson, 1971). Perhaps more importantly, the greater enzyme activity encourages the utilisation of fat rather than carbohydrate during physical activity (J.O. Holloszy, 1973); the conservation of glycogen thus realised is of help to the distance athlete, the child avoids excessive fat deposition and the obese middle-aged adult is encouraged by the mobilisation of subcutaneous adipose tissue.

Table 4.2: *In vitro* Release of Free Fatty Acids from Epididymal Tissue of Male Rats Subjected to Habitual Exercise (E), Controls (C) and Hypokinesis (H)

Condition	Age 85 days			Age 125 days		
	E	C	H	E	C	H
Spontaneous release:						
60 min incubation	192	100	80	141	100	84
210 min incubation	183	100	41	174	100	114
After adrenaline:						
100 min incubation	105	100	80	150	100	95

Source: Based on experiments of J. Pařízková (1977).

J. Pařízková (1977) studied the liberation of fat from rat epididymal tissue (Table 4.2). Habitual exercise facilitated both the spontaneous release of free fatty acids from adipocytes and also their response to adrenaline, restoring to old rats a responsiveness that almost matched that of younger animals; in the young, the response to adrenaline was curtailed by hypokinesis but was not greatly increased by added activity, whereas in older animals the reverse was true.

Much of the body cholesterol is synthesised in the liver. One might thus anticipate the blood levels of this 'risk factor' and resultant arterial wall deposition could be controlled by striking an improved balance between the total energy intake and habitual physical activity (Chapter 2). This concept has yet to be tested in the growing child. However, in young adults blood cholesterol levels change little in response to a training programme, provided that the total intake of energy is sufficient to sustain body mass (R.C. Goode *et al.*, 1966). From the viewpoint of atherosclerosis (W.P. Castelli *et al.*, 1977; T. Gordon *et al.*, 1977), the total cholesterol is probably less important than the ratio of high-density to low-density lipoprotein cholesterol. It may be that the HDL cholesterol competes with the LDL at the cell membranes, preventing entry of the more irritant LDL into the cells; alternatively, the HDL may act as a scavenger, carrying excess cholesterol back to the liver before it has opportunity to cause vascular damage (P.D. Wood, 1979). There have been a number of reports indicating that concentrations of HDL cholesterol are positively correlated with regular participation in regular aerobic exercise (for example, L.A. Carlson, 1967; E.B. Altekruse & Wilmore, 1973;

A. Lopez *et al.*, 1974; P.D. Wood *et al.*, 1976; A.S. Leon *et al.*, 1977; G.H. Hartung *et al.*, 1978; A. Lehtonen & Viikari, 1978). However, the magnitude of the response is small (15–18 per cent increase), and no change is observed when middle-aged subjects participate in such moderate activities as a six-month industrial fitness programme (R.J. Shephard *et al.*, 1980b). Triglyceride readings are reduced by a regular daily programme of vigorous activity (R.C. Goode *et al.*, 1966), but it is uncertain how far a high triglyceride reading contributes to the risk of ischaemic heart disease, once allowance has been made for the associated influence of high serum cholesterol levels.

Physical activity has both acute and chronic effects upon the secretion of hormones. During the acute phase of activity, lipid mobilisation is favoured by an increased blood level of growth hormone, but the long-term effect of training seems to be a reduced secretion of growth hormone at any given rate of working (L.H. Hartley *et al.*, 1972; L. Mikulaj *et al.*, 1975; R.J. Shephard & Sidney, 1975). The level of free thyroxine is increased by an acute bout of exercise; regular activity also increases free thyroxine, but decreases total thyroxine, apparently without any effect upon the rate of basal metabolism (R.L. Terjung & Tipton, 1971; R.L. Terjung & Winder, 1975). Vigorous exercise causes an increased output of adrenaline and noradrenaline, particularly if there is associated emotional stress (E.W. Banister & Griffiths, 1972; L.H. Hartley *et al.*, 1972; U.S. Von Euler, 1973; H. Galbo *et al.*, 1975; L.H. Hartley, 1975); the response is less marked after training (L.H. Hartley *et al.*, 1972), but this may be partly because conditioning has diminished both the physical and the emotional stress associated with performance of a given work bout.

Body composition

We have already noted that training may lead to cardiac hypertrophy. Typically, there is also an increase in total blood volume, and some authors such as A. Holmgren (1967) have claimed a close correlation between total blood volume, total haemoglobin and physical working capacity. A muscle-building regimen may lead to some increase in red cell mass per unit volume of blood (R.J. Shephard *et al.*, 1977a), but often other factors such as iron loss in sweat, poor iron absorption, diminished red cell synthesis and an increased rate of haemolysis lead to a low blood haemoglobin level in the endurance-trained individual (J.F. de Wijn *et al.*, 1971; R.J. Shephard, 1980c).

Regular conditioning avoids fat accumulation in the child, and reduces adiposity in the adult, energy balance being adjusted by: (i) the appetite-suppressing effect of vigorous activity (J.A.F. Stevenson, 1967); (ii) the energy cost of the added activity; (iii) the energy cost of muscle building; and (iv) possible energy losses in ketosis (W. O'Hara *et al.*, 1979). Although scorned by many clinicians, vigorous exercise can lead to a rapid and substantial loss of body fat in a sedentary, middle-aged adult, particularly if it is performed in a cold environment (W. O'Hara *et al.*, 1977). Furthermore, once the habit of regular exercise is established, the fat loss is sustained, in marked contrast with the poor long-term effects of most programmes of dietary restriction (K.H. Sidney *et al.*, 1977). Reports that denigrate exercise are usually based on a search for 'weight loss'. In fact, regular daily activity provides an effective means of avoiding fat accumulation, and although body mass often remains unchanged over the course of a training programme, the reason is that excess fat becomes replaced by a similar mass of skeletal muscle. The type of activity most effective in controlling the percentage of body fat is sustained moderate work. There are two main reasons for this: (i) since fat combustion requires oxygen, the proportion of fat that is burnt is greatest at levels of activity that allow full perfusion of all active muscle fibres; and (ii) it is easier to burn a substantial amount of energy through an hour of moderate activity than through five minutes of all-out effort.

The lean body mass generally shows some increase with training, although the response is larger with weight-lifting and isometric programmes than with endurance-type activity. The practical consequence of such hypertrophy is that the muscle groups affected are able to exert a greater maximum force. In some instances, very rigorous programmes of endurance training such as those adopted for marathon and ultra-marathon contests lead to a loss of protein from less active regions of the body including the arms and the upper part of the trunk (R.J. Shephard, 1978a).

Relevance of Training Responses to Prevention of Ischaemic Heart Disease

General changes

Some of the benefits of a regular exercise programme are very general in nature, and arise almost independently of the intensity or amount of activity that is undertaken. The individual becomes health conscious and shares advice on prudent living with fellow enthusiasts; particularly if activity is followed on a group basis, matters such as smoking habits, diet and attitudes to daily work receive frequent discussion (S.M. Fox *et al.*, 1972). Many participants, particularly the women, value the camaraderie that develops in a group setting (R.J. Shephard *et al.*, 1980a), and the resultant psychological support may buttress the individual against life stresses that are a frequent precipitant of cardiac attacks (T.H. Holmes & Rahe, 1967). Class members also speak enthusiastically about an elevation of mood, although this is hard to document by formal psychological tests (K.H. Sidney & Shephard, 1977a). Transient effects probably arise from the increased secretion of catecholamines and the added input to the reticular formation of the brain stem; if so, the mood change would be greater with vigorous than with light effort. There has been much discussion of the possible role of physical activity in the release of tension and pent-up aggression. The concept of catharsis had its origins in ancient Greece (R.J. Shephard, 1978c), where the dramatic portrayal of violence with appropriate punishment of the evil-doer was held to purge an audience of dangerous emotions. Freud applied this concept to physical activity, but in more recent times some sports psychologists have tended to the view that violent games breed as much excitement and aggression as they release (J.E. Kohanson, 1970; M. Gluckman, 1973). However, G. Rivard *et al.* (1977) found that boys participating in an international hockey tournament had above average teacher-ratings for such items as group integration and participation (team work). The contest itself had no immediate effect on frustration scores, whether the participant's team won or lost. Much presumably depends upon the nature of the activity, the manner in which it is pursued and the attitude of team-mates and coach (if any). Non-competitive walking, cycling or jogging is less likely to arouse excitement, tension or hostility than competitive sports such as ice-hockey, tennis or squash. Nevertheless, many coronary-prone individuals have the type of personality that turns any activity into an aggressive act; they are determined to beat their opponent at tennis, and equally insist upon walking further and faster than others of their own age, sometimes to the point of provoking a coronary attack while they are exercising (Chapter 3). E.M. Layman (1970) distinguishes hot-tempered anger, induced by and directed towards an external stimulus ('reactive aggression') and the coldly calculated but equally fierce aggression of a body check ('instrumental anger'). Violence can perhaps restore physiological equilibrium following hot anger, although this seems unlikely to occur if the external stimulus is removed from the sports arena or gymnasium (for example, a problem of home, office or classroom); instrumental aggression, in contrast, seems likely to breed further aggression.

Cardiovascular changes

There is normally a linear relationship between heart rate and oxygen consumption or the equivalent power output of the body during sub-maximal exercise. Training leads to a substantial rightward shift in this relationship, due largely to: (i) the decrease of resting heart rate; (ii) the increased maximum rate of working; and (iii) some decrease of maximum heart rate. Other possible (but less firmly established) contributory factors include: (i) habituation to the various stresses of vigorous activity; (ii) a reduction in skin blood flow (heat dissipation being facilitated by a reduction of subcutaneous fat and an earlier onset of sweating); (iii) other improvements in blood flow; (iv) more ready perfusion of the working muscles (due to an increase in their maximum voluntary force); (v) better maintenance of stroke volume (due to an increase in blood volume and an increase in cardiac contractility; and (vi) an increased arterio-venous oxygen difference (related to an increase in red cell mass, a resultant increase in arterial oxygen content and a reduction in mixed venous oxygen content attributable to either more effective distribution of cardiac output or more complete extraction of oxygen in the active muscles). The net result of the slower heart rate is a considerable decrease in the cardiac work rate at any given level of oxygen consumption, so that, for a given coronary blood flow, myocardial ischaemia is less likely to arise.

The systemic blood pressure is also reduced by training; the resting values show only a minor change, but there are larger decreases during the performance of a given sub-maximal task. The latter changes reflect both alterations in central regulatory mechanisms and also a strengthening of the working muscles, since one function of the exercise-induced hypertension is to sustain the perfusion of muscle fibres that are contracting at more than 15 per cent of their maximum voluntary force (A.R. Lind & McNicol, 1967). The lesser rise of blood pressure during exercise reduces the cardiac work rate required for a given external effort. Moreover, myocardial efficiency is improved, since that component of work performed against tension in the ventricular wall does not contribute to the pumping of blood around the circulation.

Other possible cardiac responses to training could further improve the precarious balance between cardiac work rate and coronary oxygen supply, as follows:

(i)   myocardial hypertrophy might facilitate cardiac perfusion by reducing the tension per unit cross section of ventricular wall;

(ii)   reduction of systolic reserve might, through the LaPlace relationship, reduce wall tension for a given intraventricular pressure;

(iii)   lessening of the sympathetic drive to the heart might decrease myocardial contractility and thus myocardial O_2 consumption at any given external work rate;

(iv)   lengthening of the diastolic phase of the cardiac cycle (when left ventricular perfusion occurs) might increase the average coronary blood flow over a cardiac cycle;

(v)   possible widening of the arterio-venous oxygen difference in the coronary circulation (through an increase in red cell mass, or an increase in myocardial enzyme activity) might increase oxygen delivery per unit of coronary blood flow.

The possible impact of endurance training upon the coronary vasculature has already been noted. Animal experiments suggest the potential for both an enlargement of the coronary arterial tree and a development of collateral anastomoses. There have been no related studies of primary prevention in man, although the middle-aged adult apparently fails to respond in this way when he participates in the usual type of mild training programme arranged for his age group. Nevertheless, there are mechanisms whereby regular physical activity can reduce the obstruction associated with partially formed intravascular lesions. Fibrinolysis is promoted, at least in the period immediately after an exercise bout (J.D. Cash & McGill, 1969; B. Berkada *et al.*, 1971; V. McAlpine *et al.*, 1971; T. Åstrup, 1973). There may also be an acute decrease in the stickiness of the platelets (G. Lee *et al.*, 1977), although increases in the platelet count and in some of the plasma clotting factors (A. Pelliccia, 1978) leads to an increase in the coagulability of the blood with exercise (J.R. Poortmans *et al.*, 1971; K. Korsan-Bengtsen *et al.*, 1973). Habitual endurance activity apparently curtails the increase in blood coagulability following a fatty meal (G.A. McDonald & Fullerton, 1958), but it is still disputed whether it can decrease the blood coagulability of fasting subjects (H.J. Montoye, 1960; K. Korsan-Bengtsen *et al.*, 1973).

Respiratory changes

The training-induced increase in anaerobic threshold, reduced oxygen cost of breathing and increase in maximum exercise ventilation all tend to improve oxygen transport to the heart and the active muscles. Oral augmentation of breathing may also be avoided during submaximal exercise, on account of the greater efficiency of ventilation;

this lessens the chances of provoking reflex bronchial and coronary arterial spasm in a cold and dry atmosphere.

A sub-normal vital capacity is possibly linked to risk of ischaemic heart disease through a mutual association with cigarette smoking. Endurance training could thus improve both lung function and prognosis by encouraging abstinence from cigarettes. On the other hand, the extent of physical activity necessary to break an established smoking pattern seems to be quite large (P. Morgan *et al.*, 1976).

Metabolic changes

The increase in muscle enzyme activity with conditioning has at least two practical consequences. The ability to metabolise fat during exercise is enhanced; conceivably, this could reduce not only the accumulation of fat in peripheral depots, but also the fatty infiltration of the blood vessels. There is also some possibility of increased oxygen extraction from blood perfusing the working tissues; such a change would diminish the cardiac output needed to sustain a given power output in the active muscles.

A few authors have noted an increase in electron transport in cardiac muscle following endurance training (for example, H. Kraus & Kirsten, 1970; M.J. Hamilton & Ferguson, 1972); unfortunately from the viewpoint of preventing myocardial ischaemia, these findings have not been confirmed by other investigators (L.B. Oscai *et al.*, 1971; P.D. Gollnick & Ianuzzo, 1972; G.L. Dohm *et al.*, 1972).

The blood-lipid profile may be modified by a training programme, particularly if the required exercise is vigorous and prolonged, with a negative energy balance. A high total cholesterol, a high triglyceride level and a low HDL cholesterol are well-accepted risk-factors for the development of ischaemic heart disease; control of blood lipids from early childhood is plainly advantageous, but there is less evidence that correction of the lipid profile in middle age will improve ultimate prognosis.

It is easier to ascribe primary and/or secondary preventive value to some of the hormonal responses to increased physical activity. Excessive blood levels of catecholamines are plainly a factor contributing to ventricular dysrhythmias, and the training-induced reduction of noradrenaline and adrenaline secretion at any given work-rate should thus diminish the likelihood of developing a ventricular tachycardia or fibrillation. Fat deposition is reduced and fat mobilisation is enhanced by both the greater sensitivity of the adipocytes to catecholamines (Table 4.2) and the vigorous secretion of growth hormone during acute bouts of physical activity. The development of maturity-onset diabetes seems linked to lack of exercise, and the condition is often corrected by a programme of progressive activity (B.P. Björntorp et al., 1972); again, the onset of diabetes is recognised as a risk factor for subsequent ischaemic heart disease (F.H. Epstein, 1974), but it is less certain that the late (secondary) control of glucose intolerance will restore a normal prognosis. Lastly, the increase of free thyroxine levels during acute bouts of exercise may help to control fat accumulation by burning excess energy, although any increase of metabolism is of relatively short duration.

Body composition

Cardiac hypertrophy has several conflicting effects upon the relative oxygen supply to the myocardium. Usually, the capillary blood supply increases roughly in proportion with the increase in cross section of the myofibrils. However, if the mean radius of the ventricle is increased, the wall tension is augmented, as would be predicted from the LaPlace relationship. Fortunately, this tendency is offset by the increase in wall thickness, so that the tension per unit of cross section is diminished.

Any rise in red cell mass is also a mixed blessing. While the increase in oxygen carriage per unit volume of blood lessens the cardiac output needed to sustain a given external power output, any large increase in red cell count can lead to a substantial augmentation in both the viscous resistance to blood flow and the coagulability of the blood.

Skeletal-muscle hypertrophy reduces the force that must be exerted by unit cross section of muscle at any given intensity of activity. This lessens the perception of exertion (and associated psychological stress); it also facilitates perfusion of the working muscles, reducing the need for compensatory hypertension with resultant loading of the heart.

A reduction in subcutaneous fat, if associated with a decrease in body mass, increases the relative aerobic power (oxygen transport per kilogram of body mass), and reduces the oxygen cost of most tasks that involve the raising and lowering of body parts. Furthermore, the isometric demands for body support become smaller. All of these changes reduce the cardiac loading for a given external task. Loss of subcutaneous fat also facilitates heat elimination, thus curtailing the skin blood-flow requirement when exercising in a warm environment. It is less certain how far fat loss helps the individual who already has pre-clinical atherosclerotic changes in his blood vessels; observations in patients with wasting diseases and ileal by-pass operations are encouraging (G. Weber, 1978), but if secondary changes have occurred in connective tissue, with clotting and calcium impregnation of fatty plaques, such changes are unlikely to be reversed by an increased consumption of fat.

Required pattern of exercise

The pattern of activity needed in a programme of primary or secondary prevention cannot be fully resolved until there is more agreement on the basis of such prevention. Some of the supposed general benefits of exercise — advice on prudent living, camaraderie, joie de vivre and pleasurable relaxation — stem more from the development of new interests and affiliation to a group of like-minded enthusiasts than from the vigour of the exercise that is undertaken; it is thus arguable that equal benefit could be derived from a class directed to an alternative aspect of health or even to a pleasant but sedentary hobby. Other supposed mechanisms of prevention — reduction in adiposity, control of serum cholesterol and triglyceride levels and correction of glucose intolerance — demand a substantial daily expenditure of energy, but sustained moderate exercise is a more effective method of attaining this objective than brief bouts of very vigorous activity (G. Gwinup, 1975). Intense exercise is the only likely stimulus to enlargement of the coronary arterial tree, development of the collateral circulation and habituation of the individual to the stresses of maximum effort. However, most suggested mechanisms of primary and secondary prevention (S.M. Fox *et al.*, 1972; Table 4.3) require regular endurance-type training.

Primary prevention is easier to institute than secondary prevention, since the child is more ready to learn an active pattern of behaviour than is the middle-aged adult. However, it is important that the activity habit be taught in such a way that it is maintained throughout adult life; certain school programmes with a heavy team emphasis tend to be abandoned rapidly after completion of school or university. Instruction should encompass a wide variety of endurance-type activities, so that the pupil has a chance to find an athletic discipline that is both enjoyable and suited to his body build and motor skills. The emphasis should be upon participation rather than the development of a star performance, with the development of interests that can be carried over into adult life and practised as a family. A minimum of facilities, equipment and fellow participants should be required. Suitable suggestions include distance cycling, swimming, cross-country skiing, jogging, fast walking, hill-climbing and the vigorous performance of non-mechanised household chores such as lawn-mowing and sawing logs.

Table 4.3: Possible Mechanisms by Which Physical Activity May Prevent Ischaemic Heart Disease

Light activity	Moderate activity	Intense activity	Increased energy consumption
Prudent living	Reduced cardiac workload, heart rate, blood pressure, increased myocardial efficiency	Coronary artery size enlarged	Adipose tissue decreased
Camaraderie		Collateral vessels developed	Serum cholesterol reduced
Joie de vivre	Improved O_2 transport, red cell mass, arterial O_2 content, blood volume, blood flow distribution, tissue enzyme activity	Habituation	Serum triglycerides reduced
Relaxation			Glucose tolerance improved
Correction of 'stress'	Hormonal changes, neurohormonal balance, catecholamine secretion, growth hormone, thyroid hormone		
	Blood coagulability, fibrinolysis, platelet stickiness improved		

Source: After S.M. Fox et al (1972), but classified in terms of activity pattern required.

There have been a number of longitudinal studies of exercise programmes in children (for example, T.K. Cureton, 1964; H.H. Clarke, 1971; R. Bauss & Roth, 1977; R. Mirwald *et al.*, 1977; R. Renson *et al.*, 1977; R.J. Shephard *et al.*, 1977b). Physical condition has generally improved as a result of training, with gains of maximum oxygen intake, muscle strength, and physical performance. J. Pařízková (1977) also observed a reduction in body fat in boys attending a special summer camp, but other investigators have found surprisingly little effect of increased classroom activity upon the percentage of body fat in free-living students (R.J. Shephard *et al.*, 1977b). There is plainly a need for studies that commence in childhood and continue throughout the adult life-span. However, practical problems have prevented the initiation of such a project. Indeed, most of the investigations completed to date have continued for insufficient time to allow the effects of school-age programmes upon the health and behaviour of the young adult to be assessed. One exception is a follow-up study of Swedish female swimming champions, carried out five years after ceasing competition. This demonstrated that the physical condition of the swimmers had on average regressed to the point where the maximum oxygen intakes were less than in sedentary housewives of the same age (P.O. Åstrand *et al.*, 1963). While the protagonists of exercise programmes must be discouraged by this information, it should be stressed that the individuals concerned had been obliged to undertake gruelling competitive training. It thus remains possible that the moderate activity appropriate to a programme of primary prevention may build up more favourable attitudes, with permanent acceptance of an active lifestyle.

Animal Experiments

General considerations

In view of the dearth of long-term primary preventive trials in man, particular interest attaches to the results obtained from longitudinal animal experiments. Through specific manipulation of diet, physical activity and hormonal balance, the time course of atherosclerosis can be accelerated by a factor of 20-30, coronary narrowing can be surgically induced and specimens can be taken freely for histological examination. Furthermore, activity and dietary patterns are more readily controlled than in human studies.

Spontaneous atherosclerosis is a well-recognised feature of zoo and domesticated animals (M. Sherman, 1964). This is apparently due in part to an inappropriate diet; 80 per cent of laboratory dogs that are

Table 4.4: Some Characteristics of Animal Models Used in the Study of Atherosclerosis

Model	Characteristics of atherosclerotic model
Dog	Produced by thyroid depression and atherogenic diet. Cardiovascular system, lipid and cholesterol metabolism differ from man
Fowls (chicken, pigeon)	Produced readily by atherogenic diet, but plaques differ from human, as do anatomy, lipid and cholesterol metabolism. Picture sometimes complicated by cholesterol accumulation in reticulo-endothelial system
Rabbit	Produced readily by atherogenic diet, but plaques differ from human, as to topography of lesions, lipid and cholesterol metabolism. Lesions resistant to regression
Monkey	Advanced atherosclerosis readily produced by atherogenic diet; lesions, anatomy and biochemistry similar to man, but animals are expensive, hard to handle and procure
Pig	Plaques difficult to produce without special manipulation but anatomy, physiology and biochemistry similar to man, plaques similar, large size permits arteriography, open heart surgery and measurements of cardiac functions

Source: R.W. Wissler and Vesselinovitch (1977).

fed a commercial dry dog food have a serum cholesterol reading of $200 \text{ mg} \cdot \text{dl}^{-1}$ or less, whereas 67 per cent of more liberally fed household pets show a cholesterol value of over $200 \text{ mg} \cdot \text{dl}^{-1}$, and in ten per cent of animals values are greater than $300 \text{ mg} \cdot \text{dl}^{-1}$.

Atherosclerotic lesions can be produced experimentally in a variety of species, including monkeys, pigs, rabbits and fowls (D. Kritchevsky, 1974; M.L. Armstrong, 1976; H.C. Stary *et al.*, 1977; R.W. Wissler & Vesselinovitch, 1977). However, the relevance of such models to human disease has been questioned (H.C. McGill, 1965; E.P. Benditt, 1977). The appearance and distribution of the atherosclerotic plaques sometimes differs substantially from that observed in human ischaemic heart disease, and there are inevitable inter-species differences in vascular anatomy, physiology, biochemistry and lipid metabolism, including the characteristics of the various lipoproteins (Table 4.4). Furthermore, the 'accelerated' lesions that are so convenient for rapid experimentation appear only if the animal is exposed to a markedly atherogenic diet, hormonal manipulation such as thyroid extirpation and/or a severe restriction of physical activity (H. Montoye, 1960).

Primary prevention

The preventive value of exercise is suggested by the fact that atherosclerosis is more common in domesticated species than in their wild (and presumably more active) counterparts. Among the fowls, for example, atherosclerosis is seen in the turkey and the chicken, but is less evident in birds that fly regularly; certain varieties of domesticated pigeon are markedly affected, but in racing pigeons the condition does not progress beyond a slight fatty streaking of the great vessels (M. Sherman, 1964).

Prospective experimental studies, reviewed by Sherman, have yielded conflicting results (N.H. Warnock *et al.*, 1957; A.L. Myasnikov, 1958; F.F. McAllister *et al.*, 1959). When cockerels were fed a high-fat diet, exercise corrected elevation of the serum cholesterol (N.H. Warnock *et al.*, 1957). On the other hand, hens that were exercised on a treadmill five days per week for twelve weeks showed as much atherosclerosis as non-exercised birds. One study of rabbits suggested that regular physical activity failed to inhibit deposition of cholesterol in the heart and aorta, perhaps because exercised animals ate more than the controls (A.L. Myasnikov, 1958). A second study of the same species noted that exercise decreased the severity and extent of experimental atherosclerosis without decreasing the serum cholesterol level (S.D. Kobernick *et al.*, 1957). It was thus speculated that physical activity in some way hampered the escape of cholesterol from the blood stream.

Studies of longevity have been carried out in rats (D.W. Edington *et al.*, 1972). The influence of physical activity upon lifespan apparently depends upon the age at which it is initiated. In young animals, the effect is favourable, but in 'middle-aged' animals (400 days or more from a 600-day lifespan) the prognosis is worsened by a daily training programme.

J.T. Flaherty *et al.* (1972) have emphasised the role of mechanical stress in determining the location of lesions within the vascular tree. In their experiments, lesions were potentiated when blood flow was increased by a surgical arterio-venous anastomosis. Exercise plainly leads to an increase in both aortic and coronary blood flow, and it is thus arguable that wall stress is augmented during the acute phase of physical activity. However, from the viewpoint of atherosclerosis, the crucial information is presumably the average wall stress for a 24-hour period, and there is at present little evidence whether this is increased or decreased by a regular programme of activity.

Secondary prevention

From the viewpoint of secondary prevention, it is encouraging to observe the regression of experimental atherosclerotic lesions when an atherogenic diet is replaced by hypolipidic foods (D. Vesselovitch *et al.*, 1974; G. Weber *et al.*, 1975; M.L. Armstrong, 1976; R.J. Friedman *et al.*, 1976; A.S. Daoud *et al.*, 1977; R.G. De Palma *et al.*, 1977; H.C. Stary *et al.*, 1977). To the extent that physical activity improves the lipid profile, it presumably has a similar effect to the hypolipidic diet.

Coronary circulation

It is difficult to visualise the coronary circulation in man, and much of the evidence concerning exercise and myocardial blood flow is thus derived from animal experiments. Unfortunately, the data are far from consistent. Acute bouts of physical activity can have an adverse effect if they are linked with experimental narrowing of the coronary vessels. P.L. Thompson & Lown (1975) developed a pattern of coronary occlusion that was tolerated by resting dogs. When the same procedure was given to exercising animals, it was often lethal, eight of ten dogs dying of ventricular fibrillation within 24 hours. Occlusion immediately following exercise also worsened prognosis (two sudden deaths and four further deaths among ten animals over a 24-hour period). However, if exercise was undertaken more than one hour after occlusion, the activity did not lead to ventricular fibrillation or death.

Wild species have a better myocardial oxygen supply than their domesticated counterparts (O. Poupa *et al.*, 1970). A regular programme of daily activity enlarges the coronary arterial tree of the rat (J. Tepperman & Pearlman, 1961; J.A.F. Stevenson, 1967), particularly if there is cardiac hypertrophy (A. Kerr *et al.*, 1968; A.S. Leon & Bloor, 1970). It also augments the capillary/fibre ratio of the myocardium (T. Petren *et al.*, 1936; R.J. Tomanek, 1970; R.L. Rasmussen *et al.*, 1978) at least in young animals (where hyperplasia occurs; O. Poupa *et al.*, 1970), but it may decrease the ratio in older animals where there is simple hypertrophy (J. Hakkila, 1955; O. Poupa *et al.*, 1970). Prior training increases survival after experimental narrowing of the coronary vessels (R.W. Eckstein, 1957) or infarction (B.C. Wexler & Greenberg, 1974). On the other hand, regular exercise does not seem to protect an animal against subsequent occlusion of its coronary vessels (J.J. Burt & Jackson, 1965; E. Kaplinsky *et al.*, 1968; T.M. Sanders *et al.*, 1978).

Summary

Animal experiments generally support the view that regular physical exercise will inhibit the development of atherosclerosis, increasing longevity (at least in young animals) and enhancing the formation of coronary collaterals (at least where there is already some narrowing of the coronary vessels). Furthermore, there is some evidence that established lesions can be reversed by a sustained programme of physical activity. Nevertheless, these findings must be accepted with caution, since there are some discordant reports, and in any event there are significant differences in the atherosclerotic process between man and most of the commonly used experimental animals.

5 EXERCISE AND THE SECONDARY PREVENTION OF ISCHAEMIC HEART DISEASE

Evidence concerning the value of physical activity in the secondary prevention of ischaemic heart disease is largely epidemiological in type (J.O. Holloszy, 1973; W.L. Haskell & Fox, 1974; R.J. Barnard, 1975; V.F. Froehlicher, 1976; G.H. Hartung, 1977; H.J. Montoye, 1977). After a brief discussion of the epidemiological method and problems of direct experimentation, we will examine available experimental data. Information garnered from studies of ethnic populations, athletes and groups differing in occupational or leisure activities will then be reviewed in the light of Bradford Hill's postulates for a 'causal' association between two variables.

Epidemiology versus Direct Experimentation

Epidemiology examines associations between events as they occur in free-living populations. The associations observed may have a high level of statistical significance but, unless a direct experimental step is undertaken, it is generally difficult to establish a cause and effect relationship between two variables.

One of the earliest epidemiologists was a physician named John Snow (1855). He practised in the Soho district of London at a time when epidemics of cholera were commonplace. The wisdom of the period attributed this disease to mysterious miasmata, spreading from the creeks of central London during episodes of dense fog. However, John Snow patiently traced the relationship between an outbreak of cholera and the drinking of water from a specific source, the Broad Street pump. Microscopic examination of the water in question showed the presence of many 'animalicules', and further enquiry established that a sailor with obvious symptoms of cholera had taken up residence in a public house adjacent to the pump shortly before the disease became prevalent. The distance separating the privy of the hotel from the well was only a few feet. Cause and effect was indicated more clearly than in many subsequent epidemics, yet the crucial step in John Snow's research was experimental rather than epidemiological — the outbreak of cholera was checked when he removed the handle from the offending pump. (Purists may note that this does not provide categoric proof. In fact, the handle was removed from the pump at a time when the epidemic was waning from natural causes.)

The hypothesis that exercise is of benefit in the secondary prevention of ischaemic heart disease rests largely upon a series of epidemiological associations. The crucial experimental proof is lacking. In essence, no-one has found a way to 'take the handle off the pump'. The problem lies in the area of logistics. Coronary events in normal middle-aged men are sufficiently rare that given a 25 or 50 per cent benefit from an increase in physical activity, the usual experiment with random allocation of subjects to exercise and control groups would require an unmanageably large sample in order to have a reasonable chance of demonstrating a significant effect (Table 5.1). The required number of subjects is further increased by sample attrition (Table 5.2). One pilot trial concluded that, even if attention was focussed upon a population with a number of coronary 'risk factors', the cost of a definitive experiment would be US $31 million, measured in 1962 currency (H.L. Taylor *et al.*, 1966; R.D. Remington & Schork, 1967). The likely drop-out rate would be 50 per cent over the first six months of exercise (J. Ilmarinen & Fardy, 1977), with further defections over the remaining four to five years of observation; the residual sample would thus be small and atypical of the original population from which it was drawn, making valid conclusions impossible. The British Cardiac Society (Joint Working Party, 1976) likewise concluded that while a randomised controlled trial of exercise in the secondary prevention of ischaemic heart disease was a theoretical possibility, it was not practical.

As we shall see in the next chapter, prospective assessments of exercise therapy have been attempted in patients with a recent myocardial infarction. Such individuals have a substantial motivation to increased physical activity from their 'critical event', but even when using this type of population, results are inconclusive because of: (i) a high drop-out rate; (ii) poor compliance with the required exercise programme; (iii) contamination of control subjects with an interest in physical activity (R.J. Shephard & Kavanagh, 1978b); and (iv) simultaneous changes in other health habits.

According to current thinking, lack of physical activity remains one probable risk factor in the causation of ischaemic heart disease, but other variables such as smoking habits, systemic hypertension and serum cholesterol levels are of at least equal importance. Having regard to both the high cost of a definitive trial and the multifactorial nature

Table 5.1: The Size of Random Sample Needed for a 90 Per Cent Chance of Demonstrating a 25 and a 50 Per Cent Reduction in the Incidence of Myocardial Infarction ($P < 0.05$) as a Result of Increased Physical Activity

Age of sample (years)	Annual incidence (5-year study per 1,000 subjects)	Sample size		Annual incidence (10-year study per 1,000 subjects)	Sample size	
		25% reduction	50% reduction		25% reduction	50% reduction
40–49	3.2	14,800	3,200	3.8	6,100	1,300
45–54	4.6	10,200	2,200	5.3	4,300	925
50–59	6.6	7,050	1,550	7.5	3,000	650
55–64	9.5	4,900	1,050			

Source: H.L. Taylor *et al*. (1966).

Table 5.2: The Size of Random Sample Needed for a 90 Per Cent Chance of Demonstrating a 50 Per Cent Reduction in the Incidence of Myocardial Infarction ($P < 0.05$) in Relation to Drop-out Rate and Incidence of Disease in Control Subjects

Incidence in control group (one year, per 1,000)	Sample size versus drop-out rate		
	10% of residue per year	25% of residue per year	50% of residue per year
7.5	2,600	5,500	21,000
10.0	2,000	4,200	15,000
15.0	1,300	2,800	11,000
20.0	1,000	2,100	7,600
40.0	500	1,100	3,900
80.0	260	720	2,100

Source: R.D. Remington & Schork (1967).

of the disease, the present generation of secondary preventive trials are thus adopting the technique of multiple risk-factor modification. Such an approach may well cure the disease without indicating whether an increase in physical activity has made a useful contribution to therapy.

Table 5.3: Changes in Coronary 'Risk Factors' with One-year and Ten-year Participation in a Lifestyle-modification Programme

Variable	One year	Ten years
Participation (%)		
Non-smokers	96.4	71.8
Smokers	92.3	49.7
Energy intake		
(10-year average, % baseline)	—	−25.7
Total fat intake		
(10-year average, % baseline)	—	−19.1
Animal fat intake		
(10-year average, % baseline)	—	−32.4
Cholesterol intake		
(10-year average, % baseline)	—	−48.6
Decrease in body mass		
(%, continuing participants)	− 5.5	− 4.7
Serum cholesterol		
(% change, continuing participants)	−10.8	− 7.3
Diastolic pressure		
(% change, continuing participants)	− 5.0	− 4.3
On-job activity		
(arbitrary units, continuing participants)	+ 0.1	− 0.6
Leisure activity		
(arbitrary units, continuing participants)	+ 0.4	+ 0.5
Cigarette smoking	About a half of continuing participants stopped smoking by 6 years	

Source: J. Stamler (1978).

Experimental Trials of Secondary Prevention

Chicago Programme

In 1957, J. Stamler (1978) initiated a lifestyle-modification programme in central Chicago. His subjects were deliberately selected in terms of coronary risk factors such as a high serum cholesterol level, an excessive body mass relative to actuarial tables, a diastolic pressure higher than 95 mm Hg, non-specific changes in the T wave of the electrocardiogram and cigarette smoking. The retention of study participants was remarkably successful, 71.8 per cent for non-smokers and 49.7 per cent for smokers over a ten-year period of observation (Table 5.3). As in data from Toronto (R.J. Shephard & Cox, unpublished), a seven-day diet recall sheet indicated a suspiciously large reduction in energy, fat and cholesterol intake over the course of the programme. Presumably, the collection of nutritional information led to a temporary

Table 5.4: Influence of Chicago Programme of Lifestyle Modification on Prognosis

	N	Ten-year mortality (per 1,000) All causes	Coronary heart disease
Chicago programme	519	54	23
adjusted data*	519	64	27
US 'Pooling Project'	2,896	85	36
Life insurance standard risk, age 50		119	—
Life table — US white males, age 19-70		134	—

* Adjusted to allow for age and risk factors, relative to data of US 'Pooling Project'.

Source: J. Stamler (1978).

modification of diet during the week of observation. Nevertheless, continuing study participants showed useful changes in a number of risk factors, including a decrease of body mass, serum cholesterol and diastolic pressure, an increase of leisure activity and the cessation of smoking in about a half of those who initially had a cigarette habit.

It is difficult to assess the impact of the programme upon prognosis, since the subjects were volunteers rather than a random sample of the Chicago population. After adjustment for age and the various risk factors observed on entry to the study, the ten-year mortality from coronary heart disease was some 25 per cent below the average for subjects enrolled in five US prospective epidemiological studies (the 'Pooling Project'; D. McGee & Gordon, 1976). However, this could reflect the initial selection of subjects willing to enrol in a ten-year health study rather than a specific response to the subsequent programmed lifestyle modification (Table 5.4).

Other studies in the US

Subsequent prospective studies in the US have examined dietary modification (National Diet-Heart Study Research Group, 1968; L. Mojonnier *et al.*, 1979), reduction in body mass (A. Keys & Parlin, 1966; MRFIT, 1977), control of hypertension (Hypertension Detection Follow-up Programme, cited by H. Blackburn, 1979),

Table 5.5: Changes in Risk Factors over a Prospective Trial of Exercise (Three One-hour Sessions per Week)

Variable	Change over study	
	Exercise group	Control group
Serum cholesterol (mg•dl $^{-1}$)	−5.4	−4.1
Blood pressure		
Systolic (mm Hg)	−3.1	−2.2
Diastolic (mm Hg)	−4.0	−3.6
Quit smoking (number of subjects)	4	4

Source: Based on data of H.L. Taylor *et al.* (1973).

cessation of smoking (MRFIT, 1980) and management of stress (A.P. Shapiro *et al.*, 1977; C.B. Taylor *et al.*, 1977) as possible tactics for the control of ischaemic heart disease.

The Multiple Risk Factor Intervention Trial (MRFIT) is a relatively large-scale experiment which will conclude in 1982 (R.C. Benfari, 1979). The subjects, 12,000 men aged 35–57 years, are at increased risk of ischaemic heart disease due to a high serum cholesterol, a high diastolic blood pressure and cigarette smoking. An attempt is being made to modify each of these variables over a six-year period, using dietary counselling, antihypertensive agents and various smoking cessation techniques. As yet, only a few preliminary results are available (MRFIT, 1977, 1980).

Surprisingly few of the US trials have included deliberate physical activity in their protocol. H.L. Taylor *et al.* (1973) initiated a three-centre study where 'high-risk' middle-aged men carried out three one-hour sessions of supervised exercise per week. Subjects were asked to maintain a normal lifestyle with respect to diet and smoking habits. After twelve months, the exercised group showed a greater reduction of serum cholesterol than the controls, but by 18 months the two groups showed similar small decreases in serum cholesterol, systolic and diastolic blood pressures, and a few members of each group had quit smoking (Table 5.5).

A. Leon *et al.* (1979) had greater success with a sixteen-week exercise regimen. This involved 90 minutes of supervised walking per day at a treadmill speed of 5.1 km•h $^{-1}$ and a slope of 10 per cent. Favourable changes in coronary risk factors included a loss of body fat and body mass, improved glucose tolerance, decrease of serum

Table 5.6: Effects of 16 Weeks of Walking (90 min, Five Days a Week, 5.1 km·h⁻¹, 10 Per Cent Grade) on Obese Young Men Not Subjected to Dietary Restriction

Variable	Change over 16 weeks
Body mass (kg)	− 5.6
Mass of fat (kg)	− 4.8
Mass of lean tissue (kg)	− 0.9
Skinfold readings (mm)	−10.7
Blood-glucose (mg·dl⁻¹)	−39.0
Insulin (μU·ml⁻¹)	−140.9
Plasma cholesterol (mg·dl⁻¹)	− 6.0
Plasma triglycerides (mg·dl⁻¹)	−21.0
HDL/LDL ratio	+ 0.07
Treadmill endurance (min)	+ 2.5

Source: Based on data of A. Leon *et al.* (1979).

Table 5.7: Influence of Hygienic Measures and of Hygienic Measures plus Exercise upon Frequency of Electrocardiographic Abnormalities

Variable	Hygienic measures Initial	After 6 weeks	Hygienic measures plus exercise Initial	After 6 weeks	Control Initial	After 6 weeks
Standard ECG	2.0	2.7	2.8	2.5	2.2	2.4
Isometric test	3.8	5.4	4.4	2.6	4.4	5.0
Treadmill test	2.7	1.9	1.7	3.3	3.2	2.1
Multiple waveform (%)	44	48	20	24	55	35
R on T PVCs (%)	15	15	20	12	28	17
Pairs or runs of PVCs (%)	44	44	32	28	28	31
PVC fusion, beats (%)	19	7	0	16	7	10

Source: H. Blackburn *et al.* (1976).

cholesterol and triglycerides and an increase in the ratio of HDL to LDL cholesterol (Table 5.6). As in an earlier study by K.H. Sidney *et al.* (1977), regular exercise was remarkably successful in controlling appetite and energy balance, without specific dietetic measures.

H. Blackburn *et al.* (1976) examined the possibility of controlling premature ventricular contractions by either hygienic measures (for instance, cessation of smoking, abstinence from coffee, reduced consumption of alcohol and increased hours of sleep) or a combination of such measures with a supervised programme of endurance exercise (one hour of walking and jogging three times per week). Unfortunately, the trial was concluded after six weeks, but over this period neither of the two treatment groups showed any striking improvement in their ECG tracings relative to a control sample drawn from the same population (Table 5.7).

K.H. Cooper *et al.* (1977) reviewed data for subjects attending the Aerobics Institute in Dallas, Texas. Of 9,000 men and women tested since 1971, seven had sustained a fatal myocardial infarction, 11 had experienced a non-fatal episode, and nine had undergone cardiac 'by-pass' surgery. The 27 cardiac victims were compared with 81 matched controls, chosen for their initial similarity in terms of serum cholesterol, systemic blood pressure, glucose tolerance, left-ventricular dimensions and age. It was concluded that a low level of physical fitness (as indicated by a limited treadmill-endurance time) and an abnormal stress electrocardiogram each contributed to the detection of subsequent coronary events independent of the other risk factors isolated. However, the close correlation between a low treadmill score and the development of electrocardiographic abnormalities prevented any assessment of the relative importance of these two variables.

European studies

European centres have embarked upon a number of risk-factor intervention studies (M. Miettinen *et al.*, 1972; L. Wilhelmsen *et al.*, 1972; P. Puska, 1974; P. Leren *et al.*, 1975; World Health Organization, 1977). However, with the exception of the experiment initiated by the World Health Organization European Collaborative Group, no attempt has been made to increase the physical activity of study participants.

The World Health Organization compared entire factories, matched for size, geographical location and nature of the manufactured product. In experimental factories, community advice was given on diet, smoking cessation, reduction in body mass and the treatment of hypertension, particular attention being directed to high-risk subjects.

Table 5.8: Changes in Risk Factors over Two Years of WHO European Collaborative Trial (E = Experimental Group, C = Control)

Country and sample	Serum cholesterol (mg•dl^{-1})		Systolic blood pressure (mm Hg)		Cigarettes smoked per day in smokers	
	E	C	E	C	E	C
Belgium						
Random sample	+ 5.9	+ 20.0	−7	−0.4	− 9	− 4
High-risk sample	−10.0	+ 1.0	−	−	−11	−10
Italy						
High-risk sample	− 3.0	−	−	−	−	−
UK						
Random sample	+ 2.2	+ 5.4	−4	−4	−11	+ 2
High-risk sample	− 6.0	−	−	−	−29	−17

Source: Based on data of World Health Organization (1977).

Over a two-year period of observation, serum cholesterol, systolic blood pressure and the number of continuing smokers all changed favourably relative to workers in the control factories (Table 5.8).

In Europe, as in the US, many studies have been marred by a rapid attrition of volunteers. A participation rate of some 90 per cent was achieved in North Karelia (P. Puska *et al.*, 1978), but in Gothenburg 25 per cent of the population neither answered a mailed questionnaire nor attended an initial screening examination (L. Wilhelmsen *et al.*, 1976). Careful investigation disclosed an excess of immigrants, unmarried and divorced men and cigarette smokers among the non-volunteers (L. Wilhelmsen *et al.*, 1972); non-participants also had an above-average prevalence of alcoholism and chronic disease (L. Wilhelmsen *et al.*, 1976).

P. Teräslinna *et al.* (1969) found that 58 per cent of male executives either did not respond or were unwilling to participate in an exercise training programme. Subjects with a high-risk profile were selected from the 42 per cent of positive respondents. Endurance exercise was carried out for 30–60 minutes three times per week. Over 18 months, the drop-out rate was 14 per cent, with a class-participation rate of 72 per cent; the maximum oxygen intake increased by 20 per cent relative to control subjects, but there was no significant change of serum cholesterol, body mass, systemic blood pressure or smoking habits (K. Pyörälä *et al.*, 1971). Three years after completion of the study, the majority of the subjects had reverted to a sedentary lifestyle (J. Ilmarinen & Fardy, 1977).

Conclusion

Logistics have to date prevented effective long-term trials of exercise in the secondary prevention of ischaemic heart disease. Physical activity of sufficient vigour induces favourable changes in a number of coronary risk factors. However, such a response is not always observed with the relatively mild exercise programme usually arranged for the middle-aged adult. Furthermore, high drop-out rates cast doubt upon the practicality of exercise as a means of secondary prevention in the absence of greater social acceptance of physical activity as a normal component of leisure.

Cross-cultural Comparisons

Rationale

Cross-cultural comparisons identify regional and ethnic populations with coronary risk profiles that differ substantially from those of the typical 'white' North American.

Body fat content

Many 'primitive' people are extremely thin (R.J. Shephard, 1978a). For example, a double fold of skin and subcutaneous tissue measures only 6–7 mm in the Canadian Eskimo, as compared with 12–16 mm in an average 'white' person. On the other hand, measurements of total body fat suggest that the internal stores of the Eskimo are not proportionately reduced (R.J. Shephard *et al.*, 1973). Furthermore, because of a short stature and well-developed musculature, the traditional Eskimo has a substantial excess body mass relative to actuarial standards for the 'white' population. The low percentage of body fat is related to continued acceptance of a traditional lifestyle, and there is a positive correlation between the thickness of subcutaneous fat and indices of 'acculturation' to our western civilisation (R.J. Shephard, 1978a). In Alaska, skinfold readings have increased from six to twelve millimetres over 15 years of urbanisation (P.L. Jamison & Zegura, 1970). Two other indigenous populations with substantial obesity (the Maoris and the Polynesians of Hawai) now show a high prevalence of coronary arterial disease (D.R. Bassett *et al.*, 1966; I.A.M. Prior & Davidson, 1966).

Table 5.9: Lipid Profile of Greenlandic Eskimos and Danes

	Eskimos	Danes
Total lipid (g•l^{-1})	6.18	7.15
Cholesterol (mmol•l^{-1})	5.91	7.27
Triglyceride (mmol•l^{-1})	0.57	1.23
Chylomicrons (g•l^{-1})	0.27	0.19
Pre-β-lipoprotein (g•l^{-1})	0.43	1.29
β-Lipoprotein (g•l^{-1})	4.45	5.21
α-Lipoprotein (g•l^{-1}) .	4.00	5.34

Source: Based on data of H.O. Bang *et al.* (1976).

Blood lipids

When different populations are compared, the rank-order correlation
between the prevalence of atherosclerotic lesions and an elevation of
serum cholesterol levels is as high as 0.76 (N.S. Scrimshaw & Guzman,
1968; A. Keys, 1970). There is little question that the serum cholesterol
is low in most underdeveloped nations, although the relative
contribution of vigorous daily activity and restricted diet to this
situation remains uncertain. Traditional Eskimos have a favourable lipid
profile (Table 5.9) despite a very high fat diet (H.O. Bang *et al.*, 1976;
H.H. Draper, 1976; J. Sayed *et al.*, 1976); nevertheless, much of the
ingested fat may be unsaturated in type (A. Keys, 1975). Somali camel-
herders (V. Lapiccirella *et al.*, 1962) and East African Masai (G.V.
Mann *et al.*, 1965) eat much milk, meat and blood, yet maintain a low
serum cholesterol and a low incidence of ischaemic heart disease.
Although this has been attributed to high levels of daily energy
expenditure, other possible contributory factors include a low total
intake of energy (A. Keys, 1975), efficient inhibition of cholesterol
synthesis (K. Biss *et al.*, 1971) and the presence of a specific cholesterol
inhibitor in fermented milk (G.V. Mann, 1977). Other studies from
Africa (R.F. Scott *et al.*, 1966), Israel (J.H. Medalie *et al.*, 1968), India
(I.J. Pinto *et al.*, 1970) and the Pacific (I.A.M. Prior & Evans, 1970) all
show favourable lipid readings in 'primitive' groups, although there
remains an association between serum cholesterol and the likelihood of
myocardial infarction even when average values for the population are
very low (I.J. Pinto *et al.*, 1970). As a 'western' lifestyle is adopted,
serum cholesterol concentrations increase. Thus Alaskan Eskimos in
general (K. Ho *et al.*, 1972; J.E. Maynard, 1976), Canadian Eskimos

living in Montreal (R. Carrier *et al.*, 1972), and Greenlandic Eskimos living in Denmark (H.O. Bang *et al.*, 1976) all show relatively 'normal' cholesterol readings, with a corresponding increase in cardiovascular disease relative to their counterparts who conserve a traditional life-style (S.A. Feldman *et al.*, 1972; O. Schaefer, 1973; J.E. Maynard, 1976). Even within India, there is a trend to increasing cholesterol values (I.J. Pinto *et al.*, 1970), and much higher figures are encountered in wealthy Indians who have migrated to East Africa (R.F. Scott *et al.*, 1963).

Habitual activity

It has often been suggested that a high level of physical activity is necessary for survival in a 'primitive' community. However, formal measurements of 24-hour pulse rates (L. Hermansen & Ekblom, 1966) and energy expenditures (O.G. Edholm *et al.*, 1973; G. Godin & Shephard, 1973b; R.J. Shephard, 1978a) do not always confirm this supposition. In the pleasant climate of Easter Island, many of the native people undertake very little physical activity (L. Hermansen & Ekblom, 1966). Ugandan farmers work no more than 3½ hours per day (W.H. Boshoff, 1965), and the activity of East African nomads is reported as no more than 'moderate' (A.G. Shaper, 1970). Relatively few 'primitive' people exhibit high levels of energy expenditure or aerobic power (R.J. Shephard, 1978a). The ceremonial runners of the Tarahumara Indians are one notable exception (D. Groom, 1971). High daily energy expenditures are also encountered in traditional Canadian Eskimos (range 10.6-18.6 MJ per day, average 15.3 MJ. 'Acculturated' Eskimos who spend most of their time at wage-earning work in permanent settlements have a lower average energy usage (13.7 MJ per day), with a parallel loss of aerobic power and an increase in skinfold thickness (A. Rode & Shephard, 1971a). There seems to be an increased incidence of ischaemic heart disease with decreasing physical activity, even in underdeveloped nations. V.V. Shah *et al.* (1968) found that ischaemic heart disease was more frequent among sedentary Indian workers than in those with active occupations, while S.G. Sarvotham & Berry (1968) did not find a single case of cardiac disease among Indian heavy manual workers. In general, statistics for ischaemic heart disease favour underdeveloped societies, but it is by no means proven that physical activity is responsible for this advantage; other possible contributing factors (R.J. Shephard, 1974a) include genetic constitution, differing types and intensities of emotional stress, differences in the amount and type of tobacco consumed, differences in blood coagulability, differences in the prevalence of hypertension, differences in diet and drinking water (hard versus soft water) and inherited differences in glucose tolerance.

Apparent ethnic differences

Substantial ethnic differences in the prevalence of ischaemic heart disease have been observed between populations living in the same region. While it is well-recognised that constitutional factors contribute to 'coronary' susceptibility (M.M. Gertler & White, 1954; R. Cederlöf et al., 1967; T.M. Allan & Dawson, 1968), lifestyle factors are probably responsible for many of the apparent ethnic differences. H.C. McGill (1968) compared men of Caucasian and African descent living in New Orleans, São Paulo and Puerto Rico. In each of these locations, postmortem examination showed that the men of African origin had less coronary arterial stenosis than the Caucasians. Data on men of American Indian ancestry were unfortunately obtained from other cities (Caracas, Calin and Lima), but coronary arterial stenosis in such subjects was less severe than that observed in either Caucasians or Africans.

Studies of migrants

European-born men predominated among Israelis showing scars of myocardial infarction and coronary thrombosis following traumatic death (I. Mitrani et al., 1967). A prospective study of 10,000 male civil-service employees (J.H. Medalie et al., 1968) showed significant differences in the prevalence of angina pectoris, myocardial infarction and ischaemic heart disease according to the area of birth. Age-adjusted rates were highest for Jews from eastern or central Europe, intermediate for those born in Israel or southern Europe and lowest for those from Africa and other parts of the Middle-East (Table 5.10).

The importance of community lifestyle is strongly supported by other studies of migrants. Native-born Australians have a mortality from arteriosclerotic and degenerative heart disease of 1.69/1,000 over the age range 40–9 years. Italians resident in Australia for up to six years have a mortality of only 0.16/1,000 over the same age span; however, with 7–19 years of residence the figure rises to 0.51/1,000, and with more than 20 years of residence it is 1.30/1,000 (Table 5.11). Equally, United Kingdom, Norwegian, Irish and Japanese migrants to the United States have shown an increase in ischaemic-heart-disease mortality, with increased cigarette consumption accounting for only a part of the worsening of prognosis (G. Rose, 1970; M.F. Trulson et al.,

Table 5.10: Prevalence of Ischaemic Heart Disease in Migrants to Israel

Country of birth	Criterion (age-adjusted prevalence, per 1,000)		
	Angina pectoris	Previous myocardial infarction	ECG changes (LBBB, probable or possible infarct)
Eastern Europe	40	28	27
Central Europe	37	26	31
Southern Europe	40	15	18
Israel	33	20	20
Middle East	24	7	12
Africa	22	9	17

Source: J.H. Medalie *et al.* (1968).

Table 5.11: Mortality from Arteriosclerotic and Degenerative Heart Disease (ISC 420–2) among Italians Migrating to Australia, Australians, and Italians Remaining in Italy

Country of birth	Years of residence	Deaths from heart disease (per 1,000 per year)		
		Age 40–9 years	Age 50–9 years	Age 60–9 years
Italy	0–6 years (Austrialia)	0.16	1.23	2.60
	7–19	0.51	1.70	3.76
	20	1.30	3.44	7.58
	Resident in Italy*	0.80	2.40	6.80
Australia	Resident in Austrialia	1.69	5.92	14.72

* Those who remain in Italy also have a differing prognosis from early migrants; both existing disease and lifestyle factors probably influence the decision to migrate.

Source: G. Rose (1970).

cited by H.S. Ingraham, 1977).

As in more 'primitive' societies, differences in habitual activity may contribute to inter-population differences in the prevalence of ischaemic heart disease, but there seems no simple method of separating the effect of this variable from other lifestyle-related influences.

Studies of Ischaemic Heart Disease in Athletes

Studies of ischaemic heart disease in athletes have two principal attractions — the individuals concerned have engaged in more rigorous training than could be expected of the general population, and they have maintained this activity for months if not years.

Data on former athletes

Surveys of the incidence of ischaemic heart disease in former athletes (K. Yamaji & Shephard, 1977) have not been particularly helpful in proving or disproving the exercise hypothesis (Table 5.12). Early studies compared former university athletes with the general population, but it was soon realised that the advantage of longevity in ex-athletes was due to their favoured socio-economic status rather than to the physical activity involved in competitive sports. Comparisons were next made between those who represented their university for a particular sport and other members of the same academic community; this approach overcame socio-economic inequalities, but was nevertheless fallible, since it was rarely established that the 'non-athletes' were inactive while at university; some control series were indeed locker-holders in an athletic facility.

P. Fardy *et al.* (1976) found that, in later life, former athletes maintained some advantage of both activity pattern and myocardial function relative to non-athletes. However, other studies noted that many of those classed as athletes ceased to participate in their chosen sport some years before reaching the period of manifest coronary disease (Figure 5.1); when compared with their contemporaries, the so-called athletes were less active, more likely to be regular cigarette smokers and drinkers of alcoholic beverages and more likely to have sustained a large increase in body mass (Figure 5.2; H. Montoye *et al.*, 1956).

Data on continuing athletes

Where athletes have continued with vigorous endurance activity into

Table 5.12: Causes of Death among Former Athletes

Author	Heart and vascular disease	Genito-urinary disease	Cancer and tumours	Influenza, pneumonia, bronchitis	Tubercu-losis	Accidents, war, death, homicides, suicides
Wakefield (1944):						
Athletes	16.3		—	10.5	13.8	34.0
Controls	16.3		—	11.5	20.9	17.3
Rook (1954):						
Athletes	36.4	5.2	13.9	8.9	—	12.0
Controls	41.5	7.1	12.8	10.5	—	7.0
Pomeroy & White (1958):						
Athletes	37.9	4.6	12.6	10.3	—	24.1
Controls	49.0	3.7	13.6	4.8	—	7.5
H. Montoye *et al.* (1956):						
Athletes	66.0		12.0	2.0	—	10.0
Controls	56.0		14.0	5.8	—	13.0
Poldenak & Damon (1970):						
Major athletes	38.0	—	12.0	7.2	—	5.4
Minor athletes	42.5	—	12.3	3.9	—	7.4
Non-athletes	40.0	—	9.7	4.8	—	5.0
Schnor (1971):						
Athletes	34.7	5.6	23.6	3.5	—	9.1
Controls	36.7	4.1	25.1	1.2	—	7.7
Poldenak (1972):						
Major athletes	39.6	—	14.4	5.4	—	6.2
Minor athletes	42.6	—	13.3	4.0	—	7.6
Non-athletes	41.7	—	11.7	5.0	—	6.6

Source: Based on data accumulated by K. Yamaji & Shephard (1977).

their middle and later years, they have sometimes lived several additional years relative to (presumably) less active fellow citizens. M.J. Karvonen *et al.* (1974) studied cross-country skiers (mainly participants in the Oulu races of 1889–1930); mortality was compared with the general male population of Finland, using a life-table analysis. On average, the skiers lived 73.0 years, while the longevity of the reference population was 68.7 years. However, there is no proof that there were not initial differences of health favouring the ski champions, and their endurance sport necessarily fostered other health habits, including a

Figure 5.1: Current sports participation of former 'athletes' and 'non-athletes'; note that the sample size is small for the oldest age group.

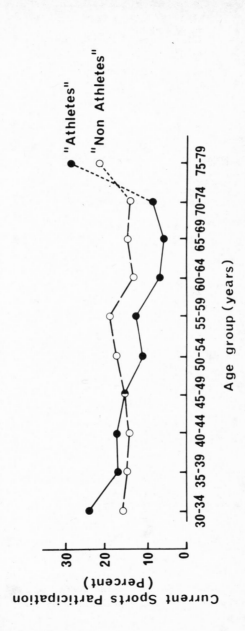

Source: Based on data of H.J. Montoye et al. (1957).

Figure 5.2: Percentage of subjects smoking and drinking regularly in middle age in relation to athletic 'letter' earnt while at University.

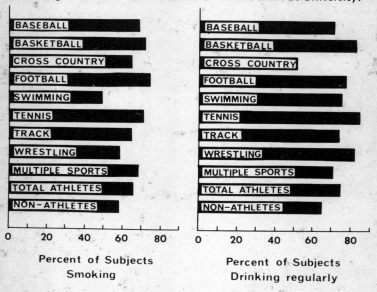

Percent of Subjects
Smoking

Percent of Subjects
Drinking regularly

Source: Based on data of H.J. Montoye *et al.* (1957).

lifetime aversion to cigarette smoking. A study of former long-distance runners and champion skiers (K. Pyörälä *et al.*, 1967a, b) revealed a lower blood pressure than in controls (137/87 mm Hg, compared with 147/92 mm Hg); symptoms of ischaemic heart disease were also less frequent, but nevertheless electrocardiographic abnormalities had a similar prevalence in atheletes and non-athletes.

The Bassler hypothesis

T.J. Bassler (1977) has repeatedly advanced the hypothesis that the running of marathon distances protects the heart against what he has described as coronary heart disease, ischaemic heart disease, fatal myocardial infarction, loafer's heart and coronary atherosclerosis. He has attributed the supposed protection in part to the rareness of cigarette smoking in the distance runner, and in part to the metabolic consumption of fat, which is the major fuel used in marathon running. Unfortunately for the Bassler hypothesis, T. Noakes *et al.* (1977) have now described six cases of myocardial infarction in well-trained

Table 5.13: Resting Systemic Blood Pressures (mm Hg) for Participants in Masters' Track and Field Competitions, Compared with Data of A. Master *et al.* (1964) for the General Population

Age group (years)	Masters' athletes						Sedentary normals	
	(T. Kavanagh & Shephard, 1977a)		(M.L. Pollock, 1974)		(K. Asano *et al.*, 1978)		(A.M. Master *et al.*, 1964)	
	Syst.	Diast.	Syst.	Diast.	Syst.	Diast.	Syst.	Diast.
< 40	124	79	—	—	—	—	127	80
40–50	120	77	117	76	117	70	130	82
50–60	127	77	129	81	132	79	137	84
60–70	128	77	122	78	135	82	143	84
> 70	140	83	141	83	157	78	146	82

Source: Based on data collected by T. Kavanagh & Shephard (1977a).

marathon runners, four of the six cases having coronary arterial disease demonstrated by angiography. P. Milvy (1977) has further stressed that the number and age of marathon runners (total sample of 9,958 in the US in 1975) are such that, even if running conferred no protection, no more than one death would be anticipated in any two-year period.

Observations on Masters' athletes

Findings for Masters' athletes have been reviewed by T. Kavanagh & Shephard (1977a). In their study, twelve of 135 Masters' contestants had a heart volume of more than $14 \ ml \cdot kg^{-1}$, compared with the anticipated value of $10-11 \ ml \cdot kg^{-1}$ for sedentary men of the same age. The resting systemic blood pressure was also slightly less than in the general population (Table 5.13). Some authors have reported a high prevalence of ST segmental depression in the exercise electrocardiogram of former endurance competitors (A. Holmgren & Strandell, 1959), but others have found a normal or even a low prevalence of abnormalities (K. Pyörälä *et al.*, 1967b; B. Saltin & Grimby, 1968). T. Kavanagh & Shephard (1977a) noted ventricular premature systoles in 17 of 135 competitors at rest, but the abnormal rhythm disappeared during exercise in all except two of the group. Fifteen of 135 tracings showed ST segmental depression of more than 0.1 mV when subjects were exercising at 75 per cent of aerobic power; having regard to their

Table 5.14: Prevalence of Abnormal Electrocardiogram (ST Depression > 0.1 mV) when Exercising at 75 Per Cent of Aerobic Power for Masters' Track and Field Athletes, as Compared with Normal Sedentary Canadians

Age group (years)	Masters' competitors		Sedentary Canadian men
< 40	2/8	(25%)	2%
40–50	4/64	(6.3%)	7
50–60	6/34	(17.6%)	17
60–70	3/18	(16.7%)	30*
70–90	0/4	(0%)	—

* Age 60–5 years.

Source: Data of T. Kavanagh & Shephard (1977a) for Masters' athletes and of G. Cumming (1972) for sedentary Canadians.

advanced age, this was possibly a smaller proportion of abnormal records than would have been anticipated in the general Canadian population (Table 5.14). Possible explanations of any favourable findings in the Masters' athletes include a development of collateral blood flow to the myocardium, a lesser hypokalaemia of effort and a reduction of workload per unit mass of myocardium secondary to hypertrophy and other changes of myocardial dimensions.

The problem of self-selection

Self-selection is perhaps the most serious criticism of all studies of athletes. Almost by definition, the competitor is an atypical member of the population from which he is drawn. He is necessarily in good initial health, and is committed to a health-conscious lifestyle. Selection for specific sports occurs on the basis of body type, and this also is a factor with a powerful influence upon prognosis. The ectomorphic cross-country skier or distance runner is inevitably at a lower risk of ischaemic heart disease than his mesomorphic or endomorphic counterpart, and this explains part of the substantial difference in longevity between endurance athletes and other classes of sportsmen (Table 5.15; K. Yamaji & Shephard, 1977). Finally many reports do not indicate the cause of death, and while heart disease may be less common in athletes than in the general population, this potential advantage is often masked by an increase in violent deaths from accident, suicide, homicide and war (Table 5.12).

Table 5.15: Mean Lifespan of Various Sportsmen, Excluding Those Dying at War or by Accident

Sport	Dublin (1928) (expected)	Rook (1954) (years)	Poldenak (1972) (years)	Largey (1972) (years)
Track & field	91.8	67.4	66.9	71.3
Cricket	—	68.1	—	—
Crew	94.1	67.1	66.8	—
Rugby football	—	68.8	—	—
American football	88.3	—	66.6	57.4
Baseball	98.0	—	65.2	64.1
Boxing	—	—	—	61.6
Two or more sports	78.3	—	67.2	—

Source: Based on data accumulated by K. Yamaji & Shephard (1977).

Such problems make it clear that the exercise hypothesis can be neither proven nor disproven by studies of champion athletes.

Occupational Surveys

Occupational surveys also have the attraction that a given level of physical activity is usually sustained for many years. Historically, the intensity of occupational effort has ranged from completely sedentary employment to tasks demanding quite vigorous physical activity. Epidemiologists were thus quick to compare the cardiac health of workers in jobs that demanded differing levels of energy expenditure (F.G. Pedley, 1942; J.A. Ryle & Russel, 1949; J.N. Morris *et al.*, 1953; O.F. Hedley, 1959).

Types of analysis

Early studies were retrospective in nature, but more recently there have been examinations of disease prevalence (J. Stamler *et al.*, 1960; H.L. Taylor *et al.*, 1962; J. McDonough *et al.*, 1965) and substantial prospective investigations (J.M. Chapman & Massey, 1964; J.N. Morris *et al.*, 1966; R. Paffenbarger & Hale, 1975). Bases of comparison have included: (i) the annual incidence of deaths from ischaemic heart disease; (ii) the annual incidence of sudden deaths; (iii) the annual

Table 5.16: The Influence of Physical Activity upon Various Indices of Ischaemic Heart Disease, Expressed as the Ratio of Incidence for Active and Inactive Populations

Index of ischaemic heart disease	Mean ratio	Range	Number of studies
Myocardial pain	0.48	0.21—0.68	8
Angina pectoris	1.36	0.65—1.98	7
Myocardial infarction	0.56	0.33—0.98	9
Coronary heart disease			
Attack rate	0.60	0.17—1.03	16
Mortality	0.66	0.28—1.22	21
Vascular pathology	0.76	0.51—1.00	7

Source: Based on data accumulated by S. Fox & Haskell (1968a).

incidence of myocardial infarctions; (iv) the annual incidence of freshly diagnosed cases of angina; and (v) some combinations of these statistics. A few authors have also examined the prevalence of electrocardiographic evidence of myocardial ischaemia (J. McDonough *et al.*, 1965; J.N. Morris, 1975) and the extent of pathological changes visible at post-mortem examination (myocardial scarring and fibrosis, coronary atherosclerosis; J.N. Morris & Crawford, 1958; D.M. Spain & Bradess, 1960b; G. Rose *et al.*, 1967).

Typical findings

The majority of surveys (16 of 20 listed by H.H. Clarke, 1972) have shown a higher incidence of deaths, sudden deaths and infarctions among those working in relatively sedentary occupations (Table 5.16). The remaining studies, sometimes described as negative, have generally shown similar trends. Nevertheless, the benefits of exercise have not always been statistically significant, as a result of an inadequate cohort size — a problem in the studies of J. Stamler *et al.* (1960) and of A. Keys (1970); transfer of subjects from active to inactive jobs with the recognition of disease — a problem merely noted in the negative study of H. Kahn (1963), but allowed for in the positive study of R. Paffenbarger *et al.* (1977); and inadequate categorisation of either occupation or infarction (I.M. Moriyama *et al.*, 1958; O. Paul, 1969).

One study of accident victims found that ischaemic changes (calcification, fatty streaking, raised lesions and coronary narrowing) were more common in light than in heavy occupations (V. Rissanen, 1976). However, others report coronary atheromata and narrowing as being equally prevalent in men from all job categories (J.N. Morris & Crawford, 1958; G. Rose *et al.*, 1967). Further, anginal pain is more common among active than inactive workers (J.N. Morris *et al.*, 1953; W.B. Kannel *et al.*, 1971a, b). It has thus been reasoned that, if occupational activity does indeed improve prognosis, this is not by preventing the development of ischaemic heart disease, but rather by making the individual aware of his condition and giving him a greater ability to live with it.

Social class differences

One major problem when interpreting occupational data is an association of the energy requirements of work with social class and related variables such as smoking and drinking habits. The first report from the Gothenburg study of 'men born in 1913' found a significant influence of occupational activity upon the likelihood of subsequent coronary events (L. Wilhelmsen & Tibblin, 1971). A second analysis from the same study (D. Elmfeldt *et al.*, 1976) is sometimes said to 'prove' that occupational activity has no influence upon the likelihood of a subsequent coronary event. In fact, there were differences of income, housing, nutrition and health habits between those tabulated as having 'high' and 'low' levels of occupational activity, and such confounding factors may well have obscured any benefit of exercise. Similar problems have arisen in a number of US studies, some of which have failed to show a significant association between physical inactivity and cardiovascular disease. Manual workers have generally been of a lower social class than sedentary employees, and sometimes there have also been differences of milieu (urban versus rural; H.L. Taylor *et al.*, 1962) or race (J. McDonough *et al.*, 1965) between the two groups. While rural 'blacks' living in the US have less coronary disease than their 'white' counterparts (J. Cassel *et al.*, 1971), the negroes of the urban ghettos (J.M. Chapman & Massey, 1964; J. Stamler *et al.*, 1960) (who preponderate among the blue-collar workers) have a high incidence of ischaemic heart disease, linked to their propensity for obesity and cigarette smoking. J.M. Chapman & Massey (1964) observed no difference in the incidence of ischaemic heart disease with social class, but it may be that in the sample investigated the adverse health habits of the blue-collar workers were counterbalanced by the added energy expenditure of their work. Among studies with a reasonable matching of socio-economic status, we may mention comparisons of

London bus drivers and conductors (J.N. Morris *et al.*, 1953, 1966), postal clerks and mail carriers (J.N. Morris & Raffle, 1954; H. Kahn, 1963), and office and field workers of the Jewish kibbutzim (D. Brunner & Manelis, 1971).

Influence of emotional stress

It has been argued that sedentary employees are exposed to greater emotional stress than those in physically active employment. In the case of the London bus drivers, this hypothesis was explored and rejected through a comparison of men operating city and rural routes (J.N. Morris *et al.*, 1966). Other attempts to demonstrate an effect of occupational stress upon the incidence of ischaemic heart disease have generally been unconvincing (Chapter 2), one exception being managers with upward social mobility (L. Hinckle *et al.*, 1968).

Intensity of occupational activity

Occupations that demand more than two to three times the resting metabolic rate are now a rarity, and a heart rate 'ceiling' of 115 beats·min^{-1} is common for 'heavy' industry. On the other hand, most physiologists suggest that a young adult should reach a minimum heart rate of 140 beats·min^{-1} in order to improve his physical condition (M.L. Pollock, 1973; R.J. Shephard, 1975, 1977a). Even in a 65-year-old worker, conditioning is unlikely with a heart rate of less than 120 beats·min^{-1} (K.H. Sidney & Shephard, 1978). Admittedly, physiologists are still uncertain how to equate 30 minutes of training at a heart rate of 140 beats·min^{-1} and 8 hours of industrial activity at a heart rate of 115 beats·min^{-1}. Nevertheless, it seems likely that the majority of North Americans now find their main source of physical activity outside of their daily employment (H. Montoye, 1975), confounding the whole concept of classifying habitual activity by occupation.

Many retrospective occupational studies have used very 'soft' data. Occupational classifications have been crude, and there has been no guarantee that the small minority sustaining heart attacks were working at a level typical of their category. Reports have often referred to the period immediately prior to the heart attack, ignoring the possibility that warning symptoms such as angina pectoris may have led a man to change from active to sedentary employment. Where occupation has apparently had no effect upon prognosis, this may thus reflect difficulties of classification rather than a true absence of relationship.

Self-selection

As in studies of athletes, the major criticism of occupational surveys is the problem of self-selection. In general, people choose their mode of employment. In a classical paper subtitled 'The epidemiology of uniforms', J.N. Morris *et al.* (1956) showed that, at the time of recruitment to the London Transport bus system, the drivers had a larger average abdominal girth than the conductors. They also had a higher serum cholesterol, a higher systemic blood pressure (J.N. Morris *et al.*, 1956) and a greater body mass (R.M. Oliver, 1967), giving them an increased initial risk of ischaemic heart disease. A large occupational survey from Eire (N. Hickey *et al.*, 1975) showed a similar negative association between heavy work and coronary risk factors at the time of commencing employment.

The bias becomes exaggerated over a longitudinal study, since those with symptoms of ischaemic heart disease leave the labour force or are transferred from the active to the sedentary group (H.L. Taylor *et al.*, 1962; H. Kahn, 1963). This could explain why heavy work seems protective for young but not for older workers (R. Paffenbarger *et al.*, 1970, 1977). One statistical remedy is to reclassify workers annually according to their currently reported job assignment (R. Paffenbarger & Hale, 1975; R. Paffenbarger *et al.*, 1977); however, this tactic is rendered ineffective if the union insists that a worker retain a high-paying job classification even though he is unable to function at the required intensity of effort.

D. Brunner & Manelis (1971) maintained that, in the Jewish kibbutzim, difficulties of self-selection were eliminated, since the type of employment was determined by a central committee. If they are correct in this view, their data has great importance, for the field workers encountered the same diet, income and living conditions as those whose employment involved sitting for at least 80 per cent of the day. The two groups had comparable values for body mass, serum cholesterol and triglycerides, yet the physically active workers had a much lower incidence of ischaemic heart disease. Unfortunately, it is hard to believe that the kibbutz committee was uninfluenced by initial health and physique when assigning an individual's duties. Almost inevitably, such factors must have determined both initial placement and subsequent annual reallocation of jobs; indeed, the medical history probably influenced job selection more than in a free-market economy.

Multivariate analyses

Perhaps the most sophisticated of the occupational surveys is that reported by R. Paffenbarger (1977). He examined 3,686 Californian longshoremen over a 22-year period, from 1951 to 1972. Employment categories were well-defined by the union concerned, and a part of the sample had a very high energy expenditure at work (22–31 kJ·min^{-1}); the intensity was sufficiently high that union regulations limited each hour to 55 per cent labour and 45 per cent rest periods. Note was taken when a fatal heart attack was certified as the underlying cause of death, and the data were sorted into sudden deaths (within one hour of the onset of symptoms) and delayed deaths on the basis that premonitory symptoms might have caused a change of job classification in the latter group of subjects.

Table 5.17: Initial Self-selection of Job Category by Californian Longshoremen, Expressed as Age-adjusted Per Cent of Sample

Variable	Occupational energy expenditure	
	Low	High
Cigarettes (> 1 pack·day^{-1})	39.1*	34.2*
Systolic blood pressure ($\geqslant$ mean)	44.3	45.3
Diastolic blood pressure ($\geqslant$ mean)	47.2	48.7
Diagnosed heart disease	17.0	18.2
'Weight for height' ($\geqslant$ mean)	48.0*	45.9*
Abnormal glucose tolerance	4.1	4.0
Serum cholesterol ($\geqslant$ mean)	48.4	42.8

* Significant difference ($P < 0.05$).

Source: Based on data of R. Paffenbarger (1977).

Two factors of initial self-selection were noted (Table 5.17). There were less pack-a-day smokers among the heavy than among the moderate and light workers, partly because the former were not allowed to smoke except in specified 'rest areas'. Also, a smaller proportion of the heavy workers had an above average 'weight for height'. However, Paffenbarger argued that these differences were not sufficient to invalidate his subsequent data analysis.

A lesser energy output at work (6–22 kJ·min^{-1}), the smoking of more than a pack of cigarettes per day and a systolic blood pressure equal to or greater than the mean all made independent contributions

Table 5.18: Relative Risk of Fatal Heart Attack, Adjusted for Age and Other Two Principal Risk Factors for California Longshoremen

Type of death	Low energy output	Cigarettes ($\geqslant$ 1 pack·day^{-1})	Systolic blood pressure ($\geqslant$ mean)
Sudden	3.3	1.6	2.7
Delayed	1.6	2.1	1.4
Unspecified	1.7	2.5	2.2
All	2.0	2.1	2.1

Source: Based on data of R. Paffenbarger (1977).

to the risk of cardiac death; in the case of the lower energy output, the effect was much greater for sudden than for delayed deaths (Table 5.18). Serum cholesterol had surprisingly little influence upon risk, possibly because most categories of longshoremen had a higher level of energy expenditure than that required in ordinary modern occupations.

The incidence of deaths from cerebrovascular disease was also related to a lesser energy output at work, but exacerbation of disease was relatively specific to the cardiovascular system; deaths from cancer, accidents and suicides were unrelated to the activity level at work.

Paffenbarger used multivariate statistics to estimate the health benefits that would accrue from a modification of the three prime risk factors that he had identified. Acting singly, an increase of energy output would reduce the cardiac death rate by 31–67 per cent. The smoking of less than a pack of cigarettes a day would reduce the risk 20–36 per cent, while reduction of the systolic blood pressure below the population mean would reduce the risk by 21–37 per cent. If all three changes were effected, the cardiac death rate would drop by a dramatic 70–100 per cent (Table 5.19).

In marked contrast with Paffenbarger, R.H. Rosenman *et al.* (1977) had essentially negative findings in a four-year prospective survey of US Federal employees living in the San Francisco Bay area. Significant differences were seen between those classed as having light, moderate and heavy energy expenditure at work (Table 5.20). However, there was a substantial influence of social class upon smoking habits, relative body mass and serum cholesterol levels (Table 5.21). A multivariate analysis that allowed for socio-economic status revealed no effect of occupational activity upon either risk factors or the

Table 5.19: Hypothetical Reduction in Risk of Fatal Heart Attack with Change of Health Behaviour

Health behaviour modified	Fatal heart attacks per 1,000 man-years with adverse behaviour	Potential reduction in risk (%)	
1. Low energy output	6.97	48.8	(30.6—67.0)
2. Cigarettes ($\geqslant$ 1 pack•day^{-1})	9.43	27.9	(20.1—35.7)
3. Systolic blood pressure ($\geqslant$ mean)	8.91	28.8	(20..6—37.0)
4. 1 + 2	9.57	64.7	(44.5—84.9)
5. 1 + 3	9.15	73.5	(56.9—90.1)
6. 2 + 3	16.16	50.3	(39.7—60.9)
7. 1 + 2 + 3	15.19	88.2	(70.2—100.0)

Source: Based on data of R. Paffenbarger (1977).

Table 5.20: Correlations between Intensity of Vocational Activity (Light, Moderate or Heavy) and Other Risk Factors for Ischaemic Heart Disease at Beginning of Prospective Study

Variable	Age 35-9 years			Age 40-9 years			Age 50-9 years		
	Light	Mod.	Heavy	Light	Mod.	Heavy	Light	Mod.	Heavy
Current smokers (%)	27.9	39.6*	37.0*	26.0	37.7	42.4	35.9	37.3	41.4
Relative body mass (% predicted)	99.8	97.5	106.1*	100.4	101.1	102.6*	100.6	101.5	101.6
Serum cholesterol (mg•dl^{-1})	237	240	253	247	245	260*	247	242	259*
Blood pressure:									
Systolic (mm Hg)	133	133	137	134	135	137	140	141	141
Diastolic (mm Hg)	84	84	87	86	86	87	89	88	89

* Statistically significant difference from light-activity group.

Source: Based on data of R.H. Rosenman *et al.* (1977).

Table 5.21: Influence of Socio-economic Status (High, Medium, Low) upon Level of Risk of Ischaemic Heart Disease at Beginning of Prospective Study

Variable	Age 35–9 years			Age 40–9 years			Age 50–9 years		
	High	Med.	Low	High	Med.	Low	High	Med.	Low
Current smokers (%)	24.2	42.3*	46.2*	31.6	37.4*	44.3*	31.8	37.7*	40.5*
Relative body mass (% predicted)	98.5	99.2	103.6*	99.1	103.0*	102.3*	99.5	103.1*	101.4
Serum cholesterol (mg•dl^{-1})	237	246	244	243	249*	255*	248	238*	251
Blood pressure:									
Systolic (mm Hg)	132	134	136	133	133	138	139	141	142
Diastolic (mm Hg)	83	86	87*	85	86	88*	87	89	89

* Statistically significant difference from high-status group.

Source: Based on data on R.H. Rosenman *et al.* (1977).

incidence of clinical manifestations of ischaemic heart disease. Specific differences from the Paffenbarger experiment included a more heterogeneous population, a less clear-cut indicator of disease, a lower intensity of physical activity in most of the 'active' population and a less certain categorisation of activity. On the other hand, the adjustment for socio-economic status covered effects of the latter upon cigarette consumption, relative body mass, serum cholesterol level, diastolic blood pressure and non-occupational activity, factors that could have contributed to the apparent association between occupation and disease in the Paffenbarger study.

C.L. Rose & Cohen (1977) made a multivariate analysis of longevity, using as their data-base 500 white male deaths reported to Boston City Hall in 1965. Factors such as age-appearance, smoking habits, mother's age at death, sense of humour, urban-versus-rural residence, intelligence and worries were all related more closely to the age at death than was leisure activity, while this in turn was also a better indicator of longevity than was activity at work. Interestingly, the assessed vigour of activity both on and off the job decreased progressively as the individual became older (Figure 5.3).

Figure 5.3: Influence of age upon mean physical activity scores at work and during leisure

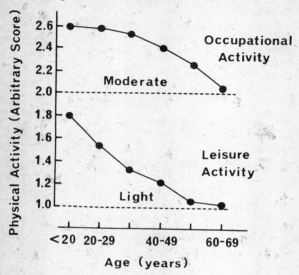

Based on data of C.L. Rose & Cohen (1977).

Conclusion

While some of the evidence from occupational surveys supports the exercise hypothesis, the verdict is by no means unanimous. Interest in organising further studies is waning, since: (a) with increasing automation the city-dweller must look to his leisure hours rather than his work in order to increase his habitual activity; and (b) observations relating occupation to the incidence of ischaemic heart disease can never provide conclusive proof that exercise has preventive value.

Leisure-activity Patterns

Problems of methodology

Problems in surveying leisure activity include the poor reliability of most physical activity questionnaires (W.J. Zukel *et al.*, 1959), and a denial of disability by those who have already suffered a myocardial infarction (V. Froehlicher & Oberman, 1972). If a whole community is studied (for example, D. Elmfeldt *et al.*, 1976), the analysis is further complicated by a positive correlation between vigorous voluntary

Table 5.22: Vigorous Leisure Exercise among Married Men Age 17 and Older Living in London area

Type of activity	Per cent participants by social class		
	I	III	IV & V
Swimming	34	20	8
Football (soccer)	6	8	5
Tennis	8	2	0
Squash	7	2	0
Athletics	2	1	0
Average number of sports	1.1	0.6	0.3

Source: Based on data of M. Young & Willmot (1973).

Table 5.23: Socio-economic Status (High, Medium, Low) and Habitual Physical Activity

Age (years)	Physical activity ($h \cdot wk^{-1}$)					
	Occupational status			Leisure status		
	High	Medium	Low	High	Medium	Low
35–9	4.6	12.6	19.3	8.9	9.4	9.6
40–9	5.3	10.9	17.5	9.3	9.5	8.4
50–9	5.2	11.9	17.1	9.7	8.7	8.7

Source: Based on data of R.H. Rosenman *et al.* (1977).

activity and social class (M. Young & Willmot, 1973; R.H. Rosenman *et al.*, 1977; Tables 5.22 and 5.23). Recent investigations have overcome this problem by focussing upon narrow cross sections of society.

Harvard alumnae study

R.S. Paffenbarger *et al.* (1977) made an extensive prospective study of Harvard graduates, relating the certified causes of death and the incidence of physician-diagnosed ischaemic heart disease to smoking habits and continued participation in various forms of physical activity. The sample size was large (16,936 subjects, 117,680 person-years), and for this reason it was possible to classify participants by athletic discipline (avoiding some of the problems of association between sport selection and body build, discussed above). Substantial protection against ischaemic heart disease (heart attack rate of 1.00 relative to standard figure of 1.64) was seen with an additional overall energy expenditure of 8,000 kJ•wk^{-1}, a figure reminiscent of that deduced from occupational surveys. Furthermore, the age-adjusted cardiac fatality rate showed a steep downward gradient as additional energy expenditure was increased from 2,000 to 10,000 kJ•wk^{-1}. Strenuous sports alone yielded a protection ratio of 1.00:1.38. Subjects who had commenced their sport after leaving university were protected, whereas those who had been athletes at college but subsequently become inactive forfeited their advantage. Protection ratios for the walking of at least one mile per day, and the climbing of fifty stairs per day were 1.00:1.26 and 1.00:1.25 respectively. Protection against a first heart attack was demonstrated in both high- and low-risk segments of the sample (Table 5.24). Paffenbarger's study thus supports the exercise hypothesis. Some criticisms remain with respect to self-selection of the type and vigour of habitual activity, although this source of uncertainty is reduced by the demonstration that sports participation at university has no influence upon prognosis. Again, it can be argued that endurance activity has modified other risk factors such as cigarette consumption (P. Morgan *et al.*, 1976), although protection is seen both in smokers and non-smokers.

British civil servants study

A prospective study by J.N. Morris *et al.* (1973) found a significant reduction in the incidence of ischaemic heart disease (Table 5.25), among British civil servants who engaged in: (a) more than five minutes per day of active recreation, keeping fit or 'vigorous getting about' (near maximum effort); or (b) more than 30 minutes per day of 'heavy' leisure activity (> 31 kJ•min^{-1}). Electrocardiographic abnormalities were also less frequent in the active groups (L. Epstein *et al.*, 1976). The added energy expenditure, no more than 750 kJ•day^{-1}, is substantially less than the figure calculated from eight-hour occupational surveys, and it seems more likely to commend itself to the average sedentary middle-aged person. J.N. Morris and his associates were able to exclude differences of cigarette smoking as an explanation of their data. Nevertheless, it remains conceivable that the chosen criteria (five minutes of vigorous getting about and/or 30 minutes of heavy leisure activity) served as indicators of a general attitude towards exercise and health. The total daily energy expenditure of the active civil servants may thus have exceeded that of

Table 5.24: Protection against First Heart Attack with Additional Weekly Energy Expenditure of 8,000 kJ, All Indices Being 1.00 for the Active Group and a Higher Figure for Those Who Are Less Active

Risk factor	Protection against first heart attack	
	Risk factor present	Risk factor absent
Cigarette smoking	2.22	1.55
Systolic pressure > 130 mm Hg	1.86	1.54
Diastolic pressure > 80 mm Hg	1.36	1.86
Quetelet index (mass $\times 10^3$/height^2) > 34	1.58	1.61
Parent dead	1.63	1.74
No varsity sport	1.59	1.65

Source: R. Paffenbarger *et al.* (1977).

Table 5.25: Frequency of Vigorous Exercise Reported by 239 British Civil Servants Sustaining First Clinical Attack of Myocardial Infarction Relative to Frequency in 476 Matched Controls

Type of activity	Frequency of physical activity	
	Attacked subjects (n = 238)	Matched controls (n = 476)
Active recreation	5	19
Keeping fit	3	16
Vigorous getting about*	1	21
Heavy work*	19	78
Climbing > 450 stairs•day^{-1}	0	8
Total reporting activity	25/238	120/476

* See text for definition.

Source: Based on data of J.N. Morris *et al.* (1973).

their sedentary counterparts by a larger margin than 750 kJ, while the choice of (for instance) a vigorous morning walk to the station may have been reflected in other positive health practices. Although active and inactive groups were similar in height, body mass and skinfold thickness, the active group included fewer subjects with a serum cholesterol > 6.4 mmol•l^{-1}, more subjects with a blood pressure >

150/90 mm Hg and slightly fewer smokers (26 versus 32 per cent). Finally, as with similar surveys, we are left with the obstacle of self-selection. It was the civil servants rather than Dr J.N. Morris who decided upon their daily activity patterns, and this decision was undoubtedly influenced both by initial health and constitution.

Other studies

W.B. Kannel (1967, 1979) studied cardiovascular risk factors in 5,127 men and women living in Framingham, Mass. Physical activity was assessed from a 24-hour history of usual physical activity and from a number of physiological indices (resting heart rate, vital capacity, hand grip strength and relative body mass). Coronary heart disease and mortality were found to be higher in cohorts where a sedentary lifestyle was inferred, although it was recognised that other risk factors (a high serum cholesterol, a high systemic blood pressure, cigarette smoking, glucose intolerance and ECG abnormalities) were more important determinants of prognosis than was exercise.

R.H. Rosenman (1970) examined the habits of more than 30,000 middle-aged men participating in the Western Collaborative Group Study. The prime focus of his investigation was psychological. Nevertheless, he observed a protective effect of regular exercise; this appeared in 'Type A' men (rates 9.1/1,000 and 15.0/1,000) but not in those with a 'Type B' personality (rates 5.7/1,000 and 5.3/1,000). He commented that the protective value of exercise disappeared if subjects had a high diastolic pressure (> 95 mm Hg), high fasting serum triglycerides (> 130 mg·dl^{-1}), or a low HDL/LDL ratio.

S. Shapiro *et al.* (1969) reported data for men and women aged 35-64 years who were enrolled in the Health Insurance Plan of Greater New York. Among men, those who were the least active on and off the job had twice as large an incidence of first myocardial infarctions as those who were moderately active, but no additional advantage was gained from further activity. Total infarctions were four times more frequent in the active group, but the incidence of angina was unrelated to reported physical activity.

We have noted above that, in the Gothenburg study, occupational activity had no significant influence upon the development of ischaemic heart disease. However, when leisure-time activities were explored, there was a trend towards inactivity in those who subsequently developed coronary disease (G. Tibblin *et al.*, 1975).

Coronary risk factors

H.J. Montoye (1975) examined the relationships between coronary risk factors and physical activity in 1,696 men living in the small town of Tecumseh, Michigan. When information from leisure and occupational activity was combined, the mean systolic and diastolic blood pressures and serum cholesterol levels were highest in the most sedentary of his subjects.

N. Hickey *et al.* (1975) screened 15,171 Irish workers; they found that heavy leisure activity was associated with a low blood pressure, a low serum cholesterol, a favourable relative body mass and a reduced likelihood of cigarette smoking.

Conclusion

As in the occupational surveys, there is much to support the exercise hypothesis in studies of leisure pursuits. Nevertheless, it is unlikely that conclusive proof will be obtained by further extension of such investigations. Problems arise from the need to average data over a wide range of subject ages and a substantial period of history (in which the epidemic of coronary disease has waned; B.M. Meyer, 1979). Above all, self-selection remains an insuperable obstacle to substantiating the value of physical activity.

The Bradford Hill Criteria

Given the impossibility of experimental proof, an alternative possibility is to exclude spurious and indirect associations, and then to weigh the evidence against nine criteria that A. Bradford Hill (1971) has suggested should be satisfied if a statistical association is to be regarded as causal rather than casual.

Spurious association

Several causes of spurious association must first be excluded. There is the Type I error of the statistical method — given a 0.05 level of probability, there is one chance in twenty that an association is a statistical artifact. The likelihood of such an error is reduced in the case of the exercise hypothesis, since the association has been replicated many times in differing circumstances.

Problems may also arise when one sub-group of a population has unusual characteristics. For example, when exploring leisure activity, the active group is likely to be younger and to have a higher social class than those who are inactive. Such difficulties have been overcome at the expense of some loss of generality by introducing age 'adjustments' and concentrating upon a single social class (for example, the executive category of civil servant in the study of J.N. Morris *et al.*, 1973).

On occasion, bias can be introduced by the methodology or the observer. For instance, in a retrospective survey of activity patterns, an investigator who favoured the exercise hypothesis might be tempted to class people with cardiovascular disease as physically inactive. However, such a bias can hardly have arisen in studies where activity was classified prior to the onset of disease. Bias in the selection of control subjects is least likely in studies where activity patterns have been classified for almost all members of a population. When volunteers have been more widely solicited, it is likely that even the control subjects were more active and more health-conscious than a true random sample of the general population. The observed influence of physical activity upon ischaemic heart disease is thus a conservative measure of the effect that would occur in a truly sedentary population with a poor lifestyle.

Indirect association

An indirect association is possible if both physical inactivity and ischaemic heart disease are linked to a common variable. One possible candidate would be cigarette smoking. Certainly, this influences the likelihood of ischaemic heart disease (P. Morgan *et al.*, 1976), and it may also be linked to physical inactivity. Regular exercise is also related to a healthy lifestyle, and particular sports to a characteristic body build (K. Yamaji & Shephard, 1977). The effect of such indirect associations is largely controlled in recent multivariate analyses of the relationship between physical inactivity and ischaemic heart disease.

Bradford Hill criteria

1. Strength of the association. A causal association is a strong one. The incidence of ischaemic heart disease should thus be low in the presence of physical activity, and high in its absence. In fact, the ratio is probably not much better than 1:2 (S. Fox & Haskell, 1967; R. Paffenbarger, 1977). This is much smaller than for the ratio relating cigarette smoking to lung cancer, but is of the same order as for other cardiac risk factors such as a high systemic blood pressure, an abnormal exercise electrocardiogram and a cigarette habit.

2. Consistency of the association. A causal association is reported by many investigators, studying different populations, and using different techniques. In general, this condition is met for exercise and ischaemic heart disease. Perhaps because of counteracting influences of race and socio-economic class, a few authors have not observed any benefit from physical activity, but there seem no reports of cardiovascular harm from vigorous habitual exercise (H.H. Clarke, 1972). Nevertheless, there remains the possibility of a consistent bias; for instance, most of the investigators concerned have a vested interest in physical activity, and this could have given a spurious unanimity to published reports.

3. Temporally correct association. Exposure to the putative cause must antedate the onset of disease by an appropriate period. As already noted, the latent period for the development of ischaemic heart disease has yet to be clarified. However, in many of the studies we have discussed, the habit of physical activity or inactivity has persisted for a sufficient number of years that this condition is likely to have been satisfied.

4. Specificity of the association. Ideally, existence of the causal variable should lead to occurrence of the disease. However, lack of specificity can occur if a given factor causes more than one disease, or if a condition has a multiple aetiology. In the present context, possible sequelae of inactivity include both obesity and ischaemic heart disease; furthermore, clinical manifestations of a sedentary lifestyle are more likely in a person with a congenital abnormality of lipid metabolism than in the absence of this disorder. There are thus reasonable explanations for some lack of specificity in the association between inactivity and ischaemic heart disease.

5. Biological gradient. A graded dose-response relationship is characteristic of a causal relationship. Some suggestion of a biological gradient with increasing inactivity can be seen in the comparison of rail clerks, switchmen and sectionmen (H.L. Taylor *et al.*, 1962), in the Framingham study (T. Gordon *et al.*, 1971) and in the comparison between long-shoremen with high, medium and low levels of occupational activity (R. Paffenbarger *et al.*, 1975). On the other hand, some reports postulate a 'threshold dose' of exercise for a protective effect, rather than a smooth activity-related gradient (R.S. Paffenberger *et al.*, 1977).

6. Biological plausibility. There should be at least one plausible pathophysiological mechanism whereby the postulated cause could bring about the disease. In the context of preventing cardiac disease, this question has been well reviewed by S. Fox & Skinner (1964) and by W.L. Haskell (1979). These authors suggest many (almost too many!) reasons why an increase in physical activity could protect an individual against ischaemic heart disease.

7. *Coherence.* The requirement of coherence is closely related to that of plausibility. If the association is causal, the hypothesis advanced should provide a coherent explanation of the data. This condition is unfortunately not well satisfied in the case of exercise and ischaemic heart disease. There are many points in the natural history of the disease yet to be elucidated, including the obvious scarring of the myocardium in physically active patients, and the occasional instance where a myocardial infarction is precipitated by vigorous and unusual exercise.

8. *Experimental verification.* A causal association should be susceptible to experimental proof. We have already reviewed the difficulties that have prevented such a verification of the exercise hypothesis. The suggested treatment cannot be administered in a double-blind fashion, and an increase of activity inevitably changes other health habits. Future randomised controlled trials will probably have a multifactorial basis, rather than testing simply the effects of increased physical activity (H. Blackburn, 1972).

9. *Analogy.* The final criterion of a causal association is that of analogy. It can be illustrated in terms of the relationship between cigarette smoking and lung cancer. The causal viewpoint is given credence because individual constituents of tobacco smoke induce analogous carcinogenic changes at the cellular level. However, there is as yet little evidence that some component of the exercise response has cellular effects that offer protection against ischaemic heart disease.

Conclusion

We must conclude that several of Bradford Hill's criteria of a causal relationship remain unsatisfied with respect to exercise and the secondary prevention of ischaemic heart disease. As. P.O. Åstrand has pointed out (1967), it may well take 100 years to obtain a proof of the exercise hypothesis that will satisfy statisticians. But in the meantime, we have a potential remedy that is both agreeable and non-addictive, with few serious complications. 'Moderate activity is part of balanced, satisfying living and is the safe and hygienic prescription of the thoughtful physician for his patients, the high risk and the healthy alike' (H. Blackburn, 1974).

6 EXERCISE AND THE TERTIARY PREVENTION OF ISCHAEMIC HEART DISEASE

Since the early observations of V. Gottheiner (1960, 1968), J.J. Kellerman & Kariv (1968) and H.K. Hellerstein (1968), many authors have assumed that a programme of exercise rehabilitation improves the prognosis of the patient who has already sustained a myocardial infarction. In this chapter, we shall look critically at existing information drawn from both simple longitudinal studies and randomised controlled trials, seeking answers to the following questions.

(1) Does a regimen of progressive endurance exercise reduce the likelihood of recurrent infarction and/or a fatal heart attack?

(2) If so, does exercise therapy improve prognosis for all post-coronary patients, or is there a category of individuals who should be warned against taking additional physical activity?

(3) If exercise indeed has an effect, does it act in its own right, or is it merely modifying other risk factors?

Early Longitudinal Studies

Studies in Israel

Findings from early longitudinal studies are summarised in Table 6.1. V. Gottheiner (1960, 1968) was probably the first physician to undertake a systematic programme of exercise therapy for coronary victims. His patients were advanced cautiously through a graded activity schedule. This culminated in selected sports, including an 11 km race around Mount Tabor. The competitive nature of his programme was regarded as useful in maintaining patient interest. The average death rate over five years of observation was 0.88 per cent per year; this was much less than the figure of 4.8 per cent per year for physically inactive but otherwise comparable patients who were attending myocardial infarction clinics in other parts of Israel. Gottheiner originally recruited 1,500 subjects, but only 1,103 continued to exercise for the full five years. It could thus be argued that the drop-out process biased the residual sample towards patients with minor infarctions.

J.J. Kellerman & Kariv (1968) rehabilitated 'post-coronary' patients attending the Tel-Hashomer Hospital through a hospital-based activity

Table 6.1: Some Estimates of the Value of Exercise in the Tertiary Prevention of Ischaemic Heart Disease, Derived from Cross-sectional Comparisons

Follow-up period (years)	N	Exercised group			Control group			Author
		Recurrence rate (%/yr)	Death rate (%/yr)	Cardiac death rate (%/yr)	Recurrence rate (%/yr)	Death rate (%/yr)	Cardiac death rate (%/yr)	
1.0	64	9.4	3.1	–	25.0	10.9	–	D. Brunner (1968)
5.0	1,103	–	0.88	0.72	–	4.8[1]	–	V. Gottheiner (1968)
2.0[2]	41	2.5[2]	–	–	6.9[2]	–	–	E.M. Heller (1968)
2.7	254	–	2.0	–	–	4.5–6.0[3]	–	H.K. Hellerstein (1968)
6.0[4]	150	–	–	3.3[4]	–	–	10.6[4]	J.J. Kellerman & Kariv (1968)
2.7[5]	71	2.1	0.5	–	10.5	0.8	–	E.M. Heller (1972)
5.0[6]	77	(1.0)[6]	(0.8)[6]	–	(7.3)[6]	(2.4)[6]	–	P. Rechnitzer et al. (1972)
7.0[7]	68	5.0	3.6	–	14.3	9.0	–	Ibid.

1. Controls followed up for one to four years at other clinics.
2. Estimate of average follow-up (some subjects were followed up for up to four years). 'Controls' were 36 'drop-outs' who failed to enter programme; twelve of the 36 showed cardiovascular complications.
3. Estimated experience of other patients in Cleveland area.
4. Apparently not true annual mortality rates.
5. Subjects followed up for 0.5–5.0 years; 2.7 years is estimated average period of follow-up. Sample of 71 patients included six cases with acute coronary insufficiency.
6. Not all subjects were followed up for the full five-year period. Death rates are thus underestimates of the true values. Controls drawn from a larger city.
7. Not all subjects were followed up for the full seven-year period. Data adjusted to an average study duration of 2.1 years, assuming a linear relationship between follow-up period and death rate. Controls taken from other hospitals in the same city.

programme; breathing and relaxation exercises, the lifting of light
weights and calisthenics were undertaken for 45-60 minutes three
times per week. The overall regimen brought physical working capacity
from 57 to 83 per cent of the age-related normal value. J.J. Kellerman
& Kariv (1968) further claimed that the cardiac death rate for their
sample was much lower than that for patients who did not receive
active rehabilitation. Nevertheless, it was accepted that a selected series
had been observed: 'no patients with acute cardiac or coronary
insufficiency or severe arrhythmias were admitted to the exercise
program' (J.J. Kellermann *et al.*, 1970).

D. Brunner (1968, 1973) exercised his patients on a cycle ergometer twice per week for four months. Individual training sessions were
conducted in an interval fashion, bouts of activity lasting three
to six minutes at loadings of 25-100 W being alternated with rest
intervals of four to eight minutes. The exercised group included cases of
both myocardial infarction and angina pectoris; 80 patients were
admitted to the programme, but only 64 completed the four-month
study. The 'control' series were the next 40 patients attending Dr
Brunner's clinic; they were treated with isosorbide dinitrate, 10 mg
three times per day, and over the next year they encountered much
more recurrent disease than those who had exercised.

Studies in USA

H.K. Hellerstein (1968) was an early advocate of exercise for the
patient with ischaemic heart disease. His report described 254 patients
who remained in a gymnasium-based exercise programme for an average
of 2.7 years. Over this time, eleven patients died, giving a death rate of
2.0 per cent per year. Hellerstein argued that this mortality rate compared very favourably with the usual figure of 4.5-6.0 per cent per year
for 'post-coronary' patients receiving conventional treatment in the
Cleveland area. However, Hellerstein's programme included not only
exercise but also a deliberate campaign against other risk factors
through an anti-atherogenic diet, abstinence from cigarettes and
reduction of body mass. Furthermore, patients who could not tolerate
the exercise programme were necessarily excluded from the group. It is
thus difficult to compare his sample with the general experience of
Cleveland clinics.

Early Canadian studies

E.M. Heller (1968, 1972) referred 'post-coronary' patients to the
YMHA for a paramedically supervised programme of progressive

endurance exercise. It is not possible to calculate precise recurrence rates from his reports, since the follow-up period varied from one individual to another, but nevertheless the exercised subjects were apparently at a substantial advantage relative to those who for various reasons did not enter the YMHA programme.

P. Rechnitzer *et al.* (1972) enrolled their patients in biweekly sessions of progressive endurance activity; this regimen was supplemented by mild daily home exercises and the walking of one to two miles per day. The first comparison was made between these patients, who were living in the medium-sized city of London, Ontario (population about 200,000) and other, conservatively treated patients who were living in metropolitan Toronto (population over two million). Critics immediately objected that conditions of life were very different in the two cities. For this reason, Rechnitzer and his associates went on to compare their data with results for patients treated at other hospitals in the London area. Both comparisons indicated that recurrence and death rates were considerably lower for the exercised than for the conservatively treated groups.

Early longitudinal studies thus suggested that exercise rehabilitation had a favourable influence upon prognosis. However, none of the reports cited were able to rule out the possibility that the apparent benefit of increased physical activity has arisen because subjects with less extensive disease were selected for exercise-rehabilitation programmes.

A Non-randomised Trial in Toronto

The Toronto trial was based upon a consecutive series of 688 patients who were referred to the exercise rehabilitation programme of the Toronto Rehabilitation Centre. Subjects attended the Centre for a period varying from one to eight years (an average of three years) over the period 1967–76 (T. Kavanagh *et al.*, in preparation). The data is unusual with respect to the intensity of the prescribed exercise, the compliance rate and success in obtaining 100 per cent follow-up information with respect to fatal and non-fatal reinfarctions plus deaths from other causes.

Patient selection

All of the sample had been referred to the Centre by their personal physicians following a myocardial infarction. The diagnosis was verified by the presence of at least two out of three criteria (classical chest pain, a significant rise in serum enzymes and serial electro-cardiographic changes). Over the period of observation, 80 patients received coronary arterial 'by-pass' operations; two of the eighty died, and to avoid all possibility of bias these two individuals were included in our sample. The other 78 'by-passed' patients were excluded from the study, leaving a total of 610 otherwise unselected referrals.

Exercise programme

Admission to the programme occurred a minimum of two months and an average of eight months following myocardial infarction. The programme of progressive supervised exercise was based on walking and jogging, the goal being to cover three miles in 30 or 36 minutes, depending upon age. For the first two years, the patient attended the Centre once per week, and trained four times a week on his own, using a personalised prescription that specified distance, pace and frequency of exercise. Thereafter, attendance was once in eight weeks, with repeat exercise tests once per year. Of the group, 22 continued to attend the Centre more frequently, and progressed to the point of running in marathon events (T. Kavanagh *et al.*, 1974b; T. Kavanagh *et al.*, 1977a); one patient covered the 42.1 km in as little as 190 minutes. Altogether, 428 of the patients (70.2 per cent) visited the Centre as scheduled. Although irregular in their attendance, many of the remaining patients persisted with their prescribed exercise; 505/610 (82.8 per cent) engaged in at least three sessions of training per week throughout the study, and even at the end of our investigation only a very small number of subjects (27/610; 2.8 per cent) were taking no training at all. Acceptance of the programme was indicated by substantial gains of maximum oxygen intake. The average improvement was 22.6 per cent over the three years, and there was a 77 per cent increase in readings for marathon participants.

Fatalities

A total of 35 patients died over the follow-up period. Of these fatalities, 23 were plainly a consequence of ischaemic heart disease (19 recurrences, one complicated by viral myocarditis, and four 'electrical' deaths). One patient died during coronary angiography, so that his death might also be regarded as due to cardiac disease, but the remaining eleven cases died of other causes (including four cerebro-vascular accidents). Recurrences rates were as follows:

| Time subsequent to | Recurrence rates | | | Number of |
infarction	Non-fatal (%/yr)	Fatal (%/yr)	Total (%/yr)	subjects
Year one	0.96	2.15	3.11	610
Year two	1.19	1.39	2.58	503
Years three to five	1.05	0.45	1.50	227
Years six to eight	0.00	0.81	0.81	41

In contrast with many series of conservatively treated patients, the recurrence rate diminished progressively with time subsequent to infarction. Since there was a 100 per cent follow-up, this cannot be attributed to attrition of the sample; either there was a change in the pattern of referrals as the study continued, or the beneficial effect of exercise developed progressively over the period of observation. Of the 23 patients who sustained a fatal recurrence, eight had been attending the exercise class for six months or less, and one man had participated in only one exercise session. In all, ten were exercising regularly at the time of their fatal recurrence, two were exercising sporadically, and eleven had ceased to participate in the programme. In only four of the non-exercisers was there a medical reason for non-participation. Of the 23 episodes, eight were sudden deaths, seven of which were unassociated with physical exertion. One man died while he was exercising away from the Centre; he was apparently recovering from a bout of influenza and, despite warnings to the contrary, had continued activity, even exceeding his normal exercise prescription.

Non-fatal recurrences

A total of 21 cases developed a non-fatal recurrence over the follow-up period. Three of those affected had been exercising for less than six months. Five were exercising regularly, four were participating in a sporadic fashion and twelve were not exercising at all. In only three cases were there medical reasons for non-participation (all of these men had exertional angina).

Comparison with HIP data

The results of the Toronto trial can be compared with published information for 745 male patients enrolled in the Health Insurance Plan of New York (E. Weinblatt *et al.*, 1968, 1973). The New York group had survived an average of six months following a first myocardial infarction or diagnosis of angina without infarction. There are obvious differences between Toronto and New York. Nevertheless, the HIP

data was selected for reference rather than results from the larger
Coronary Drug Trial (J. Stamler, 1975) because the prognosis of the
New York sample was specified in terms of a number of commonly
accepted primary risk factors, acting singly and in various combinations.

E. Weinblatt *et al.* (1968, 1973) cite smoothed cumulative
probabilities of death for the period 0.5–3.0 years after infarction in
relation to three prognostic factors (persistent abnormalities of the
resting electrocardiogram, hypertension and elevation of serum
cholesterol). In order to compare results with data from the 36.5-
month Toronto study, all probabilities of death were multiplied by
36.5/30.0; this adjustment is acceptable, since the overall mortality
rate in the New York study was very similar for 30 months (4.01 per
cent per annum) and for 54 months (3.88 per cent per annum). The
association between the several variables and the likelihood of death
is shown in Table 6.2, along with the expected number of fatalities.
If our sample had behaved in the same manner as the New York
population, there would have been 89 rather than 35 deaths;
furthermore, in Toronto only 66·8 per cent of deaths were attributable to a recurrence of cardiac disease, whereas the proportion of
recurrences was 81 per cent in New York.

Alternative hypotheses

It is particularly striking that the prognosis of the Toronto group
improved coincidently with the development of cardio-respiratory
conditioning. However, before postulating a causal association, several
alternative hypotheses must be weighed.

Information was necessarily collected on patients referred to the
Toronto Rehabilitation Centre, and it is possible that, because
vigorous exercise therapy was offered, a low-risk category of patient
was seen. In partial support of this view, a subsequent randomised trial
showed an annual rate of reinfarction of only 1.5 per cent per
annum in a low-intensity-exercise (control) group attending the
Toronto centre.

The average time of entry into our exercise programme was eight
months after infarction, but some patients were recruited as soon as
two to three months after the acute episode. Since mortality is
greatest in the first six months after infarction, this factor should have
increased rather than decreased the mortality in the Toronto series.

Treatment undoubtedly evolved between the New York study
(1961–5) and the Toronto experiment (1968–76). Some ten per cent

Table 6.2: A 'Risk-factor' Prediction of Death Rate for 610 'Post-coronary' Patients Treated by Vigorous Exercise Rehabilitation in Toronto

Cholesterol[1,2] (≥ 270 mg·dl⁻¹)	Risk factor present Hyper-tension[1,3] (≥ 150/100 mg Hg)	Persistent abnormalities of resting ECG[4]	Number of cases with specified characteristics	Anticipated deaths in sample of 610 subjects followed up 36.5 months
Yes	Yes	Yes	15	2.5
Yes	Yes	No	0	0
Yes	No	Yes	30	2.1
Yes	No	No	0	0
No	Yes	Yes	121	32.1
No	Yes	No	5	0.6
No	No	Yes	427	51.1
No	No	No	12	0.6
			Total	89.0

1. In order to make a conservative estimate of risk for the Toronto population, the table excludes from the high-risk category eleven patients merely reported as having a 'high' serum cholesterol and seven patients noted only as 'hypertensive'.

2. The methodology used in Toronto was internationally standardised. The proportion with a high serum cholesterol was less than in New York, probably as a result of an increase in dietary modification at the time of the Toronto study.

3. The Toronto subjects were well-habituated to the observer, and the diastolic criterion (100 mm Hg) was higher than in New York (165/90 mm Hg); the prevalence of hypertension thus tended to be underestimated relative to the comparison series.

4. Abnormal resting ECGs were more frequent in Toronto (97.2 per cent) than in New York (62.1 per cent); this reflects our more stringent requirement of myocardial infarction before admission to the trial.

Source: Based on data of E. Weinblatt *et al.* (1968, 1972) and T. Kavanagh *et al.* (in preparation).

of the Toronto group were receiving β-blocking drugs, although almost none were receiving anticoagulants. In any event, changes in treatment can hardly account for the improved prognosis of the Toronto group, since most studies suggest that β-blocking agents, anticoagulants, dietary modification and other forms of therapy have only marginal effects on late prognosis (S.H. Rinzler, 1968; O. Turpeinen *et al.*, 1968; S. Dayton *et al.*, 1969; J. Stamler, 1975; D.A. Chamberlain, 1978b).

Sample attrition cannot account for the favourable prognosis in the Toronto population, since all 610 patients were included in the data

Table 6.3: Potential Adjustments in a 'Risk-factor' Prediction of Death Rate for 610 'Post-coronary' Patients Treated by Vigorous Exercise Rehabilitation in Toronto

Variable	Adjustment made	Predicted deaths	
		Number over 36.5 months	Annual rate (%)
Serum cholesterol, hypertension and electro-cardiogram	See Table 6.2	89.0	4.80
Age	48.1 ± 7.3 years (six years younger than Weinblatt series)	64.2	3.46
Diabetes	1.6% of Toronto series taking insulin, 11.6% 'diabetics' in Weinblatt series	63.5	3.42
Blue-collar/ Jewish	Greater in Weinblatt series	No adjustment	
Cigarette smoking	35.8% of sample (compared with 38.4% in series of S. Tominaga & Blackburn, 1973)	No adjustment	
Angina	34.3% of sample had angina on admission to rehabilitation, compared with 17.8% of Weinblatt series	No adjustment	
By-pass surgery	3.9% of Toronto group (omitted from series, with exception of 2 fatalities; see text)	No adjustment	

Source: Based on data of E. Weinblatt *et al*. (1968, 1972) and T. Kavanagh *et al*. (in preparation).

analysis, irrespective of whether they had persisted with the required exercise programme.

A final possibility is that risk factors other than those noted in Table 6.2 were more prevalent in the New York than in the Toronto series (Table 6.3). In Toronto, almost all subjects were white-collar employees, whereas in New York about a half were blue-collar workers, with a high proportion (50 per cent) of Jewish subjects; however, recent Ontario data (P. Rechnitzer *et al*., unpublished) suggests that, if other factors are equal, reinfarction rates for white-collar workers who enrol in an exercise programme should be almost identical with those for a mixture of white- and blue-collar workers who do not exercise. The age of the Toronto sample was some six years younger than the HIP group, and 1.6 per cent of the Toronto series were taking insulin, compared with 11.6 per cent of 'diabetics' in New York. Allowing for these two important differences, but neglecting a larger proportion of subjects with angina in the Toronto series, the anticipated death rate of our sample would drop to 3.42 per cent per year; this must be compared with the observed overall rate of 1.88 per cent per year for the Toronto series (1.29 per cent per year due to cardiac events), and the even lower figure of 0.67 per cent cardiac and non-cardiac deaths per year for the third to the eighth year of rehabilitation.

Conclusion

There remain considerable uncertainties when attempting to compare patients living in Toronto and New York. Nevertheless, the apparent advantage of our exercised group is sufficient to encourage a further application of this approach, drawing exercised and control subjects from the same city and applying rigorous adjustments for all of the factors known to modify prognosis after myocardial infarction.

Randomised Controlled Studies

General considerations

A large-scale randomised controlled trial is theoretically the best method of deciding whether exercise rehabilitation improves the prognosis of the 'post-coronary' patient. However, in practice, the trials conducted to date have proved inconclusive, as a result of poor compliance with the required regimen, an inadequate duration of rehabilitation and correspondingly limited gains of physiological function.

Sample attrition is an inevitable source of difficulty. The health experience of the 'drop-outs' is usually averaged with, and dilutes, any response in programme adherents. Some studies have had many drop-outs from the exercised group, and controls have become contaminated by unauthorised participation in 'keep-fit' programmes. It could be argued that a high 'drop-out' rate is itself an argument against the practicality of exercise treatment. However, the Toronto experience (above) illustrates that good compliance can be sustained in a large group of patients for several years if the programme is well-organised.

Because sample attrition is a cumulative phenomenon, many authors have been content to report studies of relatively short duration. Interpretation of data is then complicated by the averaging of early mortality (where increased physical activity has not had time to produce an effect) and later mortality (where a beneficial response to exercise is conceivable). Most authors (E. Kentala, 1972; H. Sanne *et al.*, 1972; T. Kavanagh *et al.*, 1973b; L. Wilhelmsen *et al.*, 1975; T. Kavanagh *et al.*, 1977a) are agreed that relatively little training of the post-coronary patient is accomplished during the first few months of attendance at a rehabilitation centre; indeed, dramatic gains of maximum oxygen intake may not appear until the patient has been exercising for some years (Figure 6.1). This is in marked contrast to the response of healthy subjects, and it may reflect fear on the part of the patient, his family or his medical advisors. Plainly, it is unrealistic to expect a benefit from exercise until some training effect has occurred, and there may be a further lag period before the full potential health gains of the increased activity pattern are realised.

Large numbers of both patients and staff are required for a randomised controlled trial. There are corresponding difficulties in ensuring consistent and effective exercise and control regimens at all cooperating centres. Partly for this reason, and partly because of fears of overexertion, many so-called 'exercise' classes for the 'post-coronary' patient have been essentially homoeopathic, producing no real training response (Table 6.4).

Finally, even if a sufficient sample of subjects can be both recruited and retained over a random trial, constraints of practicality still leave a substantial 'beta error' (the chance of a falsely negative conclusion); this is commonly as large as ten or even 20 per cent (Table 5.1).

Gothenburg study

The Gothenburg study (H. Sanne *et al.*, 1972; L. Wilhelmsen *et al.*, 1975) was based on 315 patients under 58 years of age who sustained a myocardial infarction between 1968 and 1971. Although some 90 per cent of available patients were recruited for the investigation, the sample was nevertheless rather small to prove or disprove the exercise hypothesis. Both test and control subjects were given a general recommendation to increase their physical activity, but three months after infarction a randomly selected half of the sample were invited to attend the hospital three times per week for a 30-minute programme of calisthenics, cycling and interval running.

Unfortunately, only 73 per cent of the intended experimental group began training, and the drop-out rate was also high. After one year, only 39 per cent of the experimental group were attending the hospital, with a further 21 per cent continuing some training at home or at work.

Figure 6.1: Time course of the increases in directly measured maximum oxygen intake with vigorous training. Data of T. Kavanagh & Shephard for 13 post-coronary runners who finally participated in marathon events, along with individual curves for two subjects who made substantial gains in aerobic power.

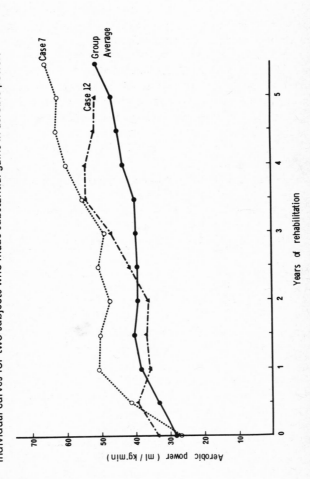

Source: Reprinted from Roy J. Shephard, 'Cardiac Rehabilitation in Prospect' in *Heart Disease and Rehabilitation*, edited by M.L. Pollock and D.H. Schmidt, by permission of the publisher.

Table 6.4: Changes of Exercise Tolerance in Selected 'Post-coronary' Rehabilitation Programmes

Author	Change of exercise tolerance
E. Kentala (1972)	20% improvement of maximal working capacity *but* seen equally in experimental and control subjects; 56% gain of maximal working capacity in sub-sample attending more than 70% of training sessions
L. Wilhelmsen *et al.* (1975)	24 W gain of working capacity in experimental subjects with no change in controls; three quarters of changes in heart-rate responses to sub-maximal exercise not significantly different in experimental and control subjects
D.A. Cunningham *et al.* (1977)	average decrease of heart rate at $\dot{V}_{O_2}$ = 1.25 l•min^{-1} 13.1 beats•min^{-1} in experimental and 0.6 beats•min^{-1} in control subjects; *but* subjects divisible into four roughly equal groups — 15% and 5% decrease of heart rate in experimental subjects and 3.6% decrease and 2.7% increase in control subjects
T. Kavanagh & Shephard	22.6% gain of predicted $\dot{V}_{O_2}$ (max) over 3 years (average for 610 patients); 77% gain over five years in marathon participants (Figure 6.1)

There was a 24-W increase in the maximum tolerated work-load of the experimental group, with no significant change in the maximum performance of the control subjects. However, the heart-rate response to sub-maximum exercise decreased both in exercise and control groups, and in three of four comparisons the difference between experimental and control subjects was not statistically significant. This reflects in part a contamination of the control group by an interest in exercise, and in part limited compliance of the experimental subjects with the intended exercise programme. Whereas the one-year gain of maximum working capacity for the entire exercise group was 14 per cent, in those 'adequately trained' it was 22 per cent.

H. Sanne *et al.* (1972) and L. Wilhelmsen *et al.* (1975) commented specifically on the issues of study duration and compliance. Over a four-year follow-up period, the mortality and morbidity were very similar for their two groups of patients — 28 deaths and 25 non-fatal myocardial infarctions in the exercised group, with 35 deaths and 28 non-fatal infarctions in the control group. Separating out patients who had participated in the study for six months or longer, H. Sanne *et al.* (1972) observed eight deaths in the training group and 19 in the control series, the difference being significant at the five per cent level of probability. When the 'six-month' patients were followed up for a total of four years, corresponding figures were 19 and 29 deaths ($P = 0.18$); this probably reflects differences in compliance since, among those who adhered to the programme for at least one year, the mortality (five of 67, seven per cent) was only half of that seen in the controls (20 of 141, 14 per cent). Interpretation of the data is complex, since more of the 'drop-outs' than the continuing exercisers were smokers (L. Wilhelmsen *et al.*, 1975).

The overall death rate for the exercise group was 3.48 per cent per annum, more than five times the figure found in the Toronto trial for post-coronary patients who were exercising hard (see above). This may reflect in part a more complete sampling of the post-coronary population in the Gothenburg study, and in part absence of an exercise response in Gothenburg due to the extensive defections from the experimental programme.

Helsinki study

E. Kentala (1972) carried out a similar study in Helsinki. Severely diseased patients were excluded from his sample but, with this proviso, 158 consecutively acutely infarcted patients younger than 65 years were allocated randomly to experimental and control groups. Again, the sample size was less than that required for conclusive examination of the exercise hypothesis.

The planned intervention was a 30-minute session of exercise conducted three times per week at the local hospital. However, after one year only ten of 79 patients were attending the exercise sessions, while a further 16 claimed to be exercising on their own. At least eleven of the control series were also exercising quite vigorously. It is thus hardly surprising that one year after the myocardial infarction there was no difference in physical working capacity between experimental and control groups.

Subjects were followed up for two years, and over this time there was no difference in either total mortality or in new ischaemic heart disease events between the supposed exercise and control groups; such findings were hardly surprising in view of the poor compliance with the intended regimen.

Oulu study

I. Palatsi (1976) initiated a home-training experiment in the Oulu region of Finland. His subjects were male and female patients under 65 years of age; those judged as having severe disease or poor motivation were excluded from the sample. A total of 180 cases (mainly city dwellers) were allocated to the training regimen, and 200 cases (mainly those living in rural areas) served as controls.

The plan involved 30 minutes of home exercises per day, reinforcing visits being made to the hospital once every month. At the end of one year, about a half of the exercisers reported that they were training between six and seven times per week, and two thirds of the group attended the last hospital session. However, the intended experimental subjects showed no improvement in physical working capacity relative to the control series.

Over a 2.5-year period of observation, twelve per cent of the exercise group and 15 per cent of the controls suffered a reinfarction, with respective mortality rates of 7 and 14 per cent.

World Health Organization study

A study initiated by the European Office of the World Health Organization (1977) involves modification of a number of risk factors including physical inactivity (Chapter 5, p. 98). Control patients are treated by their personal physicians. Analysis of one segment of this data (V. Kallio, 1978) suggests that the experimental subjects gain some protection against sudden death and coronary mortality, particularly over the first year. However, the total number of reinfarctions is higher in the exercised group.

Canadian experiments

One early controlled trial was carried out in Toronto (T. Kavanagh *et al.*, 1973b). The primary objectives were physiological, and the total sample size (31 cases) was therefore small. Over the first year of observation, patients allocated to an exercise regimen fared little better than a control group who received equal physician contact through a hypnosis class. During the second year, a proportion of the exercised group who had progressed to long-distance running showed substantial physiological and electrocardiographic gains with respect to the hypnosis group, but others, apparently those who were older and had more severe disease, still had a comparable status to the hypnotherapy controls. Over the two-year study, the recurrence rate was 2.3 per cent per annum for the exercise group, and 5.0 per cent for the controls, but the reinfarctions in the exercise group were fatal, whereas those in the hypnotherapy group were non-fatal.

A more definitive trial of morbidity and mortality was planned by P.A. Rechnitzer *et al.* (1975). A sample size of 750 patients was chosen to give a 90 per cent chance of showing a 50 per cent reduction of recurrences in the exercised group, with a probability of 0.05; this calculation was based on a recurrence rate of 23 per cent over a four-year period, with a sample attrition of 35 per cent or less. Subjects under 55 years of age were recruited three to twelve months following a well-documented attack of myocardial infarction. They were allocated in a stratified random fashion to either a regimen of vigorous and progressive endurance-type exercise, or a homeopathic recreational-exercise programme. Stratification was in terms of angina, hypertension, blue- or white-collar occupation and personality type (Friedman & Rosenmann Type A or B).

According to popular belief, the drop-out rate from an exercise programme is greatest in the first few months, and some studies have thus given their subjects several preliminary months of physical activity prior to randomisation (J. Naughton, 1978). The preliminary results of the Southern Ontario multicentre trial to date do not altogether support this view; if attrition rates are calculated as a percentage of the residual sample, losses seem at least as great in the third and fourth as in the first two years of observation; furthermore, we are now anticipating that the overall drop-out rate for the four-year study may be 60·5 per cent rather than the intended 35 per cent (R.J. Shephard, 1979c). Medical problems account for only 22 per cent of defections (N.B. Oldridge, 1979), and almost a half of these are non-cardiac problems. A further 25 per cent of subject losses are unavoidable, as a result of such factors as change of employment, leaving 42 per cent attributable to psycho-social factors and 11 per cent to other causes. The worst experience has been with blue-collar employees engaged in light work who are also smokers and inactive in their leisure time; 95 per cent of such subjects have dropped out of the study within two years. We have noted a two-fold intercentre difference in sample attrition; this seems to be related to methods of recruitment (physician referral, 43 per cent attrition, versus the combing of cardiac wards, 55 per cent attrition), socio-economic factors and differences in the personality of the clinical staff and their degree of involvement in the rehabilitation process.

The Southern Ontario trial monitored the response of subjects to training in terms of the heart rate at a directly measured or closely interpolated oxygen consumption of 1.25 l·min^{-1} STPD. On this criterion, the experimental model worked rather better than in a number of the other studies reviewed above; the heart rate decreased in those who received high-intensity exercise, but showed no significant change in the control group; nevertheless, it was possible to distinguish a substantial sub-sample of the high-intensity-exercise group who (because of poor compliance or a relatively high initial fitness level) showed little change of exercise heart rate. There was also a sub-sample of the low-intensity-exercise group who became contaminated by an enthusiasm for vigorous activity, with corresponding reductions in the exercise heart rate (D.A. Cunningham *et al.*, 1979).

As an ethical safeguard, the supervising statistician monitored cardiac events by the technique of sequential analysis (A. Wald, 1947). It was planned to halt the experiment if either the initial hypothesis was proven, or the proportion of reinfarctions in the high-intensity-exercise group exceeded 67 per cent of the sample. The sample of 750 patients was successfully recruited. A preliminary analysis of data showed that of the first 50 recurrences, 20 occurred within twelve months of recruitment (Table 6.5). It could be argued that none of these patients had been trained for sufficient time to realise the possible benefits of exercise. Theoretically, fourteen of the remaining thirty patients with recurrent disease were still enrolled in the trial. However, many were, for practical purposes, drop-outs. While the effects of training are largely dissipated by a few weeks of inactivity, it takes a minimum of two to three months to probe a patient's excuses and realise that he has dropped out of the study. Even if this problem is ignored, we have to date only 14 critical events among programme participants, ten in the high-intensity-exercise group and four in the low-intensity-exercise group. Repeated laboratory data were available for ten of these 14 subjects. An improvement in physical condition was seen in five of the six high-intensity exercisers, but there was also a significant decrease of exercise heart rate in two of the four low-intensity exercisers. As with other randomised trials, such numbers are far too small to prove or disprove the exercise hypothesis.

The statistics cited refer to the first twenty months' operation of the Southern Ontario trial, and numbers will be approximately doubled when the four-year follow-up of all patients is completed. Nevertheless, incomplete compliance with the required exercise regimen, a high attrition rate, some contamination of the control group, a slow onset of the training response and a lower frequency of reinfarction than anticipated may leave the experiment short of the statistical proof originally envisaged.

Table 6.5: Non-fatal and Fatal Recurrences among Patients Enrolled
in Southern Ontario Multicentre Exercise-heart Trial; A Preliminary
Analysis of Data in Subjects Followed for an Average Period of
20 Months

Event	Patient status	High-intensity-exercise group		Low-intensity-exercise group	
		Number of events	Reported compliance* (%)	Number of events	Reported compliance* (%)
Non-fatal recurrences	Participant > 12 months	9	76	4	83
	Participant < 12 months	9	85	5	76
	'Drop-out'	6	16	5	6
Fatal recurrences	Participant > 12 months	1	100	0	—
	Participant < 12 months	2	78	4	78
	'Drop-out'	3	8	2	0
Total recurrences	Participant > 12 months	10	78	4	83
	Participant < 12 months	11	84	9	77
	'Drop-out'	9	13	7	4

* Attendance reported for three months preceding recurrence.

Source: R.J. Shephard (1979c).
Note: A report covering the full four year study is currently being prepared by
Dr P. Rechnitzer and the Southern Ontario research team.

Conclusion

Given that all of the randomised controlled trials completed to date
have been inconclusive, what are the options for the future? To accept
empirical evidence from non-randomised trials is scientifically
unsatisfactory. Attempts to merge data from the several existing
controlled studies are also unlikely to succeed, because of differences
in populations and protocol. It is thus necessary to contemplate a larger
trial. It will be necessary first to explore carefully the factors
influencing exercise compliance, and then to recruit at least 4,000
patients willing to participate in a randomised experiment. In view of
the large sample size and the resultant cost of the investigation, this
will succeed only if organised on an international basis.

Possible Contraindications to Exercise Rehabilitation

Once infarction has occurred, the usual 'coronary' risk factors such as a high serum cholesterol, systemic hypertension and diabetes seem of less importance to prognosis. Adverse features now include a prior history of angina, a poor left-ventricular function, a wide resting arterio-venous oxygen difference, various types of dysrhythmia and left-atrial enlargement as indicated by a negative terminal force in the P wave of the electrocardiogram (E.H. Estes, 1974; E. Kentala & Sarna, 1976).

Do these 'tertiary' risk factors apply to the patient who is undergoing exercise rehabilitation? In particular, are there contraindications to deliberate exercise as shown by an increase of risk ratio relative to more conservative treatment? Information relating to these questions is available from both non-randomised and randomised trials of exercise therapy.

Non-randomised trials

T. Kavanagh *et al.* (1977c) examined factors related to fatal and non-fatal recurrence of infarction in a group of 610 'post-coronary' patients who were participating in a vigorous exercise rehabilitation programme for an average of 36.5 months. During this time, the group sustained 21 non-fatal recurrences and 23 fatal recurrences (p. 133). Calculating risk ratios (Table 6.6), the most useful indicator of a poor prognosis

Table 6.6: Method of Calculating Risk Ratios for Population of 610 'Post-coronary' Patients with 44 Non-fatal and Fatal Recurrences

Clinical status	Present	Presumed risk factor Absent	Row total
Recurrence	$(R + F)$	$44 - (R + F)$	44
No recurrence	C	$566 - C$	566
Column total	$(R + F) + C$	$610 - (R + F + C)$	610

Predictive value of positive test (P) = $(R + F)/(R + F + C)$
Predictive value of negative test (N) = $44 - (R + F)/610 - (R + F + C)$

Risk ratio = P/N
Sensitivity of risk factor = $(R + F)/44$
Specificity of risk factor = $[610 - (R + F + C)] - [44 - (R + F)]/566$

Table 6.7: Indicators of Non-fatal and Fatal Recurrence of Myocardial Infarction among 610 Patients Participating in Programme of Vigorous Exercise Rehabilitation

Variable	Frequency in subjects with recurrence		Frequency in subjects free of recurrence (n = 566; %)	Predictive value of positive (P, %)	Predictive value of negative (N, %)	Risk ratio (P/N)
	Non-fatal (n = 21; %)	Fatal (n = 23; %)				
Exercise non-compliance	57.1	47.8	0.7	85.2	3.60	23.7[4]
Medications:						
Anti-dysrhythmics	42.9	39.0	30.2	9.5	6.17	1.54
Diuretics	19.0	34.8	15.9	11.8	6.30	1.87[2]
Digitalis	9.5	39.0	11.7	14.3	5.82	2.46[2]
Still smoking[1]	47.6	43.5	34.9	10.3	5.78	1.78[2]
Angina						
Initial test	33.3	52.2	30.6	9.9	5.98	1.66
Final test	14.3	42.9	14.8	12.5	6.22	2.01[2]
Enlarged heart	4.8	13.0	3.71	16.0	6.83	2.34[2]
Aneurysm	0.0	8.7	2.12	14.3	7.04	2.05
Hypertension ($\geq$ 150/100 mm Hg)	23.8	21.7	23.1	7.09	7.25	0.98
Blood cholesterol (> 270 mg·dl^{-1})	14.3	13.0	6.89	13.3	6.72	1.98[2]
Electrocardiogram:						
Resting abnormalities	100.0	95.6	98.9	7.25	5.88	1.23
Horizontal or downsloping exercise ST $\geq$ 0.2 mV	38.1	43.5	33.4	12.4	5.59	2.22[3]
Unifocal exercise VPBs	4.8	0.0	8.8	1.96	7.69	0.25
Multifocal exercise VPBs	4.8	8.7	4.4	10.7	7.04	1.52

1. No data on 66 patients.
2. $P < 0.05$.
3. $P < 0.01$.
4. $P < 0.001$.

Source: T. Kavanagh et al. (1977c).

Table 6.8: Odds Ratios Comparing Non-compliant and Exercise-compliant Patients Enrolled in a Vigorous 'Post-coronary' Exercise Rehabilitation Programme

Risk indicator	Non-fatal recurrences	Odds ratio[1] Fatal recurrences	All recurrences
Smoking history			
Continued	∞	5.79	7.87
Reduced	13.90	—	13.89
Stopped	4.13	6.06	4.78
Never smoked	0.99	5.05	3.34
Combined odds ratio	(5.19)[2]	5.44	5.86
Z score[3]	3.65	3.52	5.37
Angina			
Both tests	2.88	9.23	5.87
Initial test	19.00	2.82	7.67
Final test	0.00	6.33	3.00
Neither test	4.13	5.23	4.91
Combined odds ratio	5.06	5.43	5.85
Z score	3.57	3.86	5.57
ST depression			
ST < 0.2 mV	3.51	13.57	7.48
ST > 0.2 mV	7.97	1.82	4.12
Combined odds ratio	4.82	(5.44)[2]	5.86
Z score	3.44	4.19	5.73
Complications			
Nil	4.66	4.51	5.00
Enlarged heart	∞	8.00	16.00
Aneurysm	—	∞	∞
Combined odds ratio	(5.12)[2]	(5.73)[2]	(5.99)[2]
Z score	3.61	3.99	5.70

1. Odds ratio = [(number of recurrences in non-compliant group)/(number without recurrence in non-compliant group)] × [(number without recurrence in compliant group)/(number of recurrences in compliant group)].

2. It is not strictly possible to calculate a mean for this category because of sample heterogeneity.

3. A Z score of 1.96 would have a chance probability of 0.05.

Source: R.J. Shephard *et al.* (1979a).

Table 6.9: Relationship between Exercise Compliance and Other Risk Factors

Variable	Exercise compliance				Significance
Smoking habits	Continued 70.5%	Reduced 84.2%	Stopped 85.5%	Never 83.2%	n.s.
Angina	Both tests 73.5%	Initial test 80.0%	Final test 83.3%	Neither 86.0%	(0.05)
ST depression	> 0.2 mV 80.1%	< 0.2 mV 84.2%			n.s.
Complication	Enlarged heart 73.9%	Aneurysm 69.2%	Nil 84.0%		n.s.

Source: Based on data of R.J. Shephard *et al*. (1979a).

was failure to comply with the prescribed exercise regimen (Table 6.7). Among the 27 subjects who had ceased exercising at the end of the study, the risk of recurrence was 23.7 times the standard figure ($P <$ 0.001). Furthermore, there was some evidence for the view that lack of exercise was responsible for the progression of disease rather than the converse. Of the 27 non-compliers, 15 were uninterested in exercise or had encountered family opposition, three had been told not to exercise by their family physicians and only nine had a medical reason for stopping exercise (angina, orthopaedic problems, mental disorders and alcoholism). Taking data for a larger group of 105 subjects who finally were exercising less than three times per week, the 'odds ratio' for either a fatal or a non-fatal recurrence was five or six to one when such poorly compliant subjects were compared with the 'compliant'. This disadvantage was independent of smoking habits, but was obscured in subjects with ST segmental depression of more than 0.2 mV during exercise at a target rate equal to 75 per cent of aerobic power (Table 6.8; R.J. Shephard *et al.*, 1979a). There was a slight suggestion that a poor exercise compliance was linked to continued smoking, the presence of angina at both tests, ST segmental depression of more than 0.2 mV and complications such as enlarged heart or an aneurysm; however, with the available sample of 46 recurrences, the only significant trend was for angina (Table 6.9).

The risk ratios of Table 6.7 suggest an adverse prognosis with several other findings, including persistent cigarette smoking, the use of digitalis or diuretics (both presumably indicators of cardiac failure), the presence of angina at the final exercise test, radiographic evidence of cardiac enlargement, a horizontal or downward-sloping depression of the ST segment of the exercise electrocardiogram and a serum cholesterol greater than 270 mg·dl^{-1}. The majority of the items noted had a fair sensitivity but (with the exception of exercise non-compliance, persistent cigarette smoking and exercise ST segmental depression) a rather low specificity; for calculation of sensitivity and specificity, see Table 6.6.

We may thus conclude that many of the secondary and tertiary risk factors encountered in sedentary individuals still apply in the 'post-coronary' patient who is engaged in vigorous physical activity.

It is now necessary to make a comparison between the risk ratios for active and sedentary individuals (Table 6.10). In many instances, the statistics are surprisingly similar. However, the risk ratio is some 50 per cent greater for active patients who have an exercise-induced ST segmental depression, and the question thus arises as to whether this

Table 6.10: A Comparison of Simple Risk Ratios for Active and Sedentary 'Post-coronary' Patients

Variable	Risk ratios*		Authors of data for sedentary patients
	Physically active patients	Sedentary patients	
Exercise non-compliance	74.9	—	R.J. Shephard *et al.* (1980)
Continued smoking	1.30	2.00	L. Wilhelmsen *et al.* (1975)
Angina (final exercise test)	1.93	1.93	S. Tominaga & Blackburn (1973)
Aneurysm	2.05	1.80	A.V.G. Bruschke *et al.* (1973)
Enlarged heart	2.40	2.32	S. Tominaga & Blackburn (1973)
Serum cholesterol $\geqslant 270$ mg•dl^{-1}	1.98	1.49	S. Tominaga & Blackburn (1973)
		0.80	E. Weinblatt *et al.* (1973)
		1.09	S. Tominaga & Blackburn (1973)
Hypertension $\geqslant 150/100$ mm Hg	0.98	2.55	E. Weinblatt *et al.* (1973)
Persistent resting ECG abnormalities	1.02	2.47	E. Weinblatt *et al.* (1973)
Exercise ST depression $\geqslant 0.2$ mV	1.82	1.23	J.R. Margolis *et al.* (1975)
Polyfocal VPBs (> 3 in 10 seconds' exercise	1.53	1.61	S. Tominaga & Blackburn (1973)
		~1	E. Kentala & Sarna (1976)

* Events in group with abnormality relative to events in group without abnormality.

Source: Based on data accumulated by T. Kavanagh *et al.* (1979).

group should be cautioned against participating in an exercise-centred rehabilitation programme. J.O. Parker *et al.* (1966) have described how exercise can induce cardiac failure in the ischaemic myocardium. Nevertheless, in the Toronto series the overall fatality rate for the exercisers was so low that the absolute prognosis was apparently improved relative to conservative tretament, even in those patients who exercised despite ST segmental depression (recurrence rate for this group 4.08 per cent per annum, cardiac fatality rate 2.27 per cent per annum).

Randomised controlled trials

Similar investigations are being carried out on patients enrolled in the Southern Ontario multicentre randomised controlled trial of exercise rehabilitation. After an average of 20 months observation, 51 of 751 participants had sustained a recurrence. Some 24 per cent of the new cardiac episodes were closely associated with various types of physical activity, and in a further 22 per cent of recurrences vigorous exercise (sometimes of an unusual nature) was noted a few hours prior to reinfarction (R.J. Shephard, 1979a). These findings could not have arisen by chance unless the subjects were physically active for six hours per day. The majority of patients had sedentary forms of employment, so that even allowing for the effect of the prescribed activity, a more reasonable expectation would have been 1½ hours of activity per day. It would thus appear that physical activity increased the immediate likelihood of reinfarction by a factor of at least four.

Since a half of the group were enrolled in a high-intensity-exercise programme, and the other half were undertaking homeopathic recreational activity, it was possible to make a comparison of 'risk factors' between the two groups (Table 6.11). The importance of continued cigarette smoking and recent angina as determinants of prognosis was confirmed. Some 36.5 per cent of the overall sample were smokers, but percentages of 55.5 and 73.6 per cent were observed among members of the high- and low-intensity groups who developed a recurrence. Likewise, 25.6 per cent of the overall sample showed angina of effort, but figures were 50.0 and 71.4 per cent for those of the high- and low-intensity-exercise groups who sustained a recurrence. There was a slight suggestion that the high-intensity-exercise programme protected continuing smokers and those with recent angina against non-fatal recurrences. On the other hand, there was a suggestion that a high serum cholesterol level was a greater risk factor for those who exercised vigorously, and as in the non-randomised trial an exercise ST segmental depression of more than 0.2 mV was significantly associated with the likelihood of a fatal recurrence in the vigorously exercised group.

Data from this survey were analysed further in the search for characteristics of those who developed a recurrence of their disease during physical activity (Table 3.2). The main features of those who

Table 6.11: Risk Factors in Post-coronary Rehabilitation — A Comparison between Patients Allocated to a Progressive High-intensity-Exercise Programme and Patients Allocated to a Homeopathic Recreational Programme

| Risk factor and type of recurrence | Incidence of risk factor in patients with recurrence | | Significance |
	High-intensity-exercise programme (%)	Recreational-exercise programme (%)	
Smoking habits			
Current smokers:			
Non-fatal recurrence	47.6	76.9	$0.1 > P > 0.05$
Fatal recurrence	83.3	66.7	
All recurrences	55.5	73.6	
Former smokers:			
Non-fatal recurrence	90.9	100.0	
Fatal recurrence	100.0	100.0	
All recurrences	92.8	100.0	
Recent angina			
Non-fatal recurrence	43.5	73.3	$0.1 > P > 0.05$
Fatal recurrence	71.4	66.7	
All recurrences	50.0	71.4	$0.2 > P > 0.1$
Hypertension (> 150/100 mm Hg)			
Non-fatal recurrences	4.8	14.3	
Fatal recurrences	0	20.0	
All recurrences	3.7	15.8	
High serum cholesterol (> 270 mg·dl^{-1})			
Non-fatal recurrences	5.2	0.0	
Fatal recurrences	28.5	0.0	
All recurrences	11.5	0.0	$0.2 > P > 0.1$
Abnormal resting ECG			
Non-fatal recurrences	52.9	72.7	
Fatal recurrences	28.5	75.0	$0.2 > P > 0.1$
All recurrences	47.8	73.3	$0.2 > P > 0.1$
Exercise ST segmental depression > 0.2 mV			
Non-fatal recurrences	17.3	26.7	
Fatal recurrences	71.4	16.7	$P < 0.05$
All recurrences	30.0	23.8	
Ventricular premature beats			
Non-fatal recurrences	4.3	6.7	
Fatal recurrences	0	0.0	
All recurrences	3.3	4.8	

Source: Based on preliminary data from Southern Ontario multicentre exercise-heart trial, published by R.J. Shephard (1979a).

succumbed during exercise were a poor exercise compliance, and a greater likelihood of an abnormal resting and exercise electrocardiogram.

As in the primary episode (Chapter 3), socio-economic factors sometimes contributed to the critical event. One man commented on a large promissory note that he was unable to finance, and another was experiencing serious family troubles. One patient was attending the funeral of a friend, and three attacks occurred during or shortly after evening parties.

Other preliminary data from the Southern Ontario multicentre trial suggest that socio-economic factors interacted with the response to added exercise. In particular, 'blue-collar' workers with a 'Type B' personality fared significantly worse in a high- than in a low-intensity-exercise programme (P.A. Rechnitzer *et al.*, report in preparation). This may reflect an unfavourable lifestyle in the lower socio-economic groups. It is also conceivable that some of the blue-collar employees obtained sufficient physical activity at work, without an additional prescription for their leisure hours. However, this is at variance with what would be predicted from the low fitness levels of heavy workers as a class (J.G. Allen, 1966).

Implications for therapy

The frequency of recurrences during physical activity is sufficient to indicate the need for a cautious approach to exercise-centred rehabilitation. Nevertheless, more detailed analysis of individual histories suggests that the majority of cardiac episodes occurred with unsupervised effort in those who were failing to fulfill their prescription on a regular basis. An adverse response to irregular and excessive exercise is predictable, and does not necessarily prove that regular and carefully graded physical activity is harmful.

It may still be that data from a larger sample of patients will establish that exercise has an unfavourable effect upon immediate prognosis. However, at most it will be shown that physical effort has localised the timing of an impending infarction to the gymnasium session. Such an observation is quite compatible with an unchanged or even an improved overall prognosis for those who participate faithfully in an exercise programme. Furthermore, if reinfarction is imminent, it is an advantage to bring the myocardial ischaemia to the attention of an observer, so that surgical treatment can be considered. If a recurrence is unavoidable, it is also better that this develops in a gymnasium where resuscitation can be undertaken, rather than in some situation where the patient is unable to obtain assistance.

Patients with severe exercise-induced ST segmental depression may form a specific sub-group for whom vigorous and infrequently supervised exercise is contraindicated. Unfortunately, such patients have a marked impact upon the overall mortality of the post-coronary population, to the point where any benefit of exercise to the remaining subjects in a clinical trial may be obscured (R.J. Shephard, 1980d).

Exercise and Risk-factor Modification

If it is eventually established that exercise has a beneficial effect upon the overall prognosis following myocardial infarction, it is conceivable that the effect will be indirect, through a modification of the various risk factors already discussed. In these circumstances, we would need to weigh the merits of exercise therapy against other, possibly more powerful, methods of changing lifestyle.

However, current evidence gives little support to the concept of benefit through risk-factor modification alone. Over a three-year period of observation, the proportion of cigarette smokers among 'post-coronary' patients attending the Toronto Rehabilitation Centre remained almost constant at 36 per cent, only a little below the figure reported for subjects enrolled in the coronary drug trial (S. Tominaga & Blackburn, 1973), the latter being a programme that did not include deliberate exercise. Likewise, the Toronto patients showed negligible changes in body mass and skinfold thicknesses over the three-year study. The resting systolic pressure decreased slightly, possibly due to a progressive habituation to the test laboratory, but there was a small increase in the maximum systolic pressure developed during exercise as myocardial contractility improved (T. Kavanagh *et al.*, 1977c).

Two comments should be made with regard to these findings. Firstly, the typical patient who is recruited a few months after a myocardial infarction is no longer an obese individual with a high consumption of cigarettes and animal fat. Such faults of lifestyle have already been corrected while in hospital. Secondly, although exercise produces no further changes in such controllable risk factors, this is not entirely a negative conclusion. In matters of diet and smoking, recidivism is commonplace, and the ability of exercise to conserve the improved health habits established in a hospital setting is itself a major accomplishment that undoubtedly improves the prognosis for a post-coronary patient.

7 NON-INVASIVE ASSESSMENT OF THE HEART AND CORONARY CIRCULATION

The family physcian must often rely on clinical assessments of exercise tolerance. Objective scales such as those proposed by the British Medical Research Council (Table 7.1) and the American Heart Association (Table 7.2) improve the reliability of patient responses to questioning, but do not overcome the limitation that sensations are reported within the framework of the patient's habitual activity patterns and current anxiety level. There has thus been an aggressive search for simple non-invasive techniques to examine the performance of the heart and coronary circulation during graded exercise.

Before considering normal cardiac responses to physical activity and training, we shall make a brief review of these non-invasive procedures. Topics to be discussed include the measurement of overall cardiac output, regional myocardial function, overall and regional coronary blood flow, the electrocardiogram and exercise stress tests.

Cardiac Output

Direct Fick principle

The standard technique against which non-invasive measurements of cardiac output are evaluated involves a direct application of the 'Fick principle'. The usual procedure requires the steady-state measurement of oxygen intake ($\dot{V}_{O_2}$), with the collection of corresponding blood samples from a peripheral artery (oxygen content C_{a,O_2}) and the pulmonary arterial trunk (mixed venous oxygen content $C_{\bar{v},O_2}$). The cardiac output $\dot{Q}$ is then given by:

$$\dot{Q} = \dot{V}_{O_2}/(C_{a,O_2} - C_{\bar{v},O_2})$$

The catheterisation of a peripheral artery is not to be undertaken lightly, particularly during exercise. Occasional complications include haemorrhage, thrombosis and even gangrene of the distal part, such risks being greatest when the procedure has been undertaken in subjects with vascular disease. Catheterisation of the pulmonary artery is also best avoided unless necessary for clinical management. Among potential

158

Table 7.1: Classification of Exercise Tolerance

Grade	Clinical status
0	Breathing as good as other people of same age and build at work, walking and on climbing hills and stairs
1	Breathing probably as good as other people of same age and build at work, walking and on climbing hills and stairs
2	Able to walk with people of same age and build on the level, but unable to keep up on hills or stairs
3	Unable to keep up with people of same age and build, but can walk 1.6 km at own speed
4	Unable to walk more than 50-70 m without a stop
5	Obviously breathless on talking or undressing, or unable to leave home because of breathlessness

Source: J.C. Gilson & Hugh-Jones (1955).

Table 7.2: Functional Classification of Cardiac Patients Proposed by the New York Heart Association

Class	Clinical status	Likely maximum oxygen intake $(ml \cdot kg^{-1} \cdot min^{-1})$
I	Patients with heart disease, but no symptoms. Ordinary physical activity does not cause fatigue, palpitations, dyspnoea or anginal pain	> 21
II	Patients comfortable at rest, but symptoms with ordinary physical activity	13–21
III	Patients comfortable at rest, but symptoms with less than ordinary physical effort	3.5–12
IV	Patients with symptoms at rest	< 3.5

Source: Criterion Committee of the New York Heart Association (1964); American Heart Association (1972).

complications of this procedure, we may note bacterial endocarditis, perforation of the heart wall, fracture of the catheter and provocation of a dysrhythmia. Again, risks are higher in the patient with ischaemic heart disease than in an individual with a normal heart (R.J. Corliss, 1979).

Because of these problems, it is usual to make indirect determination of cardiac output in the patient with ischaemic heart disease. However, opportunity for direct measurements may arise if there is angiography of the coronary circulation as a prelude to possible by-pass surgery or cardiac catheterisation to assess the function of sclerosed aortic valves.

Dye-injection techniques

Cardiac output can be assessed by the injection of a marker substance that is rapidly removed from the circulation (W.F. Hamilton, 1962). The dye indocyanine green is commonly used for this purpose. A relatively non-invasive assessment is possible at rest; the dye is injected into a peripheral vein, and its passage through the circulation is monitored by means of a photocell attached to the ear lobe. However, during leg exercise the blood flow through the arm veins is insufficient to allow a satisfactory ('square-wave') injection of dye, and a catheter must be advanced into the right atrium before dye-concentration curves are adequate to calculate cardiac output. Furthermore, exercise leads to changes in thickness of the ear lobe and mechanical displacement of the photocell; an intra-arterial catheter is thus needed to record dye concentrations accurately. The dye method then has little advantage over use of the direct Fick principle.

Foreign-gas methods

The Fick equation may be applied to the pulmonary uptake of a very soluble foreign gas such as acetylene or nitrous oxide.

The acetylene technique was originally introduced by A. Grollman (1929), and early results underestimated the true cardiac output. The necessary gas analysis has been facilitated by the introduction of gas chromatography (R. Simmons & Shephard, 1971b) and mass spectrometry (J.H. Triebwasser *et al.*, 1977). It is now possible to use low (one per cent), relatively pleasant and non-explosive concentrations of acetylene; the modern techniques yield results that have a probable error of less than three per cent and agree well with other methods (R. Simmons & Shephard, 1971b).

While acetylene is the preferred gas (L. Cander & Forster, 1959), nitrous oxide is a possible alternative. Gas concentrations are then determined by either infrared or gas-chromatographic analysis (M. Rigatto, 1967; B. Ayotte *et al.*, 1970).

Most investigators have based their calculations upon the few (eight to ten) seconds before significant recirculation of the foreign gas occurs. Open-circuit procedures have been described (T. Hatch & Cook, 1955; R.J. Shephard, 1959; M. Becklake *et al.*, 1962), but these are cumbersome and of doubtful validity during exercise.

Carbon-dioxide rebreathing

Carbon-dioxide concentrations are very readily determined by 'breathe-through' infrared cells. For this reason, the commonest non-invasive method of cardiac-output determination applies the Fick equation to the exchange of carbon dioxide:

$$\dot{Q} = \dot{V}_{CO_2} / (C_{a,CO_2} - C_{\bar{v},CO_2})$$

The steady-state output of carbon-dioxide ($\dot{V}_{CO_2}$) is measured by an open-circuit method, any given intensity of exercise testing being sustained until the expired CO_2 concentration remains constant for two successive minutes. The arterial carbon-dioxide concentration (C_{a,CO_2}) can be estimated in specimens of 'arterialised' capillary blood, collected from the heated fingertip or ear lobe. Alternatively, the arterial carbon-dioxide tension can be estimated from a continuous record of CO_2 concentration during a rapid expiration. At rest, the concentration seen in the final portion of the expirate coincides rather closely with the arterial value, but in exercise there are substantial variations of alveolar CO_2 concentration over the breathing cycle (R.J. Shephard, 1968b); mainly for this reason, the best approximation to the arterial CO_2 tension of an exercising subject is given by the average of mid- and end-tidal readings (G. Matell, 1963). A third option is to calculate the alveolar CO_2 concentration from the expired reading by means of the Bohr equation, using a formula of N. Jones *et al.* (1966) for dead space (V_D):

$$V_D = 138.4 + 0.077(V_T)$$

where V_T is the subject's tidal volume.

The mixed venous CO_2 reading is usually obtained by rebreathing from a bag containing between five and 15 per cent carbon dioxide. In the Defares method (J.G. Defares, 1956; A. Amery *et al.*, 1977), the subject takes one breath per second. A graph relating the CO_2 content of the nth to the $(n + 1)$th breath is extrapolated to the line of identity. It is assumed that at this point the bag would have reached equilibrium with the mixed venous concentration, causing CO_2 elimination to cease.

An alternative approach (N.L. Jones *et al.*, 1975) selects a re-breathing mixture close to the anticipated mixed venous gas content. If an appropriate mixture is chosen, CO_2 is neither eliminated nor absorbed. After a few oscillations, the CO_2 concentration at the mouth reaches a 'plateau' value close to that of mixed venous blood; this is disturbed when recirculation of blood with higher CO_2 content causes an upward movement of the record (after eight to ten seconds in vigorous exercise). For reasons that are still not fully understood, the plateau reading overestimates the true mixed venous value, particularly during exercise. N.L. Jones *et al.* (1967) thus proposed 'correcting' the bag reading (P_{bag,CO_2}) according to the equation:

$$P_{\bar{v},CO_2} = P_{bag,CO_2} - [(0.24 P_{bag,CO_2}) - 1.47]$$

Unfortunately, the necessary correction may modify the estimate of arterio-venous CO_2 difference by as much as 25 per cent, and this brings the absolute determination of cardiac output into serious question. On the other hand, the CO_2 rebreathing technique is quite satisfactory for following the progress of an individual, and also for comparing his performance with that of other patients tested by the same procedure. At rest, the arterio-venous carbon-dioxode tension difference is only about 6 torr, but it rises to 30–40 torr during vigorous exercise. Since both arterial and venous CO_2 tensions have an error of 1–2 torr, the CO_2 rebreathing procedure is better suited to the measurement of cardiac output when subjects are exercising than when they are under resting conditions.

Neither foreign-gas nor CO_2 rebreathing procedures work particularly well in patients with chronic chest disease, since the permissible rebreathing period (eight to ten seconds) is too short to establish an equilibrium between poorly ventilated regions of the lungs and the rebreathing bag. There thus remains scope for the development of a non-invasive procedure that will allow the measurement of cardiac output in patients with poor gas-mixing.

Regional Myocardial Function

Cine-angiography

Direct estimates of both regional function and cardiac stroke volume can be obtained by injection of a radio-opaque dye and filming the cardiac chamber in the postero-anterior and lateral planes (S.H. Bartle & Sanmarco, 1966; J.W. Kennedy *et al.*, 1966). Computer technology now permits very sophisticated three-dimensional analysis of angiographic videotapes (P.H. Heintzen *et al.*, 1974; S.A. Johnson *et al.*, 1974; H. Sandler & Dodge, 1974), but the technique involves substantial x irradiation and the injection of a dye that occasionally precipitates cardiac arrest. Furthermore, trunk movements make it difficult to apply cine-angiography during more than very light exercise.

Ultrasound

Ultrasound has potential as a method for the estimation of cardiac stroke volume during rest and light exercise (E.I. Edler, 1965; D.H. Bennett & Evans, 1974; H. Feigenbaum, 1974; R.S. Rennemann, 1974; P. Bubenheimer *et al.*, 1980; J.L. Laurenceau *et al.*, 1980; A. Venco *et al.*, 1980). However, to the present it has been used most frequently to detect portions of the ventricular wall with weakened or paradoxical motion.

High-frequency sound waves (2-10 MHz) are directed through the chest and reflected from the ventricular walls. The relative positions of various intracardiac structures are then deduced from transit times for the sound waves. Light exercise can be performed if the subject remains supine or semi-supine. Cardiac output can be estimated from the stroke volume and heart rate, but if the arterio-venous oxygen difference is to be calculated from cardiac output and oxygen intake it is important to await a 'steady state', since the exercise 'on transients' differ for these last two variables.

Nuclear cardiology

Both non-invasive and invasive applications of nuclear cardiology are used in the management of patients with ischaemic heart disease. A static image may be obtained following the injection of technetium pyrophosphate in order to localise and determine the size of a recent myocardial infarction; the marker is selectively retained by infarcted tissue for eight to ten days following the acute episode (R.W. Parkey *et al.*, 1974).

Injection of the thallium radioisotope [201] Tl is a second possible static-imaging technique. A low thallium uptake indicates a zone with poor myocardial perfusion or prior scarring (J. Leppo *et al.*, 1979; D.H. Schmidt *et al.*, 1979). The method can be used to diagnose infarction, to assess the viability of tissue, and to document regional perfusion.

Dynamic studies use either a 'gated' camera, or the 'first-pass' approach. The gated camera records radioactivity at the end of systole and the end of diastole (R.D. Burrow *et al.*, 1977). The 'first-pass' method employs a multiple-crystal camera with a fast counting rate and a short dead time; this allows a bolus of radioactive material to be followed from the moment of its injection into a peripheral vein until it has completed a first passage through the heart. Transit times and ejection fractions can thus be calculated for both ventricles (R.C. Marshall *et al.*, 1977; N. Schad, 1977). Estimates of ejection fraction correlate quite well ($r = 0.91$) with measurements made by contrast ventriculography (D.H. Schmidt *et al.*, 1979), and assessments of regional wall motion have a 75 per cent inter-observer agreement. Further developments of this technique allow semi-quantitative determinations of cardiac output both at rest and during moderate exercise (J.S. Borer *et al.*, 1977; S.K. Rerych *et al.*, 1978).

Left-ventricular function

Direct measurements of left-ventricular function are sometimes made by catheterisation before and after coronary arterial surgery (J.C. Manley, 1979). Note is taken of the left-ventricular stroke work index (the product of ventricular stroke index, ml per beat per m^2 of body surface area, and the difference between mean aortic pressure and the left-ventricular end-diastolic pressure). This index is examined in relation to left-ventricular end-diastolic pressure. Improvement of condition following by-pass surgery may be reflected in a greater capacity to increase left-ventricular stroke work, or a lesser associated rise of end-diastolic pressure during exercise. Attempts to assess myocardial performance through resting measurements of maximum shortening velocity ($\hat{V}_{max}$), mean systolic ejection rate and maximum rate of pressure rise (dp/dt) have proven relatively unsuccessful.

Indirect assessments of cardiac contractility can be derived from angiography, echocardiography and nuclear cardiology, as noted above. More simply, data can be taken from simultaneous recordings of the electrocardiogram, heart sounds and carotid pulse wave (G.R. Cumming & Edwards, 1963; W. Raab, 1966; W.S. Harris, 1974). Possible measurements include the total duration of ventricular systole (from the Q wave of the electrocardiogram to the second heart sound, QS_2), the left ventricular ejection time (from the beginning of the carotid pulse wave to its dicrotic notch, LVET) and the pre-ejection period ($PEP = QS_2 - LVET$). Since such data vary with heart-rate-related changes of contractility, they are commonly 'corrected' to a standard heart rate (H. Montoye *et al.*, 1971; G.M.A. Van der Hoeven *et al.*, 1977). The best simple index of contractility seems to be the ratio PEP/LVET; this is reduced by training, and increased by myocardial disease. Unfortunately, it is difficult to record the carotid pulse wave during vigorous exercise; measurements are thus made immediately after cycle-ergometer work, or during isometric handgrip contractions

(W.F. Jacobs *et al.*, 1970; C. Kivowitz *et al.*, 1970; C.B. Mullins *et al.*, 1970; R.H. Helfant *et al.*, 1971; D.S. Bloom & Vecht, 1978).

Coronary Perfusion

Coronary angiography

Direct visualisation of the coronary vessels by the injection of radio-opaque materials is the standard technique against which other assessments of myocardial perfusion are compared. The contrast medium outlines vessels down to a size of some 110 microns, and local narrowing by atheromatous plaques can also be seen. The status of individual arteries is commonly reported (for example, 50 per cent obstruction of the left anterior descending branch). Such data are of value in gauging the need for by-pass surgery, although it should be stressed that the apparent narrowing of a vessel varies with its orientation towards the viewing camera. Reader-to-reader variability in assessment of angiograms also has a standard deviation of 21 per cent (L.M. Zir *et al.*, 1975). Further, exercise-induced vaso-dilatation may modify the extent of obstruction. Finally, since blood flow varies as the fourth power of vessel radius, a small error in the estimate of obstruction can have a large influence upon the presumed adequacy or inadequacy of perfusion; 50 per cent narrowing has little effect upon flow, but 75 per cent narrowing cuts maximum flow by two thirds (K.L. Gould *et al.*, 1974; S.E. Logan, 1975).

The main disadvantages of angiography are the need for cardiac catheterisation, exposure to x irradiation and the injection of a viscous, cardio-toxic contrast medium that can (and sometimes does) provoke ventricular fibrillation.

Alternative procedures

The Fick principle can be applied to the local myocardial uptake of soluble gases such as nitrous oxide (D.E. Gregg *et al.*, 1951; G.G. Rowe, 1959; R.J. Bing *et al.*, 1960; C.R. Jorgensen *et al.*, 1971). It is also possible to measure the uptake of radioactive isotopes (B.L. Zaret *et al.*, 1973) that penetrate the myocardium readily (^{43}K or ^{86}Rb). Such procedures work fairly well in animal experiments, since the radio-isotope can be injected directly into the root of the aorta, and the heart can be excised subsequently for an assessment of its radioactivity. Precordial counters have been used to measure the uptake of radio-isotopes by the human heart, but such techniques lack precision. Furthermore, the myocardial extraction of the radioisotope apparently decreases from 70 to 40 per cent as the rate of coronary blood flow rises, so that accurate measurements demand an assessment of extraction by catheterisation of the coronary sinus (D. Nolting *et al*., 1958; W.D. Love & Burch, 1959). Even with catheterisation, the value obtained is an average for most of the myocardium, so that local deficiencies of blood flow may pass undetected (F.J. Klocke & Wittenberg, 1969).

Other approaches to the study of myocardial perfusion are currently being developed by the nuclear cardiologists (D.H. Schmidt *et al*., 1979). To the present, they yield qualitative rather than quantitative results. In addition to technetium pyrophosphate injections and thallium scans, some authors have used radioactive macro-aggregates and microspheres (which become trapped in the finer blood vessels). Others have administered ^{133}Xe (which escapes preferentially into well-perfused regions of the myocardium).

Because of technical difficulties associated with these various approaches, the adequacy of myocardial perfusion is still commonly assessed from the electrocardiographic response to a standard stress test.

Electrocardiogram

Technique

The majority of electrocardiograph machines currently manufactured meet the specifications of the American Heart Association (1967); these requirements — for a 0.05-Hz cut-off and a 6-dB-per-octave roll-off — ensure an error < 0.05 mV in the early part of the ST segment, with a consistent response to high-frequency detail above 100 Hz. Older designs of ECG (Figure 7.1) may respond poorly to both high- and low-frequency signals, obscuring fine details of the record and creating artefactual displacements of the ST segment.

Vectorcardiography continues to be of theoretical interest, although it is now recognised that the hope of representing the entire information content of the electrocardiogram in three 'orthogonal' tracings is unrealistic. Valuable clues to local ischaemia of the myo-cardium can be obtained by moving a unipolar (exploring) electrode across the praecordium. In the context of physical activity and ischaemic heart disease, the usual requirement is thus for a standard twelve-lead resting ECG, with use of either a single lead (CM_5) or three leads (CM_2, CM_4 and CM_6) during physical activity (Figure 7.2). Because muscle 'noise' is increased by physical activity, the recording

Figure 7.1: To illustrate the influence of a poor low-frequency
response on the waveform of a simulated ECG signal.

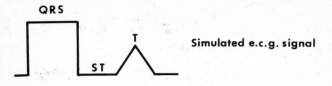

Simulated e.c.g. signal

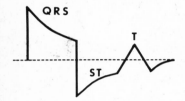

Response of e.c.g. with poor
low frequency response. Note
artefactual ST segmental depression.

Source: W.E. James & Patnoi (1974).

leads should not be attached to the limbs during exercise. The electrical
signal is best measured between the manubrium sterni and the corresponding V position on the praecordium, the neutral electrode being
attached to the back of the neck.

It remains quite difficult to obtain high-quality records during
vigorous exercise, even if chest leads are used (J. Seymour & Conway,
1969; I. Elgrishi *et al.*, 1970). H. Blackburn *et al.* (1968) asked 14
cardiologists to interpret the same series of tracings. The proportion of
abnormal records reported varied from five to 58 per cent, and on
different occasions the same physician interpreted the same tracing
differently. Reasons for inconsistency included lack of objective
criteria, uncertainty about the significance of findings such as
junctional depression and the poor technical quality of many records.
Interestingly, technical personnel were more consistent readers of the
electrocardiogram than were cardiologists. The technicians achieved
complete inter-observer agreement in 85 per cent of records, and were
also in full agreement as to those patients with clear-cut ischaemia
(more than 0.1 mV of ST segmental depression). Keys to the good
performance of the paramedical staff were the use of a magnifying lens,

Figure 7.2: To illustrate the recommended placement of electrodes for an exercise electrocardiogram (Lead CM_5). The lead labelled 'right arm' is attached over the upper part of the sternum (manubrium sterni). The lead labelled 'left arm' is attached over the apex beat (in the space between the fifth and sixth ribs, 7–10 cm to the left of the mid-line). The lead marked 'right leg' is attached at the back of the neck. Alternative placements for leads CM_2, CM_4 and CM_6 are also indicated.

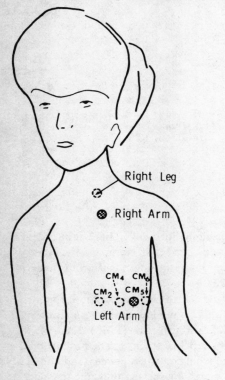

Source: From R.J. Shephard, *Endurance Fitness* (p. 136, second edition, 1977), by permission of the publisher, University of Toronto Press.

simple but standardised measuring techniques and periodic cross-checks of their interpretations against previously evaluated electro-cardiograms.

One of the main technical problems in an exercising subject is a wandering baseline. This reflects a varying electrode impedance. The phenomenon can be minimised by careful skin preparation (removal of the outer layers of the epidermis with a dental burr) and use of an amplifier with a high input impedance (D. Lewes, 1965; R. Tregear, 1965; L.A. Geddes & Baker, 1966). Electrical (60-Hz) 'noise' can be overcome by adequate grounding of the neutral electrode, screening of all cables and use of high-frequency filters with specific ('common-mode') rejection of 60-Hz signals (J. Von der Groeben *et al.*, 1969).

Measurements of the ST segment have been greatly facilitated by the development of analogue and digital averaging techniques (A. Pedersen & Andersen, 1971; P. Rautaharju *et al.*, 1971; W.E. James & Patnoi, 1974; W. Siegel, 1974; L. Jansson *et al.*, 1976; M.L. Simoons, 1976). Analogue equipment gives a visual display of the average tracing derived from 16 or 32 successive heart beats. The usual equipment allows the making up of 1,024 (2^{10}) discreet voltage readings along the length of the QRS-T complex. Noise (Figure 7.3) is thus cancelled out. The quality of the ECG signal improves as the square root of the number of cycles that are averaged; however, if too many complexes are included, a transient ST displacement may be overlooked, while slight asynchrony of the triggering process leads to a progressive rounding of the primary waveform (D.A. Winter, 1969; P. Rautaharju *et al.*, 1971). A single abnormal beat (such as a premature ventricular contraction) also gives a gross distortion of the averaged signal (L.K. Jackson *et al.*, 1969). Some investigators have programmed digital computers to give a more sophisticated solution of the same problem. The 1,024 measurements are made on each of 48 successive heart beats, and the computer program selects for averaging 16 of the 48 QRS complexes that have a mutually similar waveform. Nevertheless, problems still arise. M.L. Simoons (1977) found that in one series of 7,084 tracings incorrect averaging due to excessive drift or noise occurred in 1.8 per cent of subjects. There was also incorrect detection of the QRS complex in 0.04 per cent, P-wave detection errors in 6.5 per cent, and T-wave detection errors in 0.6 per cent. Many of the currently used systems measure ST depression at a fixed time (for example, 80 ms after the ST-T junction, or at a stated interval after the nadir of the R or S waves). Such an approach gives a simple 'packaged' apparatus for clinical purposes, but it does not allow for variations in the duration of the QRS complex and the ST segment. Alternatively, the onset of the T wave can be determined by inspection of the averaged tracing, or by electrical differentiation. Other possibilities are to calculate the slope of the ST segment (F.M. Lester *et al.*, 1967;

Figure 7.3: Components of noise distorting electrocardiogram.

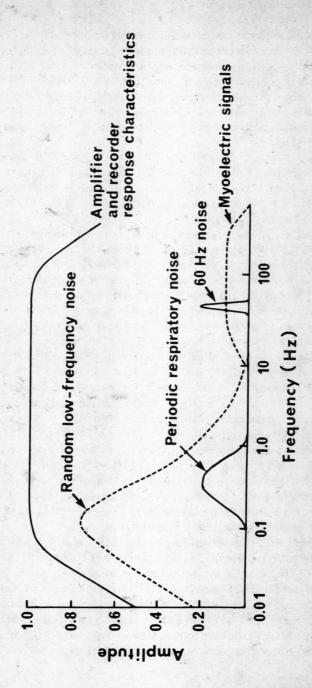

Source: Based in part on W.E. James & Patnoi (1974).

Figure 7.4: Choice of iso-electric line in assessment of ST displacement. Most authors join successive points of origin of the Q wave, although Lepeschkin has pointed out that P- and U-wave repolarisation may then cause artefactual ST depression. The shaded area is the ST integral. The point (1) is 80 ms after the onset of the ST segment, and the point (2) is the onset of the T wave as determined by inspection.

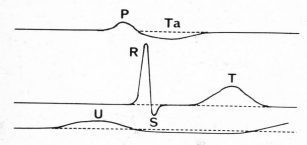

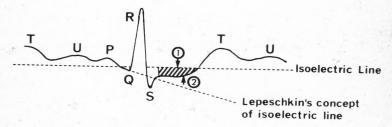

Source: Based on an illustration of E. Lepeschkin (1969).

P.L. McHenry *et al.*, 1968), or the integral of the ST segment below a pre-selected 'iso-electric' baseline (Figure 7.4).

It is not easy to establish the iso-electric ('zero') voltage line during vigorous physical activity, since repolarisation of the U and P waves may extend into the QRS complex and beyond (Figure 7.4). As a matter of convenience, most authors refer measurements to the onset of the Q wave (M. Ellestad, 1975).

Resting electrocardiogram

Many clinicians still search for evidence of myocardial ischaemia in terms of abnormalities of the resting electrocardiogram. However, even if patients have well-marked angina of effort, the resting records commonly remain within normal limits (T.W. Mattingly *et al.*, 1958). Possible clues to ischaemic heart disease include non-specific ST-T wave abnormalities, changes of electrical conduction, dysrhythmias and signs of left-ventricular hypertrophy. Occasionally, there may be ischaemic displacement of the ST segment.

Imminent or recent myocardial infarction is an important contra-indication to exercise. It may be suspected if there are prominent Q waves and elevation of the ST segment, although the latter pheno-menon is sometimes seen also in healthy athletes (S. Zoneraich *et al.*, 1977; J. Morganroth & Maron, 1977; Table 6.9). In doubtful cases, progression of the changes over several days confirms the diagnosis of infarction. If the lesion is on the posterior surface of the heart, the ST segment may be depressed rather than elevated.

Acute myocarditis also causes depression of the ST segment and inversion of the T wave. It is a second important contraindication to exercise.

Exercise should also be avoided if there is a probability of recent *pulmonary embolism*. If the emboli are small, the electrocardiogram may remain normal, but a large embolus is associated with a rapid heart rate and signs of right-heart strain (including inverted T waves over the right ventricle).

Other electrocardiographic indications for caution include dis-orders of cardiac rhythms such as premature ventricular contractions (discussed below), atrial flutter and fibrillation, and the various disturbances of electrical conduction. With *sinu-atrial block*, some of the electrical impulses arising in the sinu-atrial node fail to depolarise the atria; there are thus pauses when an entire ECG complex is missing. When this appearance is seen in athletes, hypertonia of the right vagal nerve is thought to be responsible (F. Plas, 1978; Table 7.3). However, in older adults, coronary vascular disease is often to blame and a 'sick-sinus' syndrome may limit both sinu-atrial conduction and maximum heart rate (M.I. Ferrer, 1973). Blockage of transmission at the *atrio-ventricular node* can also occur. In many athletes, the PR interval is unusually long (> 200 ms, Type I block), and in a proportion of such subjects the PR interval may become progressively extended until a beat is dropped (Wenckeback Type II block; J. Morganroth & Maron, 1977; S. Zoneraich *et al.*, 1977; F. Plas, 1978). More rarely, the PR interval remains constant until a beat is suddenly dropped (Mobitz Type II block). This variety of conduction disturbance is liable to progress to third-degree block, where the atria and ventricles

Table 7.3: Electrocardiographic 'Abnormalities' Observed in 12,000 Athletes

Abnormality	Frequency (%)
Nodal rhythm	0.325
Coronary sinus rhythm	1.15
Atrio-ventricular block	
First degree	6.16
Second degree	0.125
Third degree	0.017
Atrio-ventricular dissociation	0.117
Focal block	3.150
Right bundle-branch block	0.075
Premature ventricular contractions	1.375
Paroxysmal tachycardia	0.067
Ventricular pre-excitation	0.158
Pseudo-ischaemic abnormalities of repolarisation	0.550

Source: Based on data of A. Venerando (1979).

beat independently of each other. Marked atrio-ventricular block usually indicates some disease of the myocardium, and there is a danger of progression to a 'Stokes-Adams' attack, with complete ventricular asystole. *Left bundle-branch block* causes a leftward shift of the QRS vector, with tall and broad R waves in lead I plus deep and broad S waves in lead III. It is usually an indication of cardiac disease. *Right bundle-branch block* causes a rightward shift of the cardiac vector, with broad and late S waves in leads I and II, and a small QRS complex in lead III. It can also be pathological, although a minor degree of right bundle-branch block is a common finding in athletes (N. Hanne-Paparo *et al.*, 1976; W. Kinderman *et al.*, 1978; F. Plas, 1978; B.J.F. de Andrade & Rose, 1979; A. Venco *et al.*, 1980).

Exercise response

The main change in timing of the cardiac cycle during exercise is a shortening of the diastolic phase. However, the P-R interval is also curtailed, often to less than 0.15 seconds, and the Q-T interval is reduced in proportion to the heart rate. There is also an increase in P-wave amplitude, a decrease in T waves during exercise (probably due to sympathetic nerve activity) and an increase in T waves following exercise (possible a response to increased serum potassium concentrations).

The influence of exercise upon premature ventricular contractions and ST segmental voltages is discussed in the following sections.

Premature systoles

Premature beats can arise at any point in the conduction pathway of the electrical impulse. Although sometimes called extra-systoles, they can replace rather than supplement normal cardiac contractions.

A persistent and irregular atrial tachycardia may indicate disease, but it is also compatible with normal health and continued athletic participation (P. Fleischmann & Kellermann, 1969).

Ventricular premature contractions are usually 'ectopic', and in consequence the QRS complex has a broadened and abnormal waveform. Less commonly, a systole may arise within the normal electrical pathway, or impulse conduction may be blocked without the appearance of a visible QRS complex ('concealed conduction'). One factor contributing to premature ventricular contraction is an excessive irritability of the myocardium. This may arise from an accumulation of nicotine or caffeine in the body, or from an excessive sympathetic discharge (as in the chronically anxious person, or the athlete who is competing under intense stress). Some authors have linked emotionally provoked dysrhythmias with an increased frequency of myocardial infarction and sudden death; the effect upon prognosis is probably small (F.D. Fisher & Tyroler, 1963; N. Goldschlager *et al.*, 1973; M. Rodstein *et al.*, 1971), although there is good reason to believe that a sudden outpouring of catecholamines can sometimes contribute to sudden death during intense physical or emotional stress (R.J. Shephard, 1974b).

The premature systoles of an anxious patient usually become less frequent with effort. In other individuals, an abnormality of rhythm appears for the first time during exercise. Overdrive suppression of the abnormal rhythm does not necessarily rule out an ischaemic cause (M.H. Ellestad, 1975; P.L. McHenry & Morris, 1976; G. Koppes *et al.*, 1977). However, appearance of the premature contractions during exercise is generally regarded more seriously (P.L. McHenry *et al.*, 1972; E.F. Beard & Owen, 1973; H. Blackburn *et al.*, 1973). It is clearly associated with an increased probability of cardiac disease (ischaemia and/or scarring) (R.H. Mann & Burchell, 1952; M. Rodstein *et al.*, 1971; J.A. Vedin *et al.*, 1972; M. Ellestad, 1975; B. Surawicz, 1975). The patho-physiology is as follows.

Local hypoxia leads to inhomogeneity of repolarisation, and uni-directional conduction block develops in segments of the myocardium. This facilitates 're-entry' of the electrical impulse into regions of the ventricle that are already repolarised (Figure 1.1; A.M. Katz, 1973; L.S. Gettes, 1975). Circulating catecholamines also lower the threshold of abnormal pace-making foci. These hormones speed both depolarisation and repolarisation of the ventricle (A.M. Katz, 1977), so that non-uniformities of response to the chemical messengers provide a second basis for the 're-entry' phenomenon. The difference of prognosis between resting and exercise-induced premature ventricular contractions is an important issue, for if substantiated it implies that 24-hour tape recordings of the electrocardiogram (L. Mogensen, 1977) have less prognostic value than an exercise ECG.

A polyfocal origin (indicated by differences of QRS waveform between the abnormal beats) is associated with an increased risk of infarction or re-infarction, whereas a unifocal origin (consistent abnormal waveform) is not (T. Kavanagh *et al.*, 1977c). The premature beats are particularly dangerous if they are not only polyfocal, but also occur early in the cardiac cycle (before completion of the T wave). While such premature systoles provide a possible means of diagnosing ischaemic heart disease, it is less clearly established that they add new evidence of risk to that gained from an examination of the ST segment (below).

ST segmental changes

Concept. As the intensity of exercise is increased, the oxygen consumed by the ventricles tends to outstrip oxygen delivery via the coronary vessels. Because of differences in work rate and intramural compression of the coronary arteries, the left ventricle is more vulnerable to oxygen lack than the right. Hypoxia alters transmural potentials across individual myocardial cells (W. Trautwein, 1954; W.E. Samson & Scher, 1960) and also changes the pattern of electrical impulse conduction around the two ventricles. In consequence, there is a progressive alteration in the appearance of the ST segment of the electrocardiogram (Figure 7.5), usually seen best in the unipolar chest lead V_4 (H. Feil & Segel, 1928; S. Goldhammer & Schert, 1932; C.C. Wolferth & Wood, 1932). Depression of the S-ST junction is followed by a horizontal or downward sloping depression of the entire ST segment. Unfortunately, the phenomenon reflects nonuniform repolarisation of the ventricles rather than ischaemia *per se*, and other possible causes of ST displacement include drug-induced malfunction of the myocardial

Figure 7.5: To illustrate the possible range of appearances of ST segment: (a) normal; (b) junctional depression; (c) horizontal depression; (d) downsloping depression

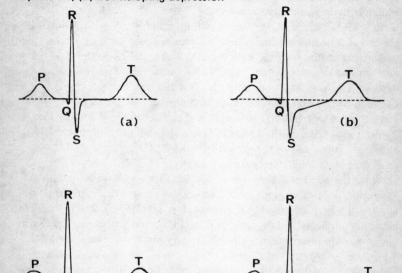

Table 7.4: Factors Influencing ST Segment Displacement during Exercise

False negative results:	Insufficient exercise intensity, resting ST elevation, use of nitroglycerine and other vasodilators, abnormalities of ventricular conduction
False positive results:	Resting ST depression, hyperventilation, cigarette smoking, use of diuretics, potassium loss, glucose and carbohydrate loading, abnormal stress on left ventricle, abnormal conduction (e.g., left-ventricular bundle-branch block), anti-dysrhythmic drugs (e.g., procaine amide, quinidine), digitalis therapy

'sodium pump' and altered concentrations of plasma electrolytes (Table 7.4).

Test format. The exercise format used by many clinicians is still the Master test (A.M. Master & Jaffé, 1941). The patient climbs backwards and forwards over a double nine-inch (22.9 cm) step for 1.5 minutes ('single' test) or three minutes ('double' test), at a rate adjusted somewhat for age, sex and body mass. The main criticisms of the Master test are: (i) reliance on a recovery electrocardiogram; (ii) use of rather mild exercise (the terminal heart rate is typically about 120 beats·min^{-1}); and (iii) a stepping rhythm that imposes a greater strain on elderly than on young subjects.

One possible alternative is to carry all tests to exhaustion, or to a 'symptom-limited' maximum (P.D. Wood *et al.*, 1950; R.A. Bruce *et al.*, 1969). Logic suggests that this will be more risky than a sub-maximum test, and some (J. McDonough & Bruce, 1969), but not all (P. Rochmis & Blackburn, 1971) of the available data support such a supposition (see below, p. 197). In the clinical setting, one disadvantage of a symptom-linked maximum test is its subjectivity. If the confidence of the patient or his examiner allows a repeat test to be pushed to a higher work rate, a misleading impression of worsening ST depression may be formed. The best approach for the clinician thus seems to record the electrocardiogram when the patient is exercising at a target heart rate corresponding to a fixed percentage, 75 per cent (R.J. Shephard, 1971) or 85 per cent (I. Åstrand, 1967) of maximum oxygen intake (Table 7.5). Some critics of this approach have pointed to the considerable range of maximum heart rates, particularly in older individuals and patients with ischaemic heart disease. However, there is a fairly close relationship between heart rate and myocardial oxygen consumption (Y. Wang, 1972), and the target reading thus provides a reasonable basis for standardising myocardial oxygen demand in patients of a given age.

The observed ST appearance depends also upon the duration of physical activity (R.J. Shephard & Kavanagh, 1978c), since an accumulation of acid metabolites in the myocardium dilates the coronary vessels, relieving the local ischaemia. If comparisons of the ST segment are to be made from one test to another, it is finally important to equate cardiac work rate, whether in terms of heart rate or some more complex measure such as the tension-time index or the triple product (see the discussion of cardiac work rate below, p. 225). It can be quite difficult to calculate the tension element of cardiac work,

Table 7.5: Approximate 'Target' Heart Rates Corresponding to 75 and 85 Per Cent of Maximum Oxygen Intake in Relation to Age

Age (years)	Target heart rate	
	75%	85%
25	160	170
35	150	160
45	140	150
55	130	140

since this depends upon the heart volume and the thickness of the ventricular wall, both factors that can vary from one test to another (K.H. Sidney & Shephard, 1977b).

Interpretation. If the coronary vasculature is healthy, there is normally no more than slight junctional depression, even in maximal exercise (R.A. Bruce *et al.*, 1969). Some authors have attached pathological significance to a marked depression of the S-ST junction (> 0.15 mV) and/or an upward sloping ST segment that remains 0.1 mV below the iso-electric ('zero') potential at the commencement of the T wave (A. Kurita *et al.*, 1977). However, false positive tests are less frequent if attention is directed simply to horizontal and downward sloping ST segments (Table 7.6). Such records are associated with as much as a ten- to 15-fold increase in the risk of future 'coronary events', including premature death from ischaemic heart disease (T.W. Mattingly, 1962; A. Rumball & Acheson, 1963; G.P. Robb & Marks, 1964; I.S. Kasser & Bruce, 1969; W.S. Aronow & Cassidy, 1975; G.P. Robb & Seltzer, 1975; G. Koppes *et al.*, 1977). A combination of ST depression with anginal pain is strong presumptive evidence of significant coronary vascular disease.

For clinical purposes it is necessary to establish an appropriate balance between the sensitivity and the specificity of the ST test criterion (Table 7.6). An increase in sensitivity decreases the number of false negative responses, but also increases the number of false positives. A false positive test may create a cardiac cripple from a healthy middle-aged adult; it may also be followed by an unnecessary angiography (a costly procedure with a significant mortality). On the other hand, a false negative test may encourage a patient to undertake excessively strenuous exertion, with a risk of ventricular fibrillation and sudden

Table 7.6: Critique of Various Procedures for Detecting Myocardial Ischaemia

Test criterion	Sensitivity (%)	Specificity (%)
Junctional depression $\geqslant 0.2$ mV	60	50
Upsloping ST segment	30	93
Horizontal or downsloping ST segment	62	91
Tesr type		
Master test (3-min duration)	33	93
Progressive exercise	59	94

Source: C.A. Ascoop (1977).

Table 7.7: Yield of Exercise Stress Tests in a Low-risk and a High-risk Population

	Ischaemia Present	Absent	Total response
(a) Low risk			
All cases	50	950	1,000
Positive stress test	40	95	135
Negative stress test	10	855	865
(b) High risk			
All cases	425	575	1,000
Positive stress test	340	58	398
Negative stress test	85	517	602

death. When undertaking the routine evaluation of an ostensibly healthy sedentary middle-aged adult, a moderate frequency of false negative tests seems acceptable. Indeed, because the prevalence of disease in the general population is quite low, a fairly high sensitivity is needed to ensure a useful yield of positive tests.

The usual criterion is a horizontal or downward-sloping ST depression of more than 0.1 mV. Given a near-maximum test, with

Table 7.8: Relationship between ECG Abnormalities and Coronary
Arterial Disease as Demonstrated at Angiography

Arteriographic status	ECG abnormalities (%)
Normal (n = 370)	8
Single-vessel disease (n = 250)	44
Two-vessel disease (n = 285)	73
Three-vessel disease (n = 367)	88
Left main vessel disease (n = 56)	91

Source: Based on data accumulated by C.G. Blomqvist *et al.* (1978).

multiple-lead recording both during and following exertion, the
sensitivity is then 70–80 per cent, and the specificity is around 90
per cent (Tables 7.6 and 7.7). Statistics depend upon the reference
criterion; this may be the angiographic appearance (Table 7.8), which
itself is subject to variability, or it may be the subsequent development of manifest ischaemic heart disease (angina, myocardial
infarction or death); in the latter case, extended clinical observation
can convert a false position to a true positive result, but it also
increases the number of false negative findings. The proportion of
abnormal records is larger if an exercise electrocardiogram is obtained
than if reliance is placed upon the recovery record alone; the latter
detects about 60 per cent of abnormalities (G.R. Cumming *et al.*, 1972;
K.H. Sidney & Shephard, 1977b), while the exercise record picks out
some 87 per cent of the ischaemic tracings encountered in exercise
plus recovery.

If a vigorous exercise test is used, some ten per cent of men over
the age of 40 years, 20 per cent of men over 60 years and an even
higher proportion of women show substantial ST segmental depression
(Figure 7.6; Table 7.9). However, not all of these individuals have myocardial ischaemia. Particularly in women (G.R. Cumming *et al.*, 1973;
K.H. Sidney & Shephard, 1977b), there is a substantial proportion of
false positive results. Taking account also of false negative findings,
some authors have maintained that the appearance of angina during
exercise provides a better indicator of adverse prognosis than does the
interpretation of ST segmental voltages (J.P. Cole & Ellestad, 1978).
Nevertheless, the development of exercise-induced ST segmental
depression in a person with a previously normal exercise electro-

Figure 7.6: Prevalence of ST segmental depression during maximum or near-maximum exercise, in published reports for middle and old age.

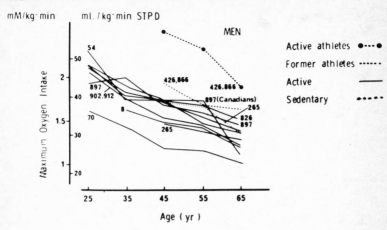

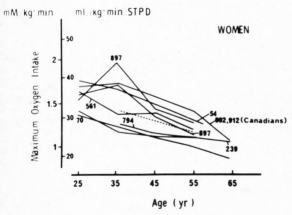

Source: From R.J. Shephard (1978b), by permission of the publishers.

cardiogram is an urgent warning of progressing coronary vascular disease (J.T. Doyle & Kinch, 1970).

Test yield. Mass screening of the general public is sometimes advocated, either in its own right, or as a prelude to the prescription of increased physical activity. However, the wholesale testing of symptomless adults is difficult to justify because of the low yield of useful information.

Table 7.9: Percentage of Elderly Subjects (Usually 60–5 Years Old) showing ECG Evidence of Myocardial Ischaemia (Usually ST Depression > 0.1 mV in Tests at > 75 Per Cent Aerobic Power)

Author*	Percentage of ischaemic records	
	Men	Women
I. Åstrand (1969)	35	55
G.R. Cumming *et al.* (1972, 1973)	37	27
J.R. Brown & Shephard (1967)	—	36
A.E. Doan *et al.* (1965)	46	—
I.S. Kasser & Bruce (1969)	25	—
T. Kavanagh & Shephard (1977a)	17[†]	—
G.R. Profant *et al.* (1972)	—	100
C.P. Riley *et al.* (1970)	32	36
K.H. Sidney & Shephard (1977b)	29	36

* For details of individual references, see Shephard (1978b).
† Masters' Class Athletes.

If 1,000 middle-aged adults are tested, some 135 will show what appears to be an ischaemic stress test, but only 40 of these will be true positive results (Table 7.7). The remainder will receive unnecessary warnings about the dangers of physical activity. A substantial demand will also be created for angiographic tests, the majority of which will prove negative. Of the 40 patients with true positive ischaemic records, perhaps a half will understand and interpret correctly the restrictions that are placed upon their physical activity. Perhaps a half of the 40 true positive tests may also be recommended for coronary by-pass surgery, but since most of them are symptom-free, they will be reluctant to accept this advice. The proportion of the initial screening sample brought to surgical treatment may thus be as low as ten per 1,000, and in the absence of symptoms the usefulness of such surgery will also remain controversial. The remaining 20 true positive patients will probably be recommended for close observation, but again because of the absence of symptoms not all patients will accept this advice. In perhaps ten of the 20, the diagnosis of myocardial ischaemia may reinforce normal medical advice with regard to an improvement of lifestyle. Nevertheless, the total number of individuals helped remains only one person for every fifty tested, so that the cost of such help

Table 7.10: Effective Cost of Helping Patients Through a
Mass-screening Programme for Ischaemic Heart Disease

1,000 stress tests at	$2.43	=	$ 2,430
135 angiographs at	$500+	=	$67,500
			$69,930
10 patients for surgery 10 patients improve lifestyle		}	cost = $3,497 per person

rises to over $3,000 per patient, a prohibitive figure for a screening
programme (Table 7.10).

The yield becomes even smaller, and the cost proportionately higher,
if tests are conducted on an annual basis. We are now looking at the
incidence rather than the prevalence of disease, in effect progression to
the point where ECG changes can be detected. Since subjects usually
survive five to ten years after the appearance of ECG changes, incidence
is only ten to 20 per cent of prevalence, with a corresponding reduction
of yield.

The proportion of positive tests could be increased by augmenting
the sensitivity of the test — for example, pushing the patient to a higher
intensity of exercise, increasing the number of ECG leads or reducing
the amount of ST segmental depression considered as abnormal.
However, this would be an unsatisfactory tactic, as it would increase
the number of individuals subjected to unnecessary, costly and
relatively dangerous angiography.

A more effective approach is to restrict the screening process to
individuals with a relatively high risk of coronary arterial disease.
R. Paffenbarger (1977) found that the incidence of fatal heart attacks
was increased by a factor of 8.5 (from 179 per 100,000 to 1,519 per
100,000) in subjects who combined a low daily energy output with
heavy cigarette smoking and a high systolic blood pressure. Assuming
that this sub-group had a similarly augmented prevalence of ECG
abnormalities, the number of positive tests would rise to 398 per 1,000,
more than 85 per cent of these being true positive tests (Table 7.7).

A further factor influencing the practicality of screening procedures
is the community participation rate. In Saskatoon, a telephone invita-
tion to attend for a free fitness test and exercise electrocardiogram
brought a participation rate of only 35 per cent (D.A. Bailey *et al.*,

1974). In Toronto, establishment of a free clinic in an office building led to participation by about 50 per cent of employees. A half of these went on to join a regular exercise programme that had been organised in the basement of the same building (R.J. Shephard & Cox, in preparation). If the ECG test is to be 'useful', the test result must have a strong impact upon the treatment plan of the physician and/or the health behaviour of the patient. Behavioural scientists have stressed that health behaviour is shaped by health beliefs (M. Becker & Maiman, 1975). In an effective screening programme, the physician or health educator thus takes time to interpret the test result in terms of health outcomes, pointing the path for change (E. Reid, 1979). At a smoking-withdrawal centre where about a third of patients were persuaded to stop smoking for at least one year, many participants commented on the importance of stress-induced ECG abnormalities and dyspnoea as factors contributing to smoking cessation (R.J. Shephard *et al.*, 1972). More recently, paramedical workers have again commented on the value of a simple step test as a motivational tool when seeking lifestyle change (R.J. Shephard, 1980a).

Exercise Stress Tests

General considerations

In the context of ischaemic heart disease, the purposes of an exercise test include: (i) prediction of prognosis; (ii) diagnosis of unusual, exercise induced symptoms; (iii) prescription of an appropriate level of physical activity for both employment and rehabilitation; (iv) monitoring of the response to exercise training; and (v) evaluating the effects of various drugs and of surgical treatment.

Traditionally, observations were confined to the recovery period because of difficulty in counting the pulse and/or recording the electrocardiogram during exercise. However, these difficulties have been overcome by modern ECG technology, and measurements are now routinely made during both exercise and the early recovery period (five to ten minutes post-exercise).

Test protocols

Tests may be made to a target heart rate corresponding to 75 or 85 per cent of maximum oxygen intake. Alternatively, exercise can be continued to a plateau of oxygen consumption (the 'directly measured maximum oxygen intake'), or the test may be 'symptom-limited', activity being halted by the appearance of symptoms such as angina

Figure 7.7: Possible test protocols for carrying a patient to a target heart rate, directly measured maximum oxygen intake or 'symptom-limited' maximum test

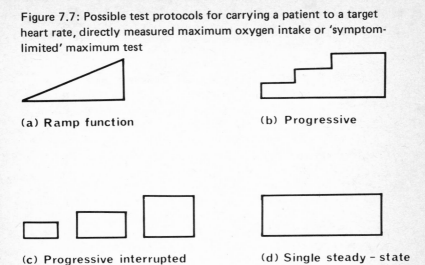

(a) Ramp function   (b) Progressive

(c) Progressive interrupted   (d) Single steady - state

or the appearance of signs (such as an ST segmental depression of more than 0.2 mV).

A variety of test protocols are used to reach these several possible end-points (Figure 7.7). With a *ramp function test*, the loading is increased continuously, or almost continuously, and no steady state is reached. An example of this procedure is the 'Stage One' test of N.L. Jones *et al.* (1975), where the bicycle-ergometer loading is increased by $100 \text{ kp} \cdot \text{m} \cdot \text{min}^{-1}$ at one-minute intervals. The average sedentary subject is carried relatively quickly (within eight or nine minutes) and with little fatigue to a point of voluntary exhaustion. Unfortunately, both heart rate and oxygen consumption lag behind the increase of work rate, so that the subject is incapable of sustaining the 'symptom-limited' power output thus defined. However, the phase lag is relatively similar for heart rate and oxygen intake, so that predictions of maximum oxygen intake based upon the oxygen scale of the Åstrand nomogram do not differ greatly from steady-state values (R.J. Shephard & Kavanagh, 1978c). Perhaps because coronary perfusion improves with a build-up of metabolites in the myocardium, the observed ST segmental depression may be greater with a ramp-function test than with a protocol where a given work rate is sustained for a longer period.

The *progressive sub-maximal test* is the procedure that we have favoured in Toronto. If a cycle ergometer is used, the subject proceeds through three or four stages, each stage augmenting the work rate by 25–50 W; three or at most four minutes are allowed per stage. Normally, this time is sufficient to allow an individual to come very close to a steady-state response of heart rate, blood pressure and oxygen intake for a given work rate, since individual increments of loading are fairly small. Some authors have expressed a fear that longer intervals are necessary to reach a steady state in patients with ischaemic heart disease. This is true of cases with advanced cardiac failure or a 'sick-sinus' syndrome, but in the average patient referred for exercise rehabilitation, the 'on transient' for the exercise-induced increase of heart rate and oxygen intake develops much as in a normal person (Table 7.11).

In the *progressive interrupted test* an interval, sometimes as long as ten minutes, is allowed between individual exercise stages (R.J. Shephard *et al.*, 1968a). The recovery period is short enough that the subject retains some 'warm-up' from one stage to the next. The main advantage of this approach is that it is possible to examine recovery from a given intensity of exercise before proceeding to a higher work rate. This is an important consideration, as dysrhythmias are often concentrated in the recovery phase. Nevertheless, the interrupted protocol is not popular with either physicians or patients, since the total test duration is inevitably extended from a few minutes to almost an hour.

The *single steady-state test* is sometimes used for the direct measurement of maximum oxygen intake. The subject must then return on several occasions to attempt exercise at slightly higher work rates. Now that it is appreciated that a similar result can be obtained by a progressive protocol (R.J. Shephard *et al.*, 1968b), few investigators persist with the single steady-state test.

Choice of ergometer

The most commonly used modes of exercise are a step test, a cycle ergometer and a treadmill (R.J. Shephard, 1977a). The *step test* is simple, inexpensive and needs no calibrating. It is well-suited to mass screening (R.J. Shephard, 1980a). Given careful skin preparation, a good-quality electrocardiogram can be obtained. It is possible to measure the oxygen cost of the activity by the usual open-circuit techniques, and a good estimate of oxygen intake can also be obtained from the rate of working (the product of body mass, step height and the number of ascents per minute). If oxygen intake is estimated rather than measured, it is important that subjects adhere to the required

Table 7.11: Rate of Adjustment to Exercise in Normal Subjects (A),
Patients Progressing Well (B), Patients Progressing Poorly (C) and
New Entrants to a Post-coronary Rehabilitation Programme (D), Given
in the Form of Three-minute Responses to Progressive Exercise
Expressed as a Percentage of Five-minute Response

Work rate	Group	Heart rate (%)	Resp. minute volume (%)	Oxygen cons. (%)	Resp. gas exch. ratio (%)	Predicted max O_2 intake
One	A	101.1	92.4	99.7	89.0	—
	B	98.7	98.8	81.2	101.7	—
	C	98.4	101.7	97.7	102.2	—
	D	100.2	103.9	96.2	105.0	—
Two	A	101.1	93.8	100.3	83.9	—
	B	97.6	92.5	88.1	102.9	—
	C	97.5	93.8	95.3	98.9	—
	D	99.0	93.9	93.4	98.7	—
Three	A	101.3	97.8	99.6	103.4	—
	B	96.8	90.0	93.2	99.1	101.9
	C	96.1	88.3	89.1	100.0	96.5
	D	98.1	94.8	97.0	100.0	97.7
Four	A	99.5	96.1	96.8	105.0	—
	B	97.5	99.1	104.5	97.5	108.7
	C	98.0	93.8	98.2	102.0	101.5
	D	95.5	90.1	94.4	100.0	98.7

Source: Based on data of R.J. Shephard & Kavanagh (1978c).

rhythm of stepping, ascending and descending the full height of the
step at each cycle. Such exercise is performed with a mechanical
efficiency of about 16 per cent (I. Ryhming, 1954; R.J. Shephard,
1967b; Table 7.12). The main disadvantage of a stepping test is that
movement of the subject impedes blood sampling, measurements of
blood pressure and cardiac-output determinations.

The *cycle ergometer* is quite expensive but, nevertheless, has
some attraction for clinical testing. The patient can remain seated

Table 7.12: Estimation of Oxygen Intake from Work Rate during Stepping Exercise

Work rate (kJ•min^{-1})	=	0.00981 X (step height, m) X (Body mass, kg) X (stepping rate per min)
Energy cost (kJ•min^{-1})	=	(100/16) X (work rate)
Oxygen cost (l•min^{-1})	=	(100/16) X (work rate) X (1/21)
Total oxygen intake (l•min^{-1})	=	oxygen cost + resting metabolism
	=	[(100/16) X (work rate) X (1/21)] + [0.3]

Table 7.13: Estimate of Oxygen Intake from Work Rate during Mechanically Braked Cycle Ergometry

Work rate (kJ•min^{-1})	=	(loading, kg) X (flywheel circumference, m) X (gear ratio) X (pedal revs per min)
Energy cost (kJ•min^{-1})	=	(100/23) X (work rate)
Oxygen cost (l•min^{-1})	=	(100/23) X (work rate) X (1/21)
Total oxygen intake (l•min^{-1})	=	oxygen cost + resting metabolism
	=	[(100/23) X (work rate) X (1/21)] + [0.3]

throughout an investigation, and data on blood pressure and cardiac output are readily collected. Unfortunately, the average coronary-prone patient has not used a bicycle for many years. He thus operates the machine in an inefficient manner and this problem can invalidate estimates of oxygen intake that are based upon the mechanical work performed. The standard test format also places a heavy load upon the quadriceps muscle (M. Hoes *et al.*, 1968), and maximum effort is determined by problems in perfusing the active fibres rather than by the performance of the heart (C. Kay & Shephard, 1969). Often, there is a substantial discrepancy between the maximum oxygen intake determined on a cycle ergometer, and that observed during uphill treadmill running (R.J. Shephard *et al.*, 1968b). If oxygen intake is estimated from the work performed (Table 7.13), there are also problems of instrument calibration. Jarring of an electrical ergometer can change dynamo characteristics (N. Jones & Kane, 1979), and supposedly automatic adjustments for variations of pedal speed may also be inappropriate, since efficiency varies with the rate of pedalling

(D. Gueli & Shephard, 1976). In both mechanical and electrical machines, a substantial proportion of unmeasured effort is lost in the pedal bearings and chain mechanism (G.R. Cumming & Alexander, 1968). In some clinical applications, the ergometer is pedalled from the supine or semi-supine position. This allows the use of such techniques as echo-cardiography, nuclear cardiology and cardiac catheterisation, but the activity is then unnatural, and firm shoulder supports are needed to operate the machine. Arm and shoulder ergometers may be used to provide additional information, particularly if a subject's employment calls for vigorous arm exercise. On occasion, a normal electrocardiographic response may be observed during leg ergometry, but during arm exercise ST segmental depression appears as the heart endeavours to pump blood through small but vigorously contracting muscles.

The *treadmill* is bulky, noisy, and expensive. It is sometimes claimed that walking is a very natural form of exercise, but this hardly applies to the task of maintaining a constant position on a narrow and inclined moving belt while breathing through a mouthpiece! Running to exhaustion on a steep and rapidly moving belt is even less natural, and can be quite a frightening experience for the novitiate. One possible advantage of the treadmill when testing a sedentary subject is that exercise is 'machine-paced'. A subject cannot slow down when he becomes tired. This makes it easier to reach the central exhaustion desired in a maximum-oxygen-intake measurement, but at the same time it poses a mechanical danger of stumbling and increases the risk of cardiac problems. Oxygen intake can be measured quite readily while running, but it is difficult to change mouthpieces for a cardiac-output measurement while using the treadmill. Rhythmic vibration of the body may cause a poor-quality electrocardiogram, particularly in a subject who is obese and has pendulous skinfolds. The standard clinical measurement of blood pressure is relatively difficult to obtain while running, and blood sampling is often unsatisfactory unless the subject has an intra-arterial catheter. The oxygen cost of sub-maximal running can be predicted from the speed and slope of the treadmill to about ten per cent (R.J. Shephard, 1968c) and, if the Bruce protocol is followed, the maximum oxygen intake can be estimated (Table 7.14) from the endurance time during a progressive, exhausting test. The treadmill is a particularly valuable tool when it is necessary to obtain a direct measurement of maximum oxygen intake. The results obtained during uphill running to exhaustion are not normally exceeded during any other form of exercise (R.J. Shephard, 1977a).

Table 7.14: Oxygen cost of Treadmill Running

(a) **Sub-maximal exercise (Shephard, 1968c)**

O_2 intake $(ml \cdot kg^{-1} \cdot min^{-1}) = [V \ (km \cdot h^{-1}) \times (2.88 + \theta \times 0.23)] + 7.7$
where θ is the treadmill slope in per cent.

(b) **Maximal oxygen intake**, as predicted from endurance time during progressive, exhausting exercise (after R.A. Bruce *et al.*, 1973)

Duration (min)	Speed $(km \cdot h^{-1})$	Slope (%)	Approximate O_2 cost $(ml \cdot kg^{-1} \cdot min^{-1})$
3	2.72	10	17.4
4	4.00	12	19.8
5	4.00	12	22.3
6	4.00	12	24.8
7	5.44	14	27.9
8	5.44	14	31.1
9	5.44	14	34.3
10	6.72	16	37.4
11	6.72	16	40.6
12	6.72	16	43.8

Measurements

Aerobic performance. The exercise test is commonly used to assess aerobic performance. As noted above, the test may be carried to voluntary or symptom-limited exhaustion. Note can then be kept of the power output (watts, measured on the cycle ergometer), the treadmill endurance time (Bruce protocol; Table 7.14), the maximum rate of climbing of a standard staircase or the distance run in a standard time (Table 7.15). Alternatively, the oxygen consumption can be measured at frequent intervals until a plateau is reached despite further increases of work rate (the 'directly measured maximum oxygen intake'). This is usually defined as an intensity of exercise where a further five per cent increase in work rate increases oxygen intake by less than 2 $ml \cdot kg^{-1} \cdot min^{-1}$ (R.J. Shephard *et al.*, 1968b). It is sometimes stated that it is dangerous to measure the maximum oxygen intake in post-coronary patients, and that the usually accepted criteria of maximum effort (R.J. Shephard *et al.*, 1968b) are obscured by such characteristics

Table 7.15: Distance Run over a Twelve-minute Interval and Maximum Oxygen Intake

Distance covered in 12 min* (km)	Maximum oxygen intake ($ml \cdot kg^{-1} \cdot min^{-1}$)
< 1.6	< 28.0
1.6–2.0	28.0–34.0
2.0–2.4	34.1–42.0
2.4–2.8	42.1–52.0
> 2.8	> 52.0

* This test requires good cooperation from the subject, a knowledge of pacing and a willingness to undertake twelve minutes of all-out effort. It is thus not suitable for unsupervised testing of newly recruited, sedentary and coronary-prone adults. However, it can be used to monitor progress after rehabilitation has commenced.

Source: Based on the data of K.H. Cooper (1968).

Table 7.16: Characteristics of Maximum Oxygen Intake in Healthy Young Normal Subjects (a), Recently Recruited 'Post-coronary' Patients (b), Successfully Rehabilitated 'Post-coronary' Patients (c), and Patients with a Limited Response to Rehabilitation (d)

Variable	Group (a) Good max.	Group (b) All	Group (b) Good max.[1]	Group (c) All	Group (c) Good max.[1]	Group (d) All	Group (d) Good max.[1]
Age (years)	26.4	45.3		42.2		48.3	
Aerobic power ($l \cdot min^{-1}$ STPD)	3.81	1.93	—	2.63	—	2.25	—
($ml \cdot kg^{-1} \cdot min^{-1}$ STPD)	49.4	24.6	26.1	36.9	36.9	29.8	29.9
Predicted aerobic power[3] ($ml \cdot kg^{-1} \cdot min^{-1}$)	45.9	26.1	27.6	35.2	37.7	27.7	29.8
Δ measured	−3.5	−0.5	−1.5	−0.6	−0.8	−2.8	+ 0.1
Max. heart rate (beats·min^{-1})	190	161	167	170	170	168	173
Δ predicted[2]	−5	−22	−17	−15	−15	−11	−8
Respiratory gas-exchange ratio	—	—	1.22	—	1.50	—	1.24
Blood lactate ($mmol \cdot l^{-1}$)	13.6	—	11.4	—	13.7	—	11.3

1. Subjects judged from observation to have made a good effort to reach exhaustion.

2. Our prediction is exigent (a linear decline of heart rate from 195 beats·min^{-1} at age 25 to 170 beats·min^{-1} at age 65).

3. Omitting observations where heart rate falls outside range permitted for use of Åstrand nomogram.

Source: Based in part on R.J. Shephard *et al.* (1968b) and T. Kavanagh & Shephard (1976a).

of the disease as a slowing of maximum heart rate, an increase in anaerobic work and a slow approach to an oxygen-intake plateau. T. Kavanagh & Shephard (1976a) examined three groups of post-coronary patients — those recently recruited, those successfully rehabilitated and those responding poorly to rehabilitation (Table 7.16). A total of 36 individuals were tested. One subject developed persistent chest pain, two had transient ventricular tachycardia and one frequent premature ventricular contractions that persisted for about a minute a quarter after exercise. The usual reasons for halting the test were exhaustion, manifested as vertigo, incoordination, a staggering gait, or weakness in the legs. However, two tests were stopped for gross ST depression (> 0.5 mV), and in one patient the limiting factor was back pain. As in normal young subjects, the directly measured maximum oxygen intake on average agreed quite closely with the value predicted from the heart rate response to sub-maximal exercise (Table 7.16). The maximum respiratory gas-exchange ratio exceeded the figure of 1.15 normally anticipated in young and healthy adults, while the terminal blood lactate of those patients who had completed successful rehabilitation was well up to the level required of younger individuals. Heart rates were apparently somewhat less than predicted values, although our predicted figures were based upon a more exigent standard than that used in many reports. These experiments demonstrated that the typical patient referred for 'post-coronary' rehabilitation can perform a directly measured test reasonably well; on the other hand, we observed some potentially dangerous test sequelae, and in view of the correspondence between directly measured and predicted maxima, it seems preferable to base the routine assessment of the post-coronary victim upon a sub-maximum test.

The Åstrand nomogram is one simple approach to sub-maximum assessment. Modifications of the nomogram now permit the prediction of maximum oxygen intake from sex-specific diagrams that need no age correction (Figure 7.8). Alternatively, the equivalent formulae can be used in computer predictions of maximum oxygen intake (R.J. Shephard, 1977a).

A third possibility is to report the heart rate at a fixed oxygen intake or work rate. For example, data from the Southern Ontario multi-centre exercise-heart trial have been interpolated or briefly extrapolated to a common oxygen intake of 1.25 l·min^{-1}, while in the Canadian Home Fitness Test a simple classification of fitness is based upon endurance time and the immediate recovery heart rate when subjects

Figure 7.8: Age- and sex-specific nomogram for the prediction of maximum oxygen intake from heart rate and oxygen intake in sub-maximum effort. In the event that oxygen intake is not measured, it may be estimated as $[0.012W + 0.3]$ l·min^{-1} (where W is the power output in watts, measured on a cycle ergometer), or $[4/3 \times (MN \times 10^{-3}) + 0.3]$ l·min^{-1} (where M is body mass in kg, and N is the number of complete ascents of a 45-cm step per minute).

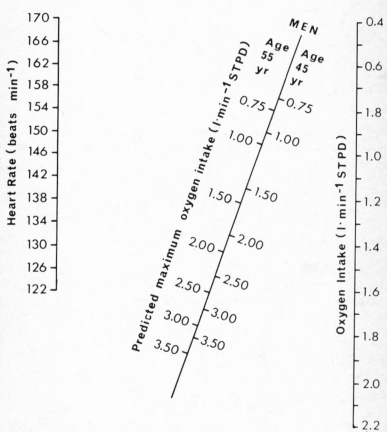

Source: R.J. Shephard (1974c).

Table 7.17: Prediction of Aerobic Fitness from Endurance Time and Immediate Post-exercise Ten-second Pulse Count*

Age (years)	Stepping rate (per min)†	First 3 min (Undesirable fitness level)	Second 3 min (Minimum fitness level)	(Recommended fitness level)
15–19	144	⩾ 30	⩾ 27	⩽ 26
20–9	144	⩾ 29	⩾ 26	⩽ 25
30–9	132	⩾ 28	⩾ 25	⩽ 24
40–9	114	⩾ 26	⩾ 24	⩽ 23
50–9	102	⩾ 25	⩾ 23	⩽ 22
60–9	84	⩾ 24	⩾ 23	⩽ 22
Warm-up for oldest group	66			

* Data for male subjects climbing 40.6-cm double step at age- and sex-specific rhythm set by a long-playing record ('Canadian Home Fitness Test'). Preliminary clearance by a medical screening questionnaire (Par-Q; D. Chisholm *et al.*, 1975) is recommended. Climbing rates are slightly lower for women, to allow for their lower aerobic power per unit of body mass.
† Each subject performs the first three minutes of exercise at a rate appropriate for someone ten years older. Assuming the resultant pulse count is not excessive, he proceeds after a 25-second interval to a rate appropriate for a person of his own age.
Source: D.A. Bailey *et al.* (1974); R.J. Shephard (1980a).

climb a domestic staircase at an age- and sex-specific rate corresponding to an anticipated 70 per cent of maximum oxygen intake (Table 7.17; R.J. Shephard, 1980a).

Difficulties with such sub-maximum assessments include uncertainties about maximum heart rate (a problem with the sick-sinus syndrome and inferior infarcts), inter-individual differences in maximum heart rate, nonlinearity of the oxygen intake/heart rate relationship, drug-induced modifications of the heart-rate response to exercise (for example, β-blocking agents, guanethidine, methyldopa), and possibly activation of ventricular-wall baro-receptors in severely diseased hearts (A.J. Wohl *et al.*, 1977).

Where the test is being conducted for clinical purposes such as exercise prescription, it may suffice to note the heart rate at which electrocardiographic abnormalities appear, setting prescribed activity at a suitable margin below this threshold. One difficulty with this approach is that the increment of blood pressure and thus the cardiac work rate differs when a given heart rate is attained by arm rather than leg exercise. If electrocardiographic abnormalities develop, it is thus preferable to limit effort in terms of some index of cardiac work rate, as discussed below.

Systemic blood pressure. The systemic blood-pressure response to exercise is monitored in order to avoid either an excessive rise or an undue fall in pressure. The pressure recorded by a standard sphygmomanometer cuff may differ from the true intravascular pressure during vigorous exercise (Marx *et al.*, 1967). Nevertheless, cuff recordings are the most practical approach when repeated assessments are required, as in a cardiac-rehabilitation programme. The cuff must be of sufficient size to encircle the arm; if this precaution is neglected, an apparent change of pressure may arise as an obese patient loses sub-cutaneous fat.

Thorough habituation to the investigator and the testing laboratory is also important, otherwise the process of familiarisation may lead to a progressive fall of blood pressure. Of the individuals told that they are hypertensive by a physician, relatively few have a high blood pressure when measurements are made in a relaxed setting (R.J. Shephard *et al.*, 1979b).

Anaerobic threshold. If the work rate is increased progressively, a point is reached where the oxygen delivery to the muscle is no longer sufficient to sustain the activity. Lactic acid begins to accumulate, and there is a disproportionate hyperventilation, with an increase in the respiratory gas-exchange ratio. It has been suggested that this anaerobic threshold bears a consistent relationship to the maximum oxygen intake, thus providing an estimate of endurance fitness that does not require maximal exertion (B. Whipp *et al.*, 1977). In practice, this hope has not been realised. The build-up of lactate varies with the test protocol (for example, step versus ramp function; Figure 7.7); the type of activity (lactate accumulates at a much lower fraction of maximum oxygen intake during cycle ergometry than during step or treadmill tests; R.J. Shephard *et al.*, 1968a); and the level of training (an individual with strongly developed muscles is better able to sustain perfusion during vigorous effort; C. Kay & Shephard, 1969; in contrast, many post-coronary patients have weak muscles, and accumulate lactate at a small fraction of their maximum oxygen intake; S. Degré *et al.*, 1972).

Cardiac work rate. Non-invasive indices of myocardial oxygen consumption include: (i) the heart rate; (ii) the product of systolic pressure and heart rate, sometimes called the tension-time index; (iii) the triple product (systolic pressure × heart rate × duration of systole; G. Blomqvist, 1974); and (iv) multiple regression models based upon systolic pressure and heart rate.

Heart rate is proportional to cardiac work rate only if ventricular pressure, stroke volume, heart size, heart shape and myocardial contractility all remain constant (R.G. Monroe & French, 1961; E.L. Rollett *et al.*, 1965; S. Rodbard *et al.*, 1959; E.H. Sonnenblick *et al.*, 1965; J. Ross, 1972). Despite these limitations, heart rate has proved quite a useful index in some animal experiments (C.R. Jorgensen, 1972; Y. Wang, 1972); this has reflected a close correlation between systemic blood pressure and heart rate in the chosen experimental model (C. Jorgensen *et al.*, 1977), a situation unlikely to prevail in the patient with ischaemic heart disease.

The validity of the systolic pressure-heart rate product and of related multiple-regression equations still depends upon the constancy of stroke volume, heart size and myocardial contractility. The index is said to correlate quite well with more direct measurements of myocardial oxygen consumption (D. Laurent *et al.*, 1956; L.N. Katz & Feinberg, 1958; S.J. Sarnoff *et al.*, 1958; R.G. Monroe & French, 1961; R.J. Ferguson & Gauthier, 1975; E.A. Amsterdam & Mason, 1977; C.R. Jorgensen *et al.*, 1977), although it can be invalidated by drugs that affect ventricular volume and contractility (particularly the β-blocking agents).

The triple product has the soundest theoretical basis, since the only interfering variables are the cardiac stroke volume and heart size. Unfortunately, there is no accurate non-invasive method of measuring systolic contraction time, and for this reason the triple product has no closer correlation with myocardial oxygen consumption than that obtained from the tension-time product (R.G. Monroe, 1964; C.R. Jorgensen *et al.*, 1977).

Test safety. The risks of exercise testing were discussed in the last section of Chapter 6. Given a coronary-prone population, there is a likelihood of one episode of ventricular fibrillation for every 10,000 sub-maximal tests, with as many as one episode for every 3,000 maximal tests. The majority of those affected have a healthier myocardium than patients who develop ventricular fibrillation while at rest. Furthermore, skilled medical attention is at hand, and the myocardium is not subjected to a long period of hypoxia. Resuscitation is thus successful in most instances. Nevertheless, the incidence of cardiac emergencies is sufficient to insist that personnel have recent familiarity with resuscitation procedures, plus the necessary equipment for cardiac massage and/or defibrillation.

Fibrillation is probably provoked by a combination of exercise and fear. Thus, the patient should be reassured before he exercises, and unnecessary frightening apparatus should be removed from view. The test itself should be conducted in a relaxed, informal manner. The safety of informal testing is illustrated by experience with the Canadian Fitness Test. This procedure has now been performed by over 500,000 people of all ages. The required intensity of stepping amounts to 70 per cent of maximum oxygen intake, yet the only known complications have been one ankle injury and a few transient faints following exertion.

How important is the preliminary screening of patients presenting for exercise? Comment has already been made upon the Physical Activity Readiness Questionnaire that is issued with the Canadian Home Fitness Test (PAR-Q; D. Chisholm *et al.*, 1975). This simple screening tool seems to be effective in excluding most of the patients with obvious contraindications to exercise, although it is somewhat over-exigent, since some 20 per cent of office volunteers respond positively to one or more of its seven questions (R.J. Shephard, 1980e). Medical screening is equally unsatisfactory; different physicians prohibit exercise testing in 0.7 to 15.6 per cent of volunteers, and apparently this decision has almost no influence upon the frequency of electrocardiographic abnormalities that develop during exercise (R.J. Shephard, 1980e). Nevertheless, certain well-recognised contra-indications to exercise can be identified at a preliminary medical examination (Table 7.18).

A second safeguard is a careful monitoring of the subject during exercise. Usually accepted indications for halting a test are shown in Table 7.19. Some authors now question the need to abort a test at an ST depression of 0.2 mV. Anginal pain is rarely sensed until there is 0.3–0.4 mV of ST depression, and on occasion subjects have been exercised with impunity to ~ 1 mV of ST depression (G. Cumming, personal communication).

Table 7.18: Contraindications to Exercise Testing

Absolute contraindications

Acute infectious disease

Unstable metabolic disorder

Significant locomotor disturbance

Excessive anxiety

Recent or impending myocardial infarction

Manifest cardiac failure

Acute myocarditis

Aortic stenosis

Probability of recent pulmonary embolism

Special precautions needed

Atrial fibrillation or flutter

Atrio-ventricular block

Left bundle-branch block

Premature ventricular excitation (Wolff-Parkinson-White syndrome)

Table 7.19: Indications for Halting Exercise

Increasing chest pain

Severe dyspnoea or fatigue

Faintness

Claudication

Signs of cerebrovascular insufficiency (pallor, cold moist skin, cyanosis, staggering gait, confusion)

Excessive rise in blood pressure

Sudden fall in systolic pressure

ST segmental depression > 0.2 mV (horizontal or downsloping)

Premature ventricular contractions (more than three in ten seconds, polyfocal, R on T)

Paroxysmal ventricular or supraventricular dysrhythmias

Conduction disturbances other than slight atrio-ventricular block

8 HEART AND CORONARY CIRCULATION IN EXERCISE

In this chapter, we shall take a brief look at normal responses of the heart and coronary circulation to exercise and training. We shall also examine possible modifications of response encountered in patients with ischaemic heart disease.

Heart Rate

Normal values

The 'resting' heart rate is normally 70–80 beats·min^{-1}, although much lower values (down to 30 beats·min^{-1}) are encountered in highly trained endurance athletes (Chapter 4). Since the resting cardiac output per unit of body surface area is relatively fixed at 3.0–3.5 l·min^{-1}·m^{-2}, measurement of the resting heart rate provides some guide to resting stroke volume:

Cardiac output = heart rate × stroke volume

In practice, it is difficult to use the resting heart rate in this manner, since the cardiac frequency is increased by anxiety, a high environmental temperature, recent food, drink, drugs such as tobacco and exercise. Two possible approaches are to take the pulse rate immediately on waking, or to measure the sleeping heart rate by means of a portable tape recorder (R.J. Shephard, 1978).

The heart rate increases with exercise, the rate of rise being a linear function of oxygen consumption between 50 and 90–100 per cent of maximum oxygen intake. The linearity of this relationship provides the basis of various procedures for predicting maximum oxygen intake from the heart rate during sub-maximum effort (I. Åstrand, 1960; J.S. Maritz *et al.*, 1961; R. Margaria *et al.*, 1965).

The maximum heart rate of a young man is normally about 195 beats·min^{-1}, with an inter-individual variation of some 5–10 beats·min^{-1}. Lower maxima (185–195 beats·min^{-1}) are sometimes seen in well-trained endurance athletes (C.T.M. Davies, 1967; B. Saltin & Åstrand, 1967; M. Lester *et al.*, 1968) and at high altitudes (threshold for an effect, 2,000 metres, with a decrease to ∼ 135 beats·min $^{-1}$ at 6,000 metres; L.G.C.E. Pugh, 1962; E.L. Buskirk *et al.*, 1967).

Aging leads to a progressive reduction in maximum heart rate. At one time it was held that the average value for a 65-year-old man was about 160 beats·min $^{-1}$ (S. Robinson, 1938; E. Asmussen & Molbech, 1959), but more recent observers have set the maximum for a sedentary 65-year old North American at more than 170 beats·min $^{-1}$ (S.M. Fox & Haskell, 1968b; M. Lester *et al.*, 1968; K.H. Sidney & Shephard, 1977c). The reason why aging has this effect is unclear. Unlike the situation at altitude, an old person cannot counteract the slowing of maximum heart rate by the inhalation of oxygen (I. Åstrand *et al.*, 1959). Possibly, the rate of diastolic filling becomes a factor limiting cardiac performance. Greater stiffness of the ventricular wall could increase filling time and modify the feedback of information to the cardio-regulatory centres. Alternatively, the sympathetic drive to the cardiac pacemaker may diminish with age.

Ischaemic heart disease

Several recent reports have suggested a sub-normal response of heart rate to exercise in ischaemic heart disease (L.E. Hinckle *et al.*, 1972; M. Ellestad & Wan, 1975; A.C.P. Powles *et al.*, 1979).

In some cases, there is a simple explanation for this. A stress test may be 'symptom-limited', exercise being halted short of an oxygen consumption plateau on account of concern on the part of the patient or supervising personnel, symptoms such as chest pain, electrocardiographic changes (K.L. Andersen *et al.*, 1971) or an excessive rise in blood pressure. The patient may be receiving β-blocking drugs such as propranolol; he may also have heart failure or an abnormal cardiac rhythm. Because ischaemic heart disease is seen mainly in heavy smokers, there is commonly some associated chronic obstructive lung disease; performance is then limited by respiratory rather than cardiac function (B.W. Armstrong *et al.*, 1967), activity being halted by extreme breathlessness at a relatively low heart rate.

In other instances, the problem lies with test methodology — for instance, maximum exercise may have been attempted on a cycle ergometer rather than a treadmill, with failure to demonstrate an oxygen plateau (A.C.P. Powles *et al.*, 1979); the heart rate is then limited by quadriceps exhaustion rather than the usual ceiling of cardiac performance.

Finally, the proportion of patients rated as having a chronotropic disorder depends markedly upon the placing of the 'normal' age/

maximum heart-rate line (T. Kavanagh & Shephard, 1976). If the data of M. Lester *et al.* (1968) is used as the normal standard, many patients will be rated as abnormal, but if the less rigorous criterion of E. Asmussen & Molbech (1959) is accepted, the proportion so classified will be much smaller. T. Kavanagh & Shephard (1976) asked 36 post-coronary patients to develop a maximum power output by uphill treadmill walking; 20 of the 36 individuals reached a true 'centrally limited' maximum oxygen intake, defined by an oxygen consumption plateau. Maximum heart-rate readings were compared with predicted norms that decreased linearly from a maximum of 195 beats$\cdot$min^{-1} at age 25 to 170 beats$\cdot$min^{-1} at age 65. The majority of those tested failed to attain this exacting standard (Table 7.16). Even among the 20 patients who satisfied objective criteria of a centrally limited maximum oxygen intake, the discrepancy between predicted and actual heart rate maxima amounted to about 14 beats$\cdot$min^{-1}. On the other hand, the observed maxima averaged only 3 beats$\cdot$min^{-1} less than the earlier age-related standards of E. Asmussen & Molbech (1959).

A.C.P. Powles *et al.* (1979) suggested that 18 of the 39 post-coronary patients that they tested had an abnormal heart-rate maximum. This interpretation was apparently based on an incorrectly plotted line of normality (R.J. Shephard, in preparation) — in fact, only four of the 39 individuals had heart rates more than two standard deviations below the line proposed by E. Asmussen & Molbech (1959). Nevertheless, Powles *et al.* made the interesting observation that the 18 subjects classed as having a low maximum heart rate also tended to show an abnormally slow heart-rate response to sub-maximum effort. Among this sub-group of 18 patients, exercise bradycardia was more marked in those with an inferior than in those with an anterior or an antero-lateral infarct, this difference being increased by vagal blockade. Since there is no great difference in the speed of adaptation to exercise in 'post-coronary' patients (R.J. Shephard & Kavanagh, 1978c; A.C.P. Powles *et al.*, 1979), exercise bradycardia cannot be attributed to a delayed 'on transient'. The most likely explanation is a local ischaemia and/or infarction of the sinu-atrial mode; oxygen lack from any cause impairs the response to both adrenergic and cholinergic stimulation (M.F. Sheets *et al.*, 1975). A further possibility is autonomic imbalance — either failure to withdraw parasympathetic tone during exercise (S. Robinson *et al.*, 1953) or a depletion of myocardial epinephrine stores secondary to cardiac failure (C.A. Chidsey *et al.*, 1965; G.D. Beiser *et al.*, 1968).

Given that at least a small proportion of 'post-coronary' patients show slow heart rates during both sub-maximal and maximal effort, what are the practical implications for exercise testing and prescription? T. Kavanagh & Shephard (1976) tested the accuracy of aerobic power predictions based upon the oxygen consumption at a target heart rate (Table 7.16). The systematic error was smaller than in healthy subjects and the standard deviation of this discrepancy (5–7 ml·kg^{-1}·min^{-1}) was similar to that encountered in normal individuals.

However, in that small sample of subjects with a 'sick-sinus' syndrome, extrapolation to an age-related anticipated maximum heart rate can give a misleading overestimate of maximum oxygen intake and maximum power output (A.C.P. Powles *et al.*, 1979), with a corresponding potential for over-prescription of exercise. There is thus virtue in carrying out at least one simple test to exhaustion on each 'post-coronary' patient; this assesses whether the anticipated age-related maximum heart rate can be reached and, in the event that it cannot, a symptom-limited maximum power output may be established.

Stroke Volume

Normal values

Under normal resting conditions, a standing or a seated subject expels some 80 ml of blood from each ventricle with every heart beat. The diastolic volume of the left ventricle is about 160 ml and around a half of this volume is emptied during systole. Stroke volume is increased with rhythmic exercise, a plateau of some 110–35 ml per beat being reached at 40–50 per cent of maximum oxygen intake. This is achieved by a greater emptying of the heart (increase of contractility and decrease of cardiac reserve). At higher work rates there may also be some increase of end-diastolic volume (L.D. Horwitz *et al.*, 1972) and pressure (J.S. Williamson *et al.*, 1978). Young adults are able to maintain the augmented stroke volume to 100 per cent of maximum oxygen intake, but in older individuals there is a tendency for stroke volume to decrease at the highest work rates (A. Granath *et al.*, 1964; M. Becklake *et al.*, 1965; G. Grimby *et al.*, 1966; J.S. Hanson *et al.*, 1968; V. Niinimaa & Shephard, 1978; Figure 8.1). It is unclear how far this impairment of myocardial performance reflects diminishing myocardial perfusion, lesser cardiac compliance or poorer ventricular contractility; other factors are reduced pre-loading (a failure of venous return) and increased after-loading (a rise in systemic blood pressure).

The maximum stroke volume is influenced by the fitness of an

Figure 8.1: Cardiac response to exercise in normal young adults (solid lines) and elderly subjects (interrupted lines). Subjects walking on treadmill at increasing slopes.

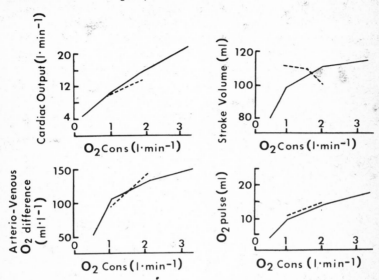

Source: Based on data of V. Niinimaa & Shephard (1978).

individual, being 20–30 ml larger in a well-trained endurance athlete than in a sedentary person. Values obtained on a bicycle ergometer are 10–15 ml lower than those seen on a treadmill (R.J. Shephard, 1977a). If exercise is performed in the supine position, the resting stroke volume is increased to ∼ 110 ml, but little augmentation of output per beat occurs during physical activity.

The largest stroke volume may be seen in the first few seconds after maximum effort, particularly if venous return is sustained by loadless pedalling during the recovery period (D.I. Goldberg & Shephard, 1980). G. Cumming (personal communication) has thus suggested that interval work is the most effective technique for increasing an individual's maximum stroke volume. With static (isometric) exercise, stroke volume shows little change, emptying of the left ventricle against the increased 'after-load' being sustained by an increase in left-ventricular force, with little increase in left-ventricular end-diastolic pressure (R.H. Helfant *et al.*, 1971; C. Kivowitz *et al.*, 1971; C.B. Mullins & Blomqvist, 1973).

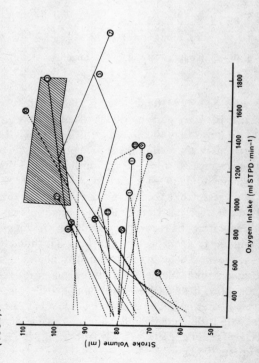

Figure 8.2: Relationship between stroke volume and oxygen intake in patients with myocardial infarction alone and in those with infarction plus angina or angina alone. Shading indicates normal response (see D.H. Paterson et al., 1979). Authors: (1) R. Malmcrona et al. (1963); (2) J.O. Parker et al. (1967); (3) B.E. Higgs et al. (1968); (4) K. Kato & Watanabe (1971); (5) R.A. Bruce et al. (1974a); (6) J. McDonough et al. (1974); (7) N. Rousseau et al. (1973); (8) O. Müller & Rørvik (1958); (9) M. Najmi & Segal (1967); (10) M.H. Frick & Katila (1968); (11) J.P. Clausen et al. (1969); (12) J.V. Messer et al. (1963); (13) R.A. Bruce et al. (1974b); (14) R.P. Malmborg (1964); (15) G.L. Foster & Reeves (1964).

Source: Based on data accumulated by D.H. Paterson.

Figure 8.3: Changes of cardiac function with three weeks of bed rest and seven weeks of subsequent training, for healthy young adults.

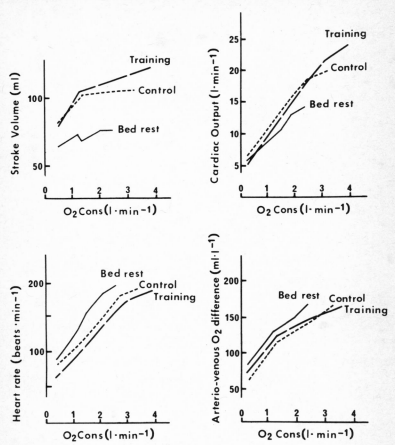

Source: Based on data of B. Saltin *et al.* (1968).

Ischaemic heart disease

Ischaemic heart disease tends to impair stroke volume for several reasons — loss of physical condition during bed rest, abnormal motion of the ventricular wall (Chapter 1) and continuing ischaemia of the myocardium (Figure 8.2).

Two to three weeks of bed rest of itself can cause a 20-30 ml decrease in both resting and exercise cardiac stroke volume (B. Saltin *et al.*, 1968). Thus, a reduced stroke volume is to be anticipated if a 'post-coronary' patient is recruited soon after infarction. In a healthy individual, the normal stroke volume can be restored by a few weeks of training (Figure 8.3; B. Saltin *et al.*, 1968). Following myocardial infarction, the exercise prescription is more cautious, but nevertheless, a gradual reversal of the bed-rest effect occurs (D.H. Paterson *et al.*, 1979).

The pumping function of the ventricular wall may be impaired by electrical-conduction delays, different segments of the wall contracting out of sequence with each other. Severely hypoxic or scarred areas of myocardium may show little or no contractile activity, and occasionally 'paradoxical' bulging of a ventricular aneurysm may occur in phase with cardiac contraction. Finally, hypoxia of the papillary muscles may cause defective functioning of the cardiac valves. Each of these problems inevitably restricts cardiac stroke volume.

More general hypoxia of the myocardium may develop as the cardiac work rate is augmented by an increase in heart rate and systolic blood pressure. There is little scope for anaerobic metabolism in the myocardium. Hence, oxygen lack impairs the regeneration of adenosine triphosphate (ATP) in heart muscle, with a decrease in myocardial contractility (F. Grögler *et al.*, 1973) and a fall in stroke volume; functional impairment can be detected with as little as eight seconds of oxygen lack in the dog heart (H.O. Hirzel *et al.*, 1973).

In practice, the average patient referred for 'post-coronary' rehabilitation has a somewhat lower stroke volume and cardiac output than a normal middle-aged man who is developing a comparable rate of rhythmic work (R.A. Bruce *et al.*, 1974; M. Rousseau *et al.*, 1974; D.H. Paterson *et al.*, 1979). This is due both to impaired contractility and slowed relaxation of the heart (W. Rutihauser *et al.*, 1973). Impaired contractility and a poor stroke volume is particularly likely in the older patient (F. Nager *et al.*, 1967) and the individual with exercise-induced angina (J.V. Messer *et al.*, 1963; G.L. Foster & Reeves, 1964; L.S. Cohen *et al.*, 1965; J.O. Parker *et al.*, 1967; E.A. Amsterdam, 1976). The energy needed for a given bout of dynamic exercise is then obtained by a broadening of arterio-venous oxygen difference and an increase in oxygen debt (Figure 8.4). If ventricular function is impaired, isometric exercise is tolerated particularly poorly, with a decrease in stroke volume and a dramatic rise in left-ventricular end-diastolic pressure.

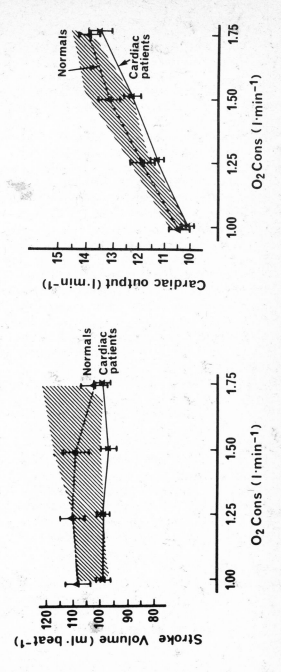

Figure 8.4: Response of 'post-coronary' patients to exercise. Based on cycle-ergometer data for 79 patients with myocardial infarction and nine normal middle-aged men. The shaded area indicates the range of normal values reported in the literature.

Source: Data from Southern Ontario multicentre trial, as repeated by D.H. Paterson et al. (1979).

Training Response

The classical response to training in the healthy person is a decrease in exercise heart rate, associated with an increase in stroke volume (Chapter 4). The maximum heart rate is unchanged, or may show a slight decrease, while the stroke volume is better sustained to maximum effort. This apparently reflects improved coronary blood flow to the active muscles with an increase of actomyosin and myosin ATPase activity (J. Scheuer *et al.*, 1977).

The response of the 'post-coronary' patient is less clear-cut, being influenced by the age of the subject, the severity of the disease process, the time that elapses between infarction and recruitment to the rehabilitation programme, the intensity of the test exercise relative to prescribed training, the rate of progression of the training programme and sometimes changes in medication such as β-blocking drugs. Almost all reports show a moderate increase in heart rate in sub-maximal exercise (Table 8.1), but several studies made over the first six months of rehabilitation show either no increase in stroke volume, or a parallel response of exercised and control subjects (Table 8.2; H. Bergman & Varnauskas, 1970; J.P. Clausen & Trap-Jensen, 1970; J.R. Detry *et al.*, 1971; D.H. Paterson *et al.*, 1979; Figure 8.5). In several of these reports, an increased oxygen delivery is realised by a widening of the maximum systemic arterio-venous oxygen difference.

The reduction in exercise heart rate could reflect: (i) a lessening of drive from the cerebral cortex to the vasomotor centre (E.E. Smith *et al.*, 1976); (ii) lesser activation of the motor cortex secondary to hypertrophy of slow-twitch muscle fibres (H. Roskamm, 1971); (iii) redirection of blood flow from skin to muscle (R.J. Shephard, 1977a); (iv) easier perfusion of the thigh muscles secondary to their hypertrophy (R.J. Shephard, 1977a); and (v) an increased peripheral extraction of oxygen secondary to an increase in the activity of skeletal-muscle enzyme systems (J.P. Clausen, 1976). D.H. Paterson *et al* (1979) found little increase in lean tissue mass over the first six months of training, and thus concluded that factors (ii) and (iv) contributed little to the early conditioning response of post-coronary patients. Blood leaving the active limb muscles also contains very little oxygen (R.J. Shephard, 1977a) so that there is limited scope for factor (v). The early decrease in heart rate with training must thus be attributed to factors (i) and (iii).

The changes of stroke volume arise from the opposing influences of a decreased sympathetic drive (which has a negative inotropic effect

Table 8.1: Effects of Training Programmes in Ischaemic Heart Disease, as Measured by Increase in Maximum Oxygen Intake or Physical Working Capacity and Decrease in Heart Rate during Sub-maximal Working

Patients Total	Myocardial infarction	Angina	Age	Training Frequency	Duration	Sub-maximal heart rate	Response Physical working capacity (PWC$_{150}$)	Maximum rate of working	Authors
(n)	(n)	(n)	(years)	(per week)	(months)	(%)	(%)	(%)	
100	92	8	–	3	24	–	–	+17	M. Wassermill & Toor (1966)
12	12	–	48	3	8	–16	–	–	J. Naughton et al. (1966)
254	–	–	–	3–5	33	–	+22 (adherents)	† (adherents)	H.K. Hellerstein et al. (1967)
5	5	3	47	2	1–2	–13	–	–	M. Frick et al. (1968)
100	66	47	–	3	33	–13	–	+17	S.H. Saltzman et al. (1969)
11	9	6	52	4	6	–	+30–40	+33	F. Kasch & Boyer (1969)
7	6	5	53	5	2	–	–	+32	J.P. Clausen et al. (1969)
9	7	–	48	3	4–6	–13	–	–	J.P. Clausen & Trap-Jensen (1970)
7	7	6	–	3	6	–	–	–	H. Bergman & Varnauskas (1970)
12	12	–	47	5	6	–23	+30	–	O. Pedersen-Bjergaard (1971)
14	14	–	48	3	3	–	–	+23	E.W. Bannister & Taunton (1971)
12	12	6	48	14	1½	–	–	+56	J.R. Detry et al. (1971)
7	7	7	51	3	2	–	–	+7	D.R. Redwood et al. (1972)
12	12	3	52	3	3	–7	–	–	S. Degré et al. (1972)
21	21	10	50	3	9	–9 to –12	+21	+15	A. Bjernulf (1973)
28	28	–	50	3	9	–8 to –12	+35	+22	H. Sanne (1973)
16	16	16	51	3	12	–	+33	–	H. Sanne (1973)
16	9	5	57	3	12	–	–	+26	R. Ferguson et al. (1973)
12	12	–	49	5	12	–	–	+17	J.D. Cantwell et al. (1973)
31	31	15	–	–	24	–	–	+35	T. Kavanagh et al. (1973b)
–	–	–	–	3	1½	–11	–	+20	T. Kavanagh et al. (1973b)
26	26	10	48	3	3	–	+24	+24	S. Degré & Denolin (1973)
26	26	13	53	5	12–18	–	–	+75	K. Bergström et al. (1974)
8	8	2	43	3	3	–13	–	+24	T. Kavanagh et al. (1974b, 1977a)
29	29	15	47	3	13	–	+33	+25	M. Rousseau et al. (1974)
14	7	7	51	5	3–24	–	+25	–	R. Ferguson et al. (1974)
12	8	7	50	3	6½	–	–	–	D. Cardus et al. (1975)
6	6	3	48	4	6½	–6	–	+41	D.R. McCrimmon et al. (1976)

Source: Based on data collected by D.H. Paterson (1977).

Table 8.2: Changes in Cardiovascular Performance over a 'Post-coronary' Training Programme, as Shown by Data for Exercising Patients

Heart rate Initial (beats/min)	Δ (%)	Stroke volume Initial (ml)	Δ (%)	Cardiac output Initial (l/min)	Δ (%)	Arterio-venous oxygen difference Initial (ml/l)	Δ (%)	Author
133	−12		0	9.5	−13	101	+9	E. Varnauskas (1966)
133	−8	110	+15	14.5	+8	107	−8	M. Frick & Katila (1968)
117	−8	104	+9	13.7	+2	96	−3	M. Frick et al. (1971)
145	−9	94	+6	11.0	+5	115	+1	J.P. Clausen et al. (1969)
131	−9	92	+14	13.0		115	−7	J.P. Clausen & Trap-Jensen (1970)
107	−14	93	+2	12.1	−9	105	+9	J.R. Detry et al. (1971)
119	−7	88	+7	9.4	−1	108	+1	H. Bjernulf (1973)
123	−13	81	+12	8.8	+2	No data		B. Kirchheiner & Pedersen-Bjergaard (1973)
114	−7	93	+10	11.3	+2	101	−3	S. Degré et al. (1972)
111	−8	100	+7	11.3	0	86	−1	S. Degré & Denolin (1973)
122	−12	94	+7	10.6	0	93	0	S. Degré & Denolin (1973)
		86	−12	10.5	−2	100	0	M. Rousseau et al. (1974)
Decreased				Decreased		Decreased		G.A. Klassen et al. (1972)
Decreased		No change		Decreased				P. Gauthier et al. (1973)
				No change				G. Avon et al. (1973)
Untrained, reference groups of 'post-coronary' patients								
126	−2	98	+8	12.4	+6	103	−4	M. Frick et al. (1971)
107	−4	85	0	9.0	−3	99	0	H. Bjernulf (1973)
115	−3	70	+9	7.5	+4	No data		B. Kirchheiner & Perdersen-Bjergaard (1973)
111	−8	91	+8	10.0	+1	100	−2	M. Rousseau et al. (1974)

Source: Based on data collected by D.H. Paterson (1977).

upon the myocardium; W.A. Neill, 1977) and an enhancement of intrinsic myocardial contractility (D.A. Cunningham & Rechnitzer, 1974). This may explain why different studies of 'post-coronary' patients have reported training responses ranging from a six per cent decrease to an 18 per cent increase in stroke volume (M.H. Frick & Katila, 1968; H. Bergman & Varnauskas, 1970; J.P. Clausen & Trap-Jensen, 1970; J.R. Detry *et al.*, 1971; A. Bjernulf, 1973; M. Rousseau *et al.*, 1974; S. Degré, *et al.*, 1977; D.H. Paterson *et al.*, 1979).

In the second six months of training, D.H. Paterson *et al.* (1979) saw a six to eleven per cent increase in stroke volume; as in other investigations, this was more marked in heavy than in light work (M.H. Frick & Katila, 1968; J.R. Detry *et al.*, 1971; J.P. Clausen, 1976; S. Degré *et al.*, 1977). It has yet to be resolved why the early training response of a normal person is delayed in the post-coronary patient. Possibly, both the patient and the supervising physician are cautious during the first six months of renewed activity, so that the exercise undertaken at this stage remains insufficient to induce an increase in cardiac stroke volume. J. Scheuer (1973) stressed that increases in myocardial ATPase activity, and thus in intrinsic myocardial contractility, demand a minimum duration and severity of training that is almost certainly lacking in the early coronary rehabilitation programme.

The response from six to twelve months of training (Figure 8.5) cannot be attributed simply to a natural correction of the asynchronous contraction seen immediately after infarction (E. Braunwald *et al.*, 1976); control patients enrolled in a homeopathic exercise programme developed a small *decrease* in stroke volume over the same period of observation. The prime explanation is probably an increase in myocardial contractility due to hypertrophy and/or changes in myocardial metabolism (B. Saltin *et al.*, 1968; J. Scheuer, 1973). However, there may also be some contribution from altered pre- or after-loading of the ventricle. Both J.P. Clausen (1973) and S. Degré *et al.* (1977) have stressed the importance of a decrease in total peripheral resistance. There are several potential mechanisms for producing such a change with training, including: (i) general reduction in sympathetic vasoconstrictor tone; (ii) enzymatic adaptations that allow more muscle fibres to participate in the required activity (thereby increasing the effective vascular bed, and reducing tension per unit of muscle cross section); and (iii) muscle hypertrophy (facilitating perfusion of the thigh muscles, often a limiting factor in cycle-ergometer work; R.J. Shephard, 1977a).

A. Bjernulf (1973) suggested that the response to training was

Figure 8.5: Influence of training upon cardiac stroke volume during exercise, based upon results for 'post-coronary' patients, allocated randomly to 'high-intensity' and 'low-intensity' exercise programmes.

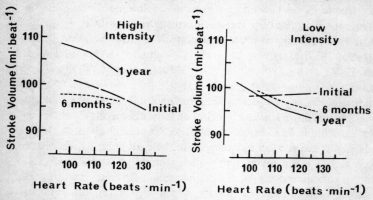

Source: Data from Southern Ontario multicentre trial as reported by D.H. Paterson *et al.* (1979).

influenced by the severity of the disease process, younger and angina-free patients being more likely to show an increase in stroke volume at a given work rate. This seems inherently probable, and indeed absence of the normal augmentation of stroke volume with exercise may be warning of an impending recurrence (R.J. Shephard, 1979a). On the other hand, neither J.R. Detry *et al.* (1971) nor D.H. Paterson *et al.* (1980) found any significant association between the size of the stroke-volume increase with training and the presence or absence of exercise-induced angina. Possibly, future investigators may have more success in relating such changes to objective criteria of hypoxia (such as exercise-induced ST segmental depression).

Cardiac failure

Cardiac failure may be suspected if end-diastolic pressure exceeds 12 mm Hg in the left ventricle or 5 mm Hg in the right ventricle. However, the relationship between diastolic volume and pressure is influenced markedly by: (1) myocardial contractility; (2) myocardial hypertrophy; and (3) fibrosis of the ventricular wall. In a normal subject, the increased stroke volume of exercise is mediated largely by an increase in contractility, with more complete emptying of the ventricle, but in heavy effort some increase in end-diastolic volume may occur (J.H. Mitchell & Wildenthal, 1971).

If the myocardial oxygen supply is inadequate, some degree of cardiac failure is likely during exercise. Initially, stroke output may be maintained at the expense of some increase in diastolic volume (compensated failure), but with a further stretching of the myocardial filaments the force that can be developed by the myosin/actomyosin cross bridges begins to decrease (decompensated failure) (B.M. Lewis *et al.*, 1953; R.M. Harvey *et al.*, 1962; J. Ross *et al.*, 1966). Increases in pulmonary artery, wedge and left ventricular end-diastolic pressures have been linked to exertional angina and low cardiac outputs during exercise (J.O. Parker *et al.*, 1966; L. Wiener *et al.*, 1968; K.P. O'Brien *et al.*, 1969; J. McDonough *et al.*, 1974). In the absence of angina, patients with ischaemic heart disease show a normal left-ventricular end-diastolic pressure during exercise (L.S. Cohen *et al.*, 1965).

Cardiac Output

Normal values

The resting cardiac output is normally 3.0–3.5 $l \cdot min^{-1} \cdot m^{-2}$, or in a person with a body surface area of 1.8 m^2, 5.4–6.3 $l \cdot min^{-1}$. During moderate exercise, the oxygen intake increases in close relationship to the increase in cardiac output, although the latter may show a lesser increase from 70 to 100 per cent of maximum oxygen intake (P.O. Åstrand *et al.*, 1964). In our studies of young adults (R. Simmons & Shephard, 1971a, b), the cardiac output at maximum oxygen intake was only marginally less than would be predicted from a linear extrapolation of the cardiac output/oxygen consumption line. Presumably, much depends on the state of training of the subject and his ability to sustain a high stroke volume against the peripheral resistance of strongly contracting leg muscles.

In a well-trained endurance athlete, cardiac output reaches a maximum of 35 $l \cdot min^{-1}$ or more, but in an older, sedentary individual a peak value of 15–20 $l \cdot min^{-1}$ is likely.

Ischaemic heart disease

Some authors have found a normal increase in cardiac output when exercise is performed by 'post-coronary' patients (J.A.L. Mathers *et al.*, 1951; C.B. Chapman & Fraser, 1954; J.V. Messer *et al.*, 1963; R.P.A. Malmborg, 1964; R. Malmcrona & Varnauskas, 1964; Figure 8.6). Others have observed a 'hypokinetic' response (K. Kato & Watanabe, 1971; R.A. Bruce *et al.*, 1974; J.S. Forrester *et al.*, 1977; D.H. Paterson *et al.*, 1979), compensated by a broadening of arterio-

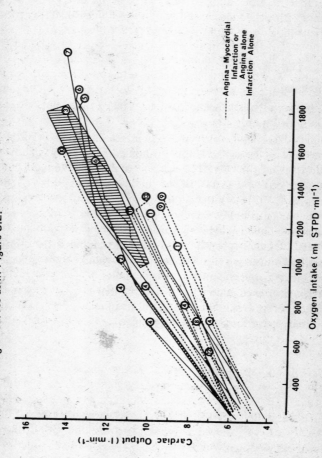

Figure 8.6: Relationship between cardiac output and oxygen intake in patients with myocardial infarction alone and in those with infarction plus angina or angina alone. Shading indicates normal response (see D.H. Paterson et al., 1979). Numbering of curves as in Figure 8.2.

Cardiac Output (l·min⁻¹)

Oxygen Intake (ml STPD·ml⁻¹)

Angina – Myocardial Infarction or Angina alone
Infarction Alone

Source: Based on data accumulated by D.H. Paterson (1977).

venous oxygen difference in sub-maximal exercise and by an increased proportion of anaerobic metabolism in maximum effort (S. Degré *et al.*, 1972). Among reasons for the discordant reports, we may note the low intensity of exercise used in some early tests, varying intervals between infarction and testing, and varying severity of both infarct and residual coronary vascular disease. Impaired myocardial performance has often been linked with exercise-induced angina (J.V. Messer *et al.*, 1963; L.S. Cohen *et al.*, 1965; G.L. Foster & Reeves, 1964; J. Parker *et al.*, 1966), although the haemodynamic limitation is usually apparent before the onset of clinical symptoms (J.A. Murray *et al.*, 1968).

Slowing of heart rate in the sick-sinus syndrome, hypoxic impairment of myocardial contractility, mechanical problems in the functioning of the ventricular pump, and a delayed 'on transient' at the beginning of exercise are all reasons why the cardiac output of a 'post-coronary' patient would sometimes be less than that of a healthy person with the same power output. However, such problems are by no means universal in ischaemic heart disease. The sick-sinus syndrome is encountered in only about ten per cent of those referred for exercise rehabilitation (A.C.P. Powles *et al.*, 1979; R.J. Shephard, 1980f). Likewise, T. Kavanagh *et al.* (1977c) noted that only 16 of their 610 'post-coronary' patients had radiographic evidence of depression of the ST segment of the electrocardiogram at a target heart rate corresponding to 75 per cent of aerobic power. R.J. Shephard & Kavanagh (1978c) reported a relatively normal exercise 'on transient' in their post-coronary patients (Table 7.11), but A.B. Ford & Hellerstein (1957) observed that an increased fraction of oxygen cost of the 1½-minute Master test was deferred to the recovery period. J.H. Auchincloss *et al.* (1974) tested oxygen consumption one minute after commencing exercise, and found a deficit of ~ 20 per cent in a half of patients with angiographic evidence of coronary arterial disease. Most of the group had severe impairment of myocardial function, with an elevation of diastolic pressure.

Arterio-venous Oxygen Difference

Normal values

The arterio-venous oxygen difference of a normal young adult increases from 40–50 ml·l^{-1} at rest to about 120 ml·l^{-1} at 40 per cent of maximum effort, with a further rise to 130–160 ml·l^{-1} in maximum effort. Higher maxima are seen in endurance athletes and in men generally, while lower maxima are found in the elderly (V. Niinimaa & Shephard, 1978).

Factors influencing the maximum arterio-venous difference include: (i) the haemoglobin level (higher in men than in women); (ii) the extent of the haemoconcentration (between five and ten per cent) induced by exercise; (iii) small effects due to a decrease in arterial pH, an increase in blood temperature and an increase in blood CO_2 content; (iv) the completeness of oxygen extraction in the active muscles (increased by augmentation of the capillary/muscle fibre ratio and by an increase in tissue enzyme concentrations); (v) the redirection of blood from viscera to the active muscles; and (vi) the demand for heat elimination via the cutaneous circulation (increased in obese and poorly trained subjects).

Ischaemic heart disease

Immediately following infarction, the arterial oxygen saturation may be limited by pulmonary oedema, collapse of the lungs (P.A. Valentine *et al.*, 1966) and a hunting of blood through poorly ventilated alveoli (G.J. Mackenzie *et al.*, 1964). This situation is normally corrected within four weeks of the acute episode. Nevertheless, if patients are recruited to an exercise rehabilitation programme some eight weeks after infarction, they may still show a 'hypokinetic' circulation, with an increased arterio-venous oxygen difference at rest and in sub-maximum effort (G.J. Mackenzie *et al.*, 1964; R. Malcroma & Varnauskas, 1964). In contrast, the maximum arterio-venous oxygen difference (130 $ml \cdot 1^{-1}$) remains at the lower end of normality (D.H. Paterson *et al.*, 1979).

In the first six months of rehabilitation, the arterio-venous oxygen difference in sub-maximum effort is unchanged (M. Frick & Katila, 1968; J.P. Clausen *et al.*, 1969; S. Degré *et al.*, 1972) or increased somewhat (E. Varnauskas *et al.*, 1966; D.H. Paterson *et al.*, 1979). Any increase may reflect a greater enzyme activity in the working muscles. At a year, the response is much as at the initial testing, with a marginal reduction of the maximum arterio-venous difference to about 127 $ml \cdot 1^{-1}$ (D.H. Paterson *et al.*, 1979).

Maximum Oxygen Intake

Normal values

The maximum oxygen intake provides perhaps the best overall estimate of cardio-respiratory performance (R.J. Shephard, 1977a). If data are expressed in units of ml O_2 STPD per kg of body mass per minute, typical values for Canadian city dwellers are as follows:

Age (years)	Men ($ml \cdot kg^{-1} \cdot min^{-1}$)	Women ($ml \cdot kg^{-1} \cdot min^{-1}$)
30-9	39.5	38.6
40-9	34.7	35.1
50-9	33.0	31.6
60-9	26.8	24.1

Rather similar standards have been proposed for the United States (American Heart Association, 1972).

The training response is influenced by the intensity of conditioning in relation to initial fitness, with lesser effects from the frequency and duration of effort and the total quantity of work performed (R.J. Shephard, 1968a, 1977a). If the training intensity is held constant, the half-time of the increase in maximum oxygen intake is about ten days. However, if the training plan is progressive, the increase in condition can extend over many weeks, particularly in older subjects with a poor initial status. The average change is about 20 per cent (R.J. Shephard, 1965, 1977a), but there are occasional reports of much larger gains.

Ischaemic heart disease

Following myocardial infarction, the peak oxygen intake for a man of 45-50 years is reduced to about 25 $ml \cdot kg^{-1} \cdot min^{-1}$ (Table 8.3), about 74 per cent of the Canadian standard, although this deficit can be made good by vigorous training (T. Kavanagh & Shephard, 1976). Angina without infarction is associated with a somewhat lower peak heart rate and peak oxygen intake. In subjects with a combination of angina and infarction, the peak oxygen intake drops to 15-20 $ml \cdot kg^{-1} \cdot min^{-1}$ ($\sim$ 50 per cent of the values encountered in sedentary Torontonians of the same age; C.G. Blomqvist & Mitchell, 1979).

A recent survey of 40 different cardiac rehabilitation experiments (D.H. Paterson, 1977) found a gain in maximum oxygen intake of up to ten per cent in nine studies, ten to 20 per cent in 22 studies, 20-30 per cent in seven studies and more than 30 per cent in the remaining two studies (Table 8.1). The typical response of the 'post-coronary' patient is thus not unlike that seen in a healthy adult. Variations of response reflect programme adherence (H.K. Hellerstein *et al.*, 1967; S.H. Saltzman *et al.*, 1969), fears of over-exertion on the part of patient or physician

Table 8.3: Exercise Tolerance in Patients with Angina Pectoris and/or Previous Myocardial Infarction

N	Age (year)	Peak oxygen intake (ml·kg⁻¹·min⁻¹)	Peak heart rate (beats·min⁻¹)	Time since infarction (months)	Functional impairment (%)*	Author
(a)	*Angina pectoris alone*					
549	52	22 (approx.)	148		27	R.A. Bruce et al. (1974a)
10	45-69	—	135		—	G.R. Dagenais et al. (1971)
19	40-58	—	119		38	R.P. Malmborg (1964)
(b)	*Myocardial infarction alone*					
21	50	25.0	150	20	17	A.M. Benestäd (1968)
16	—	26.8	163	3	11	A.M. Benestäd (1972)
249	50	25.0 (approx.)	156	—	17	R.A. Bruce et al. (1974a)
16	48	21.6	150	2-4	28	S. Degré & Denolin (1973)
15	45	24.6	161	3-5 (7-25)	18	T. Kavanagh & Shephard (1976)
(4 with angina pectoris)						
99	<57	24.9	164	3	17	H. Sanne (1973)
25	<57	26.3	169	12	12	H. Sanne (1973)
(c)	*Myocardial infarction plus angina pectoris*					
497	52	20 (approx.)	145	—	34	R.A. Bruce et al. (1974a)
7	52	—	135	—	53	J.P. Clausen et al. (1969)
10	48	15.6	135	2-4	48	S. Degré et al. (1973)
6	50	19.9	—	24	34	T. Kavanagh & Shephard (1975a)
19	40-58	—	123	—	38	R.P. Malmborg (1964)
71	<57	16.9	133	31	44	H. Sanne (1973)
27	<57	19.6	132	12	35	H. Sanne (1973)

* Relative to norms proposed by the American Heart Association (1972).

† Values are generally 'symptom-limited' rather than true plateaus of oxygen intake.

(A.J. Barry *et al.*, 1966), age (T. Kavanagh *et al.*, 1973b; K. Bergström *et al.*, 1974) and the presence or absence of exercise-induced angina (J.R. Detry *et al.*, 1971; S. Degré *et al.*, 1972; H. Sanne, 1973; M. Rousseau *et al.*, 1974; T. Kavanagh & Shephard, 1975a). In some studies (particularly those over short periods), there has been little change in control subjects (J. Naughton *et al.*, 1966; O. Pedersen-Bjergaard, 1971; T. Kavanagh *et al.*, 1973b; K. Bergström *et al.*, 1974; M. Rousseau *et al.*, 1974). In other, longer programmes, there have been similar gains in control and exercised subjects (Chapter 6; Table 8.4), implying either natural recovery of the oxygen-transport system or a contamination of control subjects by an interest in exercise. The exercised group show fairly rapid early gains, as the effects of bed rest are reversed (H. Sanne, 1973), but given a progressive regimen the response may continue for several years. Indeed, some of our patients who have participated in marathon events have not made dramatic gains of maximum oxygen intake until two or three years after infarction (T. Kavanagh *et al.*, 1977). Possibly, lack of confidence kept them from hard training in the first two years after their acute episode (A.J. Barry *et al.*, 1966). The response to training is less satisfactory in old than in younger patients (T. Kavanagh *et al.*, 1973b; Table 8.5). This is probably an expression of more severe disease and residual myocardial ischaemia in the older individuals. It is also possible that a lessening of financial and family commitments along with reduced physical expectations lessen the drive to vigorous training in an older person. If anginal pain is developed during exercise, training may give a larger than normal increase in symptom-limited performance (M. Rousseau *et al.*, 1974). On the other hand, if the response is assessed from a sub-maximum exercise test (for example, the predicted maximum oxygen intake; Table 8.6), there is plainly a very limited response of anginal patients to continuous endurance training. Nevertheless, such individuals can be treated quite effectively by a programme of modified interval training (H. Sanne, 1973; T. Kavanagh & Shephard, 1965a; Table 8.4). Gains of maximum oxygen intake are accompanied by a lesser reaction to a given intensity of sub-maximum effort (lesser increase in heart rate and respiratory minute volume, lesser increase in blood lactate; Figure 8.7).

Table 8.4: Early Recovery of Maximum Oxygen Intake Following Myocardial Infarction, Presented in the Form of Symptom-limited Maxima Expressed as Percent of Age- and Sex-specific Normal Mean Values

Time post infarction (weeks)		Symptom-limited maximum* (% of normal, mean ± range)	
3	(n = 50)	47	(25–72)
6	(n = 46)	56	(24–92)
13	(n = 38)	56	(31–97)
26	(n = 27)	58	(31–91)

* First test terminated at a heart rate of 130 beats·min^{-1} in the absence of symptoms.

Source: Based on data of A.J. Wohl *et al.* (1977).

Table 8.5: Influence of Patient Age upon Response to Endurance Training

	Maximum oxygen intake			
Group	Initial		After one year	After two years
	l·min^{-1} STPD	ml·kg^{-1}·min^{-1} STPD	l·min^{-1} STPD	l·min^{-1} STPD
All patients	1.98 ± 0.86	27.0 ± 9.4	+ 0.34 ± 0.69	+ 0.70 ± 0.63
Patients < 50 yrs	2.04 ± 0.65	26.4 ± 6.4	+ 0.32 ± 0.69	+ 0.92 ± 0.76
Patients > 50 yrs	1.89 ± 1.11	27.7 ± 12.6	+ 0.37 ± 0.73	+ 0.51 ± 0.47

Source: T. Kavanagh *et al.* (1973b).

Systemic Blood Pressure

Normal Values

Accurate measurements of systemic blood pressure are important to the assessment of: (i) myocardial performance (a sudden fall in systolic pressure during exercise is of ominous portent); and (ii) cardiac work rate.

Under resting conditions, pressures recorded from a standard sphygmomanometer cuff underestimate the true brachial systolic

Table 8.6: Response of Patients with Exercise-induced Angina to Continuous Endurance Training and Modified Interval Training

Type of patient	Predicted maximum oxygen intake, end year I[1] (ml•kg^{-1}•min^{-1})	Change induced by training year II[2] (ml•kg^{-1}•min^{-1})
Myocardial infarction		
group (a)	25.2	+ 10.7[3]
	± 5.8	± 7.8
group (b)	23.6	+ 6.4[4]
	± 7.0	± 7.3
Myocardial infarction with frequent exercise-induced angina	19.9	+ 9.0[4]
	± 7.4	± 8.1

1. During year I, all subjects attempted a progressive programme of endurance training.
2. During year II, six patients with frequent exercise-induced angina and 20 others were allocated to the interval-training programme.
3. Continuous endurance training.
4. Modified interval training.

Source: T. Kavanagh & Shephard (1975a).

pressure (recorded from in indwelling catheter) by some 10 mm Hg (1.5 kPa; S.N. Hunyor *et al.*, 1978). In contrast, the stethoscopic estimate of diastolic pressure is excessive, even if the point of disappearance of the Korotkov sounds ('fifth phase') rather than muffling ('fourth phase') is noted (J. Fabian *et al.*, 1975). From the viewpoint of cardiac work rate, aortic pressures are more important than peripheral readings, and pulse wave reflections may increase peripheral systolic values.

During exercise, much of the energy in the aorta is in kinetic form. It is important to include this component when examining myocardial performance. Kinetic energy can be detected by a centrally directed catheter and by a sphymomanometer cuff, but not by a laterally tapped or peripherally directed catheter (H.J. Marx *et al.*, 1967). The first two types of measurement indicate a progressive rise of blood pressure during exercise (Table 8.7), the magnitude of this change depending upon the type, intensity and duration of effort and the condition of the myocardium (H. Mellerowicz, 1962; I. Åstrand, 1965; P.O. Åstrand

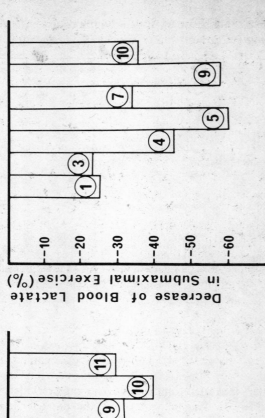

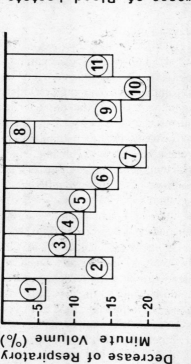

Figure 8.7: Influence of exercise rehabilitation upon respiratory minute volume and blood lactate during sub-maximal exercise, for 'post-coronary' patients. Authors: (1) E. Varnauskas (1966); (2) J. Naughton et al. (1966); (3) M.H. Frick & Katila (1968); (4) J.P. Clausen et al. (1970); (5) J.P. Clausen & Trap-Jensen (1970); (6) J.R. Detry et al. (1971); (7) S. Degré et al. (1972); (8) H. Bjernulf (1973); (9) H. Sanne (1973); (10) S. Degré & Denolin (1973); (11) M. Rousseau et al. (1974).

Source: Based on data accumulated by D.H. Paterson (1977).

Table 8.7: Increment in Systolic Blood Pressure (Δ, kPa) in Relation to Age and Work Rate

Age (years)	Work rate and Δ, kPa			
	4 Mets	6 Mets	8 Mets	10 Mets
20–9	3.3	4.8	6.3	7.8
30–9	3.3	5.3	7.2	8.9
40–9	3.5	5.7	6.8	8.1
50–9	3.9	6.4	8.5	10.5

Source: Based on data of S.M. Fox.

et al., 1965; J.S. Hanson *et al.*, 1968). The response to sub-maximal effort varies with the proportion of the maximum oxygen intake that is utilised. Increases of pressure are therefore larger in older subjects (H. Reindell *et al.*, 1960; J.S. Hanson *et al.*, 1968; G. Gerstenblith *et al.*, 1976) and in situations where there is difficulty in perfusing the active tissue (use of small muscles, particularly movements of the arms above the head; P.O. Åstrand *et al.*, 1965; S. Bevegard *et al.*, 1966; I. Åstrand, 1971; J. Schwade *et al.*, 1977; G.E. Adams *et al.*, 1978). Peripheral systolic readings of 180–240 mm Hg (24–32 kPa) may be anticipated with ten to 15 minutes of maximum effort (M. Masuda *et al.*, 1967), although the increase in central arterial pressure is smaller.

Since the maximum stroke volume and cardiac output both decrease with aging, one might have anticipated a lower maximum systemic blood pressure in an old person. However, because of loss of elasticity in the arterial walls, the pressure reached in maximum effort is often higher than in a young adult (A. Granath *et al.*, 1964; I. Åstrand, 1965; S; Julius *et al.*, 1967; I.S. Kasser & Bruce, 1969; L.T. Sheffield & Roitman, 1973). K.H. Sidney & Shephard (unpublished data) found a maximum peripheral systolic pressure of 217 ± 38 mm Hg (28.9 ± 5.1 kPa) in elderly men and 206 ± 32 mm Hg (27.5 ± 4.3 kPa) in elderly women performing maximum aerobic exercise.

Isometric effort gives a large and rapid increase both in systolic and diastolic pressures, with an accompanying tachycardia (A.R. Lind & McNicol, 1967; G.E. Adams *et al.*, 1978). Pressures first rise when the active muscles contract at more than 15 per cent of their maximum voluntary force. At intermediate intensities of effort (20–60 per cent of maximum force), the rate of rise of pressure varies with the intensity

Table 8.8: Systemic Blood Pressure at Rest and During Exercise to 75 Per Cent of Maximum Aerobic Power, Obtained in Patients before and after Three Years of Progressive Endurance Training

| | All patients (n = 553) | | Hypertensives (n = 141) | |
	Initial (mm Hg)	Final (mm Hg)	Initial (mm Hg)	Final (mm Hg)
Resting:				
systolic	133 ± 17	127 ± 15	161 ± 19	154 ± 12
diastolic	85 ± 9	87 ± 11	104 ± 9	103 ± 13
Exercising:				
systolic	169 ± 25	183 ± 29	172 ± 31	188 ± 30
diastolic	96 ± 13	96 ± 12	100 ± 12	99 ± 16
	(kPa)	(kPa)	(kPa)	(kPa)
Resting:				
systolic	17.7	16.9	21.5	20.6
diastolic	11.4	11.6	13.8	13.7
Exercising:				
systolic	22.5	24.5	22.9	25.0
diastolic	12.8	12.8	13.3	13.2

Source: Unpublished data of T. Kavanagh & Shephard.

of contraction, but the pressure at exhaustion is consistent (C.F. Funderburk *et al.*, 1974). A maximum effect is generally attained at 70–80 per cent of maximum voluntary force.

Ischaemic heart disease

Because of associated changes in the peripheral arteries (including the renal artery), many patients with ischaemic heart disease have some resting hypertension. Pulse-wave reflection is also increased, augmenting the central-peripheral pressure gradient.

Hypertension of itself may increase the rise of systemic pressure during sub-maximum exercise (A. Amery *et al.*, 1967). However, increased after-loading of the left ventricle reduces the maximum cardiac response to exercise (R. Sannerstedt, 1966; A. Amery *et al.*, 1967). Theoretically, the patient with coronary vascular disease should withstand such after-loading more poorly than a young person with essential hypertension (H.O. Wong *et al.*, 1969). In practice, the hypertension of ischaemic heart disease is often marginal, with correspondingly smaller haemodynamic consequences. Among one sample of 551 patients referred for exercise rehabilitation, T. Kavanagh & Shephard (Table 8.8) found just over a quarter of the group (141 patients) had a resting peripheral arterial pressure of over 150/100 mm Hg (20.0/13.3 kPa). The initial exercise response of the hypertensive patients was much as in those with a normal resting blood pressure. After an average of three years progressive endurance training, both groups showed a small (6–7 mm Hg) decrease in resting systolic pressure, but an increase in the systolic reading during exercise. The latter presumably reflects an increase of myocardial contractility – an expression of recovery from the acute episode plus a more specific response to prolonged endurance training (D.H. Paterson *et al.*, 1979).

Low maximum systolic pressures are commonly a warning of a deteriorating myocardium (I.S. Kasser & Bruce, 1969; L.T. Sheffield, 1974; M.H. Ellestad, 1975) and are associated with an increased risk of reinfarction (R.J. Shephard, 1979a). However, it remains difficult to disentangle a low maximum pressure due to symptom limitation of effort from a true impairment of myocardial contractility. A sudden drop in systolic pressure during the course of an exercise test is a particularly ominous sign. It suggests circulatory failure, and is an urgent indication to halt exercise while sustaining venous return (R.A. Bruce *et al.*, 1963; K.L. Andersen *et al.*, 1971).

Cardiac Work Rate

Normal values

The elements of cardiac work include 'useful' work carried out in pumping blood around the circulation and 'tension' work performed against intra-ventricular pressure (Chapter 4), plus smaller components due to basal metabolism. electrochemical reactions involved in activation of the heart muscle, the internal work of fibre shortening and energy dissipated in the heart sounds. The last four components normally account for less than two per cent of the total cardiac work, so that they can be ignored in clinical calculations (G. Blomqvist, 1974; E.F. Blick & Stein, 1977; C.R. Jorgensen *et al.*, 1977).

The useful work per heart beat $\dot{W}_a$ is given by the product of intraventricular pressure P_v and volume change ∂V, integrated between the diastolic point V_d and the systolic point V_s:

$$\dot{W}_a = \int_{V_d}^{V_s} P_v \cdot \delta v$$

To a first approximation this expression is equal to the mean ejection pressure times stroke volume. At rest, it amounts to 15 kPa (120 mm Hg) times 80 ml, or 1.2 N-m of useful work per beat. In vigorous exercise, there is an increase to perhaps 22.5 kPa (180 mm Hg) times 110 ml, or 2.5 N-m per beat in a sedentary person and perhaps 22.5 times 140 ml, or 3.2 N-m per beat in an athletic individual.

The tension work per heart beat $\dot{W}_b$ is normally much larger than the useful work. It is calculated from the tension T in the ventricular wall, integrated over the contraction phase of the cardiac cycle. A constant α is introduction into the equation so that units are the same as for useful work:

$$\dot{W}_b = \alpha \int_o^t T \cdot \delta t$$

Wall tension bears a complicated relationship to intraventricular pressure, since the myocardial fibres exhibit both helical and spherical arrangements (Streeter *et al.*, 1969; Jean *et al.*, 1972). One method of calculation modifies the formula of La Place (Chapter 4) to allow for the thickness of the ventricular walls (Mirsky, 1974):

$$T = \frac{P_v}{h} \left[\frac{R_1 \times R_2}{R_1 + R_2} \right]$$

where h is the wall thickness, and R_1 and R_2 are the principal radii of the heart. The efficiency ϵ of the heart is then given by

$$\epsilon = \frac{\dot{W}_a}{\dot{W}_a + \dot{W}_b}$$

An increase in systolic blood pressure (as occurs in prolonged isometric contraction) increases $\dot{W}_b$, thus lowering efficiency and increasing total cardiac work rate. If an increase in cardiac output is required (as in exercise), it is more economical to increase stroke volume (which has its main effect upon $\dot{W}_a$) than heart rate (which influences both $\dot{W}_a$ and $\dot{W}_b$). In practice, the effects of exercise are quite complex. There is usually an increase of myocardial contractility. The direct effect of this, demonstrated in isolated muscle, is to increase oxygen consumption per unit of time, but *in vivo* such an effect is often offset by some shortening of the contraction phase, with a decrease of diastolic volume and thus wall tension (E.H. Sonnenblick, 1971). Endurance training may lead to ventricular hypertrophy (Chapter 4), with a further reduction of tension work per unit of wall cross section.

Since tension work is difficult to measure directly, efficiency is often estimated from the ratio of useful work performed to oxygen consumed by the heart muscle. Useful work increases more than tension work during rhythmic activity. Nevertheless, the efficiency of the heart is no better than 15 per cent, even in maximum exercise (J. Scheuer *et al.*, 1974; A.M. Katz, 1977).

Simple clinical indicators of cardiac work rate were discussed in the previous chapter. Heart rate is an effective index only if work per beat remains constant (no change in stroke volume, blood pressure, contractility or heart size), while the usefulness of the rate-pressure product depends on the constancy of stroke volume, contractility and heart size; the rate-pressure product is normally an acceptable clinical tool, since tension work is the main component of cardiac work.

Attainment of a high rate-pressure product (> 35 m Hg/min) without symptoms or ECG abnormalities is a pointer to a normal coronary circulation. The limiting rate-pressure product is consistent in a given subject (B.F. Robinson, 1967), but unfortunately there is a large overlap of limiting values between subjects with and without angina pectoris (L.T. Sheffield & Roitman, 1973).

Ischaemic heart disease

The resting cardiac work rate is commonly higher in the 'post-coronary' patient than in a normal individual, as deconditioning leads to an increase in heart rate and a diminution in stroke volume. The adverse situation of the 'post-coronary' patient is also apparent during sub-maximum effort, when heart rate continues high and stroke volume low. The work-load of the heart may be further aggravated by cardiac dilatation (whether chronic, due to aneurysmal change, or acute, due to exercise-induced ischaemia of the myocardium).

During vigorous exercise, the coronary vessels of a cardiac patient are less able to dilate than in a normal individual, and there may be various symptoms and signs of local or general ischaemia (anginal pain, dysrhythmias, ST segmental depression and an output of lactate from the ventricles into the coronary circulation). The inner (endocardial) region of the ventricular wall is particularly vulnerable to oxygen lack, since: (i) the complex arrangement of the myocardial fibres creates maximal wall tensions in this zone; and (ii) the coronary arterial supply traverses a substantial thickness of contracting ventricular muscle (I. Mirsky, 1974). In consequence, myocardial infarcts are particularly frequent in the sub-endocardial zone.

At any given intensity of exercise, prolonged and vigorous rehabilitation leads to a reduction of between eight and 33 per cent in such indices of myocardial oxygen consumption as the rate-pressure product, the tension-time index and the triple product (E. Varnauskas, 1966; M.H. Frick & Katila, 1968; J.P. Clausen *et al.*, 1969; F. Kasch & Boyer, 1969; J.P. Clausen & Trap-Jensen, 1970; J.R. Detry *et al.*, 1971; M.H. Frick *et al.*, 1971; S. Degré *et al.*, 1972; B. Kirchheiner & Pedersen-Bjergaard, 1973). This reflects both a relative bradycardia and a lesser rise in blood pressure during exercise, these changes more than outweighing an increased ejection time (S.E. Epstein *et al.*, 1971). Sustained training may also increase the rate-pressure product that can be tolerated before exercise is halted by ischaemic manifestations — indeed, exercise-induced ST segmental depression sometimes disappears completely (T. Kavanagh *et al.*, 1973b).

At one time, it was hoped that a lessening of ST segmental depression might provide evidence of an improved collateral blood flow to hypoxic segments of myocardium. Unfortunately it is now realised that there are other possible explanations of such a change, including a lessening of ventricular dilatation and a reduced wall tension per unit of cross section as the myocardium hypertrophies.

Radiographic estimates of heart volume have shown no significant change with the training of 'post-coronary' patients (E. Varnauskas *et al.*, 1966; P. Rechnitzer *et al.*, 1967; M.H. Frick & Katila, 1968; J.P. Clausen *et al.*, 1969; S. Degré *et al.*, 1972; H. Sanne, 1973). However, an increase in ventricular wall thickness may be inferred from: (i) an increase in left-ventricular end-diastolic pressure measurements (M.H. Frick & Katila, 1968); and (ii) ultrasonic measurements (M.H. Frick, 1969).

Coronary Circulation

Normal values

The resting coronary blood flow of a normal young adult amounts to about five per cent of cardiac output, or 300 ml·min^{-1}. There is a correspondingly rich capillary supply (2,500–3,000 vessels per mm^2 of fibre section, compared with 200 per mm^2 in resting and 600 per mm^2 in active skeletal muscle).

Oxygen extraction within the heart wall is relatively complete, blood from the coronary sinus having an oxygen content of only 15–50 ml·l^{-1}, compared with the normal 'mixed' venous oxygen content of 150 ml·l^{-1} (E. Varnauskas & Holmberg, 1971). Although haemo-concentration allows a small increase in coronary arterio-venous oxygen difference during exercise (K. Kitamura *et al.*, 1972; R.R. Nelson *et al.*,

1974), the main adaptation to the increased oxygen demand of physical activity comes from an increase in coronary blood flow. The situation of the myocardium is somewhat precarious, since the heart cannot accumulate any significant oxygen debt (A.S. Most *et al.*, 1969; K. Wildenthal *et al.*, 1976). Measurements made upon experimental animals show a three- to six-fold increase in coronary blood flow during vigorous exercise (R. Gorlin, 1971; S.F. Vatner *et al.*, 1972; R.M. Ball *et al.*, 1975; T.M. Sanders *et al.*, 1975). In man, studies have been limited to moderate work rates, but a capacity for a five-fold increase in blood flow may be inferred from responses to vasodilator drugs such as dipyridamole (M. Tauchert *et al.*, 1972). Since the cardiac work rate increases six-fold in maximum effort, a combination of maximum vasodilatation and a small increase in coronary arterio-venous oxygen difference is essential if myocardial hypoxia is not to develop during maximum effort. Nevertheless, there seems a small margin of safety in a healthy person. The maximum heart rate and blood pressure are well sustained even if hypoxic gas mixtures are inspired during vigorous effort (L.E. Lamb *et al.*, 1969), and cardiac performance is also unaffected by the shift of blood flow from sub-endocardial to sub-epicardial tissue during vigorous activity (R.M. Ball *et al.*, 1975; T.M. Sanders *et al.*, 1975).

Ischaemic heart disease

Coronary atherosclerosis limits myocardial perfusion if the lumen of a major vessel is narrowed or blocked by an atheromatous plaque, or fibrosed, calcified vessels fail to undergo the five-fold dilatation seen in a healthy young adult.

Studies correlating coronary angiograms with clinical indices of ischaemia (anginal pain, ST segmental depression and limitations of myocardial performance) suggest that two thirds of a major vessel must be occluded before there is a serious restriction of regional blood flow. Several factors contribute to this finding: (i) obstruction usually develops in the major arteries, but the main resistance to blood flow lies in smaller vessels; (ii) flow resistance is proportional to the fourth power of vessel radius; (iii) apparent narrowing of a main artery can arise from technical problems in the angiogram (filling defects); and (iv) reversible spasm of the coronary vessels (R.C. Schlant, 1974) may develop during angiography.

Methods of evaluating the adequacy of perfusion during exercise include: (i) examination of the ST segment of the electrocardiogram; (ii) various applications of nuclear cardiology; (iii) estimation of lactate levels in coronary sinus blood (F.K. Nakhjavan *et al.*, 1975); and (iv) evaluation of myocardial function during graded exercise. Oxygen lack rapidly leads to a reduction of myocardial contractility and pump failure (A.M. Katz, 1973).

The left-ventricular systolic pressure is usually five to six times larger than that in the right ventricle. The left-ventricular wall is thus much more vulnerable to hypoxia. Its direct blood flow and any collateral supply is delivered almost entirely during diastole (S. Holmberg *et al.*, 1971; B.G. Brown *et al.*, 1972). During exercise, there is a rise in left-ventricular systolic pressure. This facilitates blood flow to the right ventricle, but increases tension in the left-ventricular wall, ensuring that perfusion is restricted to the shortened diastolic phase of the cardiac cycle. Women generally have thinner heart walls than men, but develop a similar maximum systolic pressure; the tension per unit of cross section is thus greater in the female, and this may explain their propensity to 'ischaemic' electrocardiographic appearances (G.R. Cumming *et al.*, 1973; K.H. Sidney & Shephard, 1977b; Figure 7.6; Table 7.9) despite the rarity of vascular narrowing at angiography. Both sexes usually show a sharp fall in diastolic pressure on ceasing exercise, and the resultant decrease in left-ventricular perfusion probably accounts for the frequency of ST depression and dysrhythmias during the early phase of recovery from physical activity.

A combination of exercise and cold exposure is particularly likely to precipitate myocardial ischaemia in a patient with some limitation of coronary blood flow. One possible reason is that the cold air induces a cutaneous vaso-constriction, thus increasing systemic blood pressure and cardiac work load. This general effect is augmented by a more specific cold pressor response (E.M. Glaser, 1966; J. LeBlanc, 1975). Exercise also induces mouth-breathing at a ventilation of 35–40 $l \cdot min^{-1}$ (V. Niinimaa *et al.*, 1980), and it is then possible that a reflex coronary spasm analogous to the Bezold-Jarisch reflex arises from a stimulation of vagal receptors in the air passages (J.G. Widdicombe, 1974). Certainly, the heart has a large autonomic nerve supply, although there is little evidence that sympathetic or parasympathetic nerve fibres contribute to the normal exercise-induced vasodilatation (O. Lundgren & Jodal, 1975). Some authors have thus argued that the angina experienced when jogging on a frosty morning reflects a poor coronary reserve rather than a specific reflex activation of the coronary vasomotor nerves (W.A. Neill *et al.*, 1974).

The immediate treatment of angina is commonly administration of an organic nitrite such as amyl nitrite or the longer acting glyceryl trinitrate. It was once thought that such compounds acted by dilating the coronary vessels (T.V. Brunton, 1871). However, a more important factor is the lowering of systemic pressure. This reduces the work load of the heart, and at the same time facilitates coronary perfusion by easing external compression of the coronary arteries (J.C. Krantz *et al.*, 1962).

Smoking has several adverse effects upon the myocardial oxygen supply (Chapter 2). Heart rate, and thus cardiac work rate, is increased both during rest and exercise (A. Rode *et al.*, 1972). Nicotine is also a coronary vaso-constrictor, so that exercise-induced myocardial ischaemia at a given rate-pressure product tends to be augmented by the smoking of cigarettes with a substantial nicotine delivery (W.S. Aronow *et al.*, 1968; G.R. Wright & Shephard, 1978). The associated dose of carbon monoxide reduces immediate oxygen delivery for a given coronary perfusion and, at least in high doses, a CO-induced shift in the oxyhaemoglobin dissociation curve may facilitate the formation of atherosclerotic plaques (P. Åstrup, 1977).

9 EXERCISE PRESCRIPTION AND ISCHAEMIC HEART DISEASE

We have already noted (Chapter 3) that excessive physical activity can provoke a heart attack. On the other hand, there is a threshold intensity of effort below which no training response occurs. The physician who is prescribing exercise for the 'coronary-prone' individual must thus make a nice judgement between the safety and the therapeutic effectiveness of the regimen he is advocating.

In this chapter, we shall look at appropriate activity prescriptions for the secondary and tertiary prevention of ischaemic heart disease, and will consider the issues of compliance and safety.

Exercise Prescription in Secondary Prevention

Training threshold

Possible mechanisms by which regular exercise could prevent the clinical manifestations of ischaemic heart disease are reviewed in Chapter 4. The most important aspect of training from the viewpoint of prevention and therapy seems to be the development of endurance fitness (as indicated by an increase in maximum oxygen intake). It is in this context that we shall discuss the 'training threshold'.

Many authors cite the classical experiments of M.J. Karvonen *et al.* (1957), inferring from these observations that the minimum intensity of physical activity needed to induce conditioning is that associated with a heart rate of 140 beats·min^{-1}, or an oxygen consumption that is 60 per cent of maximum. In fact, Karvonen examined one specific situation (young men running upon a treadmill for 30 minutes, four or five times per week); training was observed at a terminal heart rate of 160–180 beats·min^{-1}, but not at 135 beats·min^{-1}.

When applying such observations to a middle-aged, coronary-prone population, we must note that maximum heart rate decreases with age. A 45-year-old man thus reaches 60 per cent of maximum oxygen intake at a lower heart rate than his 25-year-old counterpart. Furthermore, initial fitness is often poor in a middle-aged person, and this probably lowers the training threshold (R.J. Shephard, 1968a). It seems logical that if exercise is rarely undertaken at 50 per cent of maximum oxygen

232

intake, this can become an effective training stimulus (R.J. Shephard, 1967a).

The nature of the interaction between the duration of activity and the training threshold is also poorly understood. P.O. Åstrand (1967) suggested that 30 minutes of activity, five times per week, was necessary to initiate training. Others have claimed that, if the intensity of exercise is substantially greater than 60 per cent of maximum oxygen intake, then the minimum period of training can be shortened, possibly to as little as five minutes per day (C. Bouchard *et al.*, 1966; K.H. Cooper, 1968; R.J. Shephard, 1968a). A brief training session is of interest to the over-worked businessman, but from the viewpoint of safety there are attractions to a more extended, low-intensity programme. Physiologists commonly examine training responses after a fixed time interval such as twelve weeks, but there is evidence that, ultimately, equal gains of physical condition can be achieved by less frequent and/or less intense activity sessions (K.H. Sidney & Shephard, 1978).

Optimum prescription

Given current ignorance about training thresholds, any exercise prescription is at best an educated guess, and it scarcely merits the mystery with which it has sometimes been surrounded.

The aim should be a gradual but steady progression of endurance activity to the point where at least 60 per cent of maximum oxygen intake is being developed for 30 minutes, four or five times per week. A simple guide to a suitable starting point for a given subject can be obtained by using the self-administered version of the Canadian Home Fitness Kit (R.J. Shephard, 1980a). The time (T, min) to cover one mile (1.6 km) is given by the formula:

$$T = 44.7 - 0.45\, V_{O_2} - 12.3H + 0.015M$$

where $\dot{V}_{O_2}$ is 60 per cent of the maximum oxygen intake as predicted from the Canadian Home Fitness Test score; H is the standing height in metres: and M is the body mass in kg. Thus, a man with a $\dot{V}_{O_2\,(max)}$ of 40 ml·kg^{-1}·min^{-1}, a height of 1.7 m and a mass of 70 kg would be required to cover 1.6 km in 14.0 min, while an older subject of the same size but with a $\dot{V}_{O_2\,(max)}$ of 20 ml·kg^{-1}·min^{-1} would be allowed 19.4 min to complete the same prescription.

Fast walking is a safe and effective method of accomplishing the required effort in an older person. It has some advantages over jogging. The dangers of slipping and ankle injury are smaller when walking, while the forces transmitted from the ground to the ankle, knee and spine are only a third or a half of those developed in jogging and running.

Other activities that involve a large proportion of the body musculature such as swimming, cross-country skiing and cycling provide useful alternative forms of exercise. However, regulation of the intensity of activity is more difficult than for walking or jogging. K.H. Cooper (1968) attempted to equate various sports in terms of their training effects, using a 'points' scheme. His system can give some guidance to the layman who is planning his own programme; nevertheless, there remains considerable uncertainty as to the relative value of brief intense activity versus more sustained but leisurely pastimes, and participants seem to earn their 'points' more easily in some sports than in others (Massie *et al.*, 1970). Other texts provide tables showing the average energy cost of various sports (Table 9.1), but again such figures can be rather misleading, since: (i) energy costs increase exponentially with the speed of movement; and (ii) there are large inter-individual differences in mechanical efficiency and thus the energy costs of most sports. Light palpation of the carotid artery during or immediately following a burst of movement provides a fair check that the intensity of activity lies in the prescriptive zone, although due note must be taken of the effects upon the exercise heart rate of: (i) isometric contractions; (ii) excitement; (iii) heat; and (iv) recent smoking. I say 'light palpation' because it has been suggested that over-vigorous palpation of the carotid artery can cause: (i) slowing of the heart rate; and (ii) loss of consciousness through compression of the carotid sinus (J.R. White, 1977). Recent reports indicate that such risks are small and outweighed by the ease of counting the carotid pulse rate during exercise (G.W. Gardner *et al.*, 1979).

Other factors to be considered in recommending activity to a patient include: (i) his skills and interests; (ii) his personality (group versus solitary pursuits); (iii) available local facilities; and (iv) possibilities for pursuit of the prescription as a family. Where possible, a substantial part of the activity should be built into the normal day — for instance, a fast 2-km walk to the subway is less easily forgotten than is the requirement to cover an equivalent distance at a gymnasium. Electrical equipment such as lawn mowers and snow-blowers can be replaced by muscle power, and stairs can be used in place of an elevator. Fardy & Ilmarinen (1975) showed that a man could increase his aerobic power substantially by deliberate climbing of at least 25 flights of stairs per

Table 9.1: Classification of Various Recreational Activities

Light activity (12–20 kJ•min^{-1})*	Moderate activity (20–40 kJ•min^{-1})*	Heavy activity (40–80 kJ•min^{-1})*
Archery	Badminton	Athletics
Billiards	Canoeing	Basketball
Bowls	Recreational cycling	Boxing
Cricket	Dancing	Climbing
Golf	Gardening	Competitive running
Table tennis	Gymnastics	Association football
Recreational volleyball	Field hockey	Rowing
Walking	Horse riding	Squash rackets
	Jogging	
	Recreational cross-country skiing	
	Downhill skiing	
	Recreational swimming	
	Tennis	

* The energy cost depends greatly on the pace of performance, and the skill of the participant and of other players. In most activities, energy expenditures also vary almost linearly with body mass. The figures cited are for a young adult, but a lower energy expenditure may be heavy effort for an older person.

Source: Based in part on data of J.V.G. Durnin & Passmore (1967).

day. A London bus conductor ascends up to 60 flights of stairs per day (J.N. Morris, personal communication), and this may be one reason why he develops less heart attacks than the driver of the same vehicle.

The average middle-aged exerciser does not normally need specific routines to develop his muscle strength. Sufficient training of the body musculature is obtained from aerobic activity. Sustained isometric effort is indeed best avoided by the middle-aged adult. Isometrics induce an undesirable immediate increase in systemic blood pressure, and may add to the long-term work of the heart by encouraging an unnecessary development of the chest and shoulder muscles.

The total exercise prescription should include a brief (between five and ten minutes) warm-up and warm-down, plus advice on other changes of lifestyle. The warm-up is intended to minimise the risk of cardiac dysrhythmia (R.J. Barnard *et al.*, 1973) and skeletal injury; it usually takes the form of progressive calisthenics, including gentle stretching exercises that improve flexibility. The warm-down sustains venous return during the early recovery period. Fluid is returned from the muscles to the central circulation, avoiding a precipitous fall in blood pressure and minimising post-exercise stiffness. Slow walking is suitable for this purpose.

Whatever form of activity is prescribed, the patient should feel no more than pleasantly tired on the following day. If there are severe residual symptoms, then the training plan is too vigorous. The coronary-prone individual with an aggressive ('Type A') personality may need strong warnings to compete only against himself, not exceeding the stipulated dose of physical activity. Because a 2-km walk is good for his health, he must not assume that a 4-km run is even better! On the other hand, the training plan must show progression, the duration and/or the intensity of exercise being increased every few weeks as the patient adapts to his current prescription. Regular assessment of fitness, whether by a paramedical professional or by the Canadian Home Fitness Test (R.J. Shephard, 1980a), provides an objective indication of the progress that has been realised. Such 'feed-back' is important to motivation of the subject and gives appropriate guidance for upward adjustment of the prescription.

Specific prescriptions

The general pattern of training discussed above should induce a substantial increase in aerobic power — at least 20 per cent in an average adult (R.J. Shephard, 1965), with larger gains in those who train exceedingly hard or who have previously lived very sedentary lives. Individual modification of the basic prescription may be needed to correct particular risk factors such as obesity, and to induce the development of specific muscle groups.

An obese patient may initially be incapable of sustaining high-intensity activity. Nevertheless, an extended programme of moderate activity (for example, progression to one hour of deliberate walking per day) may achieve a small negative energy balance, with gradual correction of the obesity. In a typical older person, an hour of deliberate fast walking four days per week for a year is sufficient to eliminate three quarters of the body fat accumulated between the ages of 25 and 65 years (K.H. Sidney & Shephard, 1978).

Deliberate muscular development is normally unnecessary for a middle-aged adult. However, if a person's work calls for the occasional performance of very heavy work by the arms and shoulder girdle, specific training of the muscles concerned will minimise the resultant rise in systemic blood pressure and thus in cardiac work rate during the activity. Specific development of the knee or the back muscles may also be helpful if there is a previous history that regular exercise was hampered by musculo-skeletal problems in these areas. The maximum isometric force of a muscle can apparently be increased by contractions lasting no longer than six seconds (T. Hettinger, 1961) and, if adequate rest intervals are allowed, isometric training can be performed without either skeletal injury or an excessive rise in systemic blood pressure.

Pulse-rate palpation

The accuracy of self-determined Canadian Home Fitness Test scores and the subsequent regulation of training intensity depend upon the ability of the ordinary middle-aged adult to count his pulse rate with reasonable accuracy (R.J. Shephard, 1980a).

In the original Saskatoon trial of the Canadian Home Fitness Test, subjects were given no specific instruction in pulse counting, and relatively large errors occurred; the coefficient of correlation between cardiotachometer readings and palpated rates was only 0.50. M. Jetté *et al.* (1976) taught their subjects to count the pulse 'until they could do this accurately'. Average readings immediately following vigorous exercise were 154 ± 22 as measured from the ECG and 147 ± 23 as obtained by palpation (difference = 7.0 ± 5.6). D. Bailey & Mirwald (1975) found a similar discrepancy (average of ECG readings, 135, average of palpated values 127 beats·min^{-1}) when they tested children aged between eleven and 14 who were used to counting their pulse (track and speed-skating contestants). In the latter experiments, the coefficient of correlation between measured and palpated readings was 0.94 for the athletes, but only 0.37 for children with no previous experience in pulse counting. We have recently observed similar results when testing office workers in Toronto (Table 9.2).

Although it is undoubtedly possible to find subjects who are inept at pulse counting (G.R. Cumming & Glenn, 1977; A. Bonen *et al.*, 1977), the majority of adults make a reasonable estimate of their heart rate. Accuracy is improved by use of the carotid rather than the radial pulse and by a modest amount of practice. Perhaps because of greater motivation, and perhaps because they have received more careful instruction, 'post-coronary' patients make a particularly valid assessment of their heart rates (W.R. Duncan *et al.*, 1968); T. Kavanagh & Shephard, unpublished data).

Table 9.2: Relationship between Heart Rate as Measured by ECG and Palpated Pulse Rate for Office Workers Carrying Out Canadian Home Fitness Test with Only the Instructions Provided on the Jacket of the Record

	ECG-measured heart rate (beats·min^{-1})*	Palpated pulse rate (beats·min^{-1})	Difference (beats·min^{-1})	Coefficient of correlation (r)
Rest	75.8 ± 10.6	75.8 ± 12.9	0.1 ± 11.3	0.55
Test stage I	125.6 ± 18.4	119.6 ± 25.8	5.9 ± 20.1	0.63
Test stage II	142.8 ± 17.2	138.8 ± 24.8	4.0 ± 18.1	0.68
Test stage III	148.7 ± 16.1	141.8 ± 19.1	6.9 ± 20.6	0.33

*　The time was measured for the ECG complexes presented during the ten-second counting interval.

Source: Shephard, Cox, Corey & Smyth (in preparation).

Exercise Prescription in Tertiary Prevention

Hospital phase

At one time, coronary patients followed a regimen of strict bed rest while in hospital. It was feared that the slightest physical activity might precipitate rupture of the weakened segment of ventricular wall. However, it is now realised that such a 'cardiac tamponade' is a rare complication of myocardial infarction. The majority of deaths occur in the first 24 hours after the acute episode, the usual cause being a dysrhythmia of sudden onset, or the progressive development of left-ventricular failure. If cardiac rhythm is normal and there is an adequate systemic blood pressure, the prognosis improves rapidly thereafter.

Exercise is best begun early, when the patient is most amenable to recommendations for a change of lifestyle. This allows hospital staff to supervise the early phases of rehabilitation. Treatment should commence within 24 hours of infarction, assuming there are no signs of heart failure, shock, intractable pain or persistent dysrhythmias (J. Acker, 1973; L.L. Brook, 1973; N.K. Wenger, 1973; L.R. Zohman, 1973).

Over the first week, activity is limited to an intensity of about 10 kJ·min^{-1}. The patient commences by sitting at 45° in his bed, feeding himself, and carrying out light exercises for individual muscle groups. By the end of the week, he is able to sit in a chair for three one-hour periods per day.

During the second and third weeks, activity is gradually increased, with occasional peaks to 16 kJ·min^{-1}. The patient attends to his personal toilet and carries out light craftwork. Walking begins, and by the third week he is covering 30 metres per trip. Each new stage of activity is initiated before rather than after a meal, and where possible it is monitored by ECG.

In the fourth week, the patient walks 0.8–1.0 km at a stretch, and returns to his home or a convalescent facility (O.A. Brusis, 1977). If progress is maintained, the pre-infarction level of activity should be reached at about eight weeks. The patient is then qualified to resume most types of daily work, and can also contemplate further training through a specific out-patient rehabilitation programme.

Outpatient phase

On recruitment to an outpatient programme, the average patient has recovered sufficient physical condition to allow performance of a standard sub-maximal laboratory stress test. This is usually carried to a target heart rate (75 or 85 per cent of maximum oxygen intake), although most patients can continue activity to a symptom-limited maximum without excessive risk (R.A. Bruce *et al.*, 1973; T. Kavanagh & Shephard, 1976). Laboratory evaluation allows the supervising physician: (i) to define an intensity of activity that is tolerated without excessive ST segmental depression or dysrhythmias; (ii) to prescribe a dose of endurance exercise appropriate for further conditioning; and (iii) to establish a 'bench-mark' for subsequent monitoring of progress.

In the first six to eight weeks of outpatient therapy, the patient should attend two or three closely monitored exercise class sessions per week. He should also exercise himself to a total of five sessions per week. In the supervised sessions, he learns the theory of walking and jogging, including such matters as an appropriate choice of clothing and footwear. The technique of pulse counting is demonstrated, and an assistant checks that the subject is recording an accurate estimate of his heart rate. If abnormal rhythms or deep ST segmental depression develop during exercise, the patient is taught to recognise the corresponding sensations, and he is counselled to halt exercise briefly until such symptoms pass. As in a healthy adult, the endurance prescription is based on both general condition and the maximum oxygen intake as determined during laboratory testing. A typical recommendation for a patient with obesity, low back-pain, osteo-arthritis of the knees or moderately impaired oxygen transport (maximum oxygen intake of less than 16 ml·kg^{-1}·min^{-1}) calls for a progressive extension of the required walking distance over the eight weeks (T. Kavanagh, 1976):

Weeks 1–2	1.6 km in 30 minutes
Weeks 3–4	2.4 km in 42 minutes
Weeks 5–6	3.2 km in 50 minutes
Weeks 7–8	4.0 km in 57.5 minutes

If the initial maximum oxygen intake is greater than $16 \text{ ml} \cdot \text{kg}^{-1} \cdot \text{min}^{-1}$, the preliminary period can be shortened to six weeks. For example, with a maximum oxygen intake of 21.4–$22.7 \text{ ml} \cdot \text{kg}^{-1} \cdot \text{min}^{-1}$, a patient aged 42 might commence by covering 1.6 km in 17 minutes; he would progress to 3.2 km in 34 minutes for weeks 3–4, and 4.8 km in 51 minutes for weeks 5–6. Starting levels for other degrees of disability are shown in Table 9.3.

The patient may move to a higher intensity of training when his existing prescription has been well tolerated for at least two weeks. Requirements include: (i) an exercise heart rate consistently below the target value (equivalent to 60 per cent of maximum oxygen intake; Table 9.4); and (ii) no signs of over-training such as muscular aches and pains, excessive tiredness or premature ventricular contractions. If maximum effort is 'symptom-limited' (anginal pain, premature ventricular contractions or deep ST segmental depression) the target heart rate is proportionately reduced (to a figure equivalent to 60 per cent of the symptom-limited maximum oxygen intake; Table 9.4) and progression to a higher intensity of effort is not attempted until the exercise heart rate has fallen at least $10 \text{ beats} \cdot \text{min}^{-1}$ below the modified target value.

When the patient has reached the fastest walking time of Table 9.3, he is ready to progress to Table 9.5. He now follows the training pattern adopted by long-distance runners — firstly a quickening of pace with some shortening of the running time, and then a lengthening of the training session at a constant running speed ($9.6 \text{ km} \cdot \text{h}^{-1}$ if under age 45 years, and $8.0 \text{ km} \cdot \text{h}^{-1}$ if over the age of 45 years). Criteria for progression follow the pattern already discussed. At a speed between 6.4 and $7.2 \text{ km} \cdot \text{h}^{-1}$ (depending on height and leg length) most patients find it convenient to pass from fast walking to jogging. Since the latter activity involves a rather different group of leg muscles to those used in walking, the change is introduced gradually at an appropriate point in the prescription. The patient begins by jogging 15 seconds out of each minute in order to make his required

Table 9.3: Relationship between Initial Maximum Oxygen Intake and Exercise Prescription for 'Post-coronary' Patients

Maximum oxygen intake (ml kg^{-1}•min^{-1} STPD)	Walking time (min)*
16.1–17.5	60
17.6–18.4	57
18.5–21.3	54
21.4–22.7	51
22.8–25.6	48
25.7–28.5	45
> 28.6	42

* All times are for a walking distance of 4.8 km; however, for weeks 1-2, 1.6 km and for weeks 3-4, 3.2 km should be covered at the same pace. An additional three minutes should be allowed if the patient is more than 45 years old.

Source: T. Kavanagh (1976).

Table 9.4: Target Heart Rate for Training of the Post-coronary Patient

Age (years)	Maximum heart rate (beats•min^{-1})	Target heart rate* (beats•min^{-1})
25	195	147
30	190	144
35	185	141
40	180	138
45	175	135
50	170	132
55	165	129
60	160	126
65	155	123

* The target is equivalent to 60 per cent of maximum oxygen intake, based on a conservative estimate of maximum heart rate (220 − age, years) and a resting heart rate of 75 beats•min^{-1}. If the resting heart rate deviates by 10 beats•min^{-1} from this standard, the target heart rate must be correspondingly adjusted upwards or downwards by 6 beats•min^{-1}. If the maximum heart rate is limited by symptoms such as angina, frequent premature ventricular contractions, or deep downward sloping ST segmental depression, the target heart rate is set at 60 per cent of this symptom-limited maximum oxygen intake. For example, if the symptom-limited heart rate at age 45 years is reduced by 15 beats•min^{-1} (160 instead of 175 beats•min^{-1}), the target heart rate is reduced by 60 per cent of 15, i.e., 9 beats•min^{-1}.

Table 9.5: Further Stages in the Training of the 'Post-coronary' Patient

Age < 45 years			Age > 45 years		
Distance (km)	Time (min)	Speed (km•h^{-1})	Distance (km)	Time (min)	Speed (km•h^{-1})
4.4	36.5	7.2	4.4	41	6.4
4.4	35	7.5	4.4	39	6.7
4.4	34	7.8	4.4	37.5	7.0
4.4	33	8.0	4.4	36.5	7.2
4.4	31	8.5	4.4	35	7.5
4.0	27	8.9	4.0	31	7.7
4.0	26	9.2	3.2	24	8.0
3.2	20	9.6	4.0	30	8.0
4.0	25	9.6	4.4	33	8.0
4.4	27.5	9.6	4.8	36	8.0
4.8	30	9.6	4.8	36	8.0
5.2	32.5	9.6	5.2	39	8.0
5.6	35	9.6	5.6	42	8.0
6.0	37.5	9.6	6.0	45	8.0
6.4	40	9.6	6.4	48	8.0
6.8	42.5	9.6	6.8	51	8.0
7.2	45	9.6	7.2	54	8.0
7.6	47.5	9.6	7.6	57	8.0
8.0	50	9.6	8.0	60	8.0

Source: T. Kavanagh (1976).

average speed. He then progresses to 30 seconds jogging and 30 seconds walking before attempting to cover all of the required distance at a jog.

Other activities may be substituted for jogging, particularly if this is made necessary by musculo-skeletal problems or by an adverse outdoor climate. An equivalent intensity of activity may be established with the guidance of data such as Table 9.1 and the resultant heart rate. If a different set of muscles are to be used (for example, a transition from outdoor jogging to indoor rope skipping), some temporary moderation of the prescription is desirable.

Class organisation

The general pattern of the 'post-coronary' exercise class is much as in a programme for a healthy person — a typical routine including five or ten minutes of calisthenics for 'warm-up' and flexibility, the prescribed endurance exercise, a 'fun' activity such as a game of recreational volleyball in order to increase motivation and a gentle warm-down. Each class is preceded by a short discussion period, when patients can review problems of training and lifestyle that are of interest to the group. Those with unusual symptoms are asked to report this to the supervising physician; they may undergo a full clinical examination and even laboratory testing before admission to the class session. One important function of the supervised class is to evaluate how the patient is reacting to his prescribed exercise. Where necessary, obscure symptoms can be evaluated by telemetry; for example, it may be necessary to distinguish the arm pain of angina from that due to osteo-arthritis. The patient must be kept under close observation not only while exercising, but also during the recovery period. Two of our patients developed ventricular fibrillation shortly after exercise, one whole standing in a hot and rather humid shower area, and the other sitting awaiting a taxi to return home. Finally, discussion periods should be arranged for the patients' wives — often spouses become more tense and anxious than the patients themselves, and they will pose many questions at such sessions, ranging from problems of dietary modification to appropriate modes of sexual expression (T. Kavanagh & Shephard, 1977b; Table 9.6).

We advise a patient who has graduated from the preparatory class to attend the Toronto Rehabilitation Centre once a week, carrying out a further four sessions of prescribed exercise on his own. This pattern of conditioning strikes a reasonable balance between the need for careful supervision of the patient and the physical problems of driving to and from an outpatient centre in a large city. Adherence to the home prescription is checked by having the patient bring an 'exercise-log' to the Centre at each visit. The log lists the walking or jogging distances actually covered each day, times, pulse rates before and after exercise and any unusual circumstances (Figure 9.1).

After a year of weekly attendance at the Rehabilitation Centre, we promote the patient to an eight-week inter-class interval. This is made necessary by problems of logistics. A visit to the Centre every two months provides an opportunity to review progress and discuss symptoms. In general, it also gives sufficient motivation to sustain the initial gains of training, although there is relatively little further progress after transfer to this type of regimen (Table 9.7). Indeed, in some patients ST segment depression is increased.

Table 9.6: Wives' Appraisal of Patients' Attitudes to Sexual Activity and to Other Socio-economic Problems

Characteristic	Normal or increased sexual activity, $n = 51$ (% showing characteristic)	Decreased sexual activity, $n = 49$ (% showing characteristic)
Patient takes less responsibility in marriage	52.9	79.5
Decrease in living standards (social, domestic or financial)	39.2	59.1
Prone to symptom claiming	27.4	57.1
Insecure in employment	15.6	38.7
Depressed	7.9	26.2

Source: T. Kavanagh & Shephard (1977b).

Table 9.7: Response of Post-coronary Patients to Infrequently Supervised Exercise

Variable	Group A (training already plateaued)		Group B (condition still improving)	
	Initial value	Change over one year[1]	Initial value	Change over one year[3]
Maximum oxygen intake:				
($l \cdot min^{-1}$)	2.02 ± 0.66	0.00 ± 0.45	2.02 ± 0.42	$+0.12 \pm 0.46$
($ml \cdot kg^{-1} \cdot min^{-1}$)	27.5 ± 8.2	-0.7 ± 6.2	25.7 ± 4.5	$+1.4 \pm 5.5$
ST depression (mV at comparable heart rate)	-0.03 ± 0.15^{2}	0.07 ± 0.13^{2}	0.01 ± 0.12	0.10 ± 0.12

1. Training sustained in 23 of 30 patients.
2. Sample initially showed small elevation of ST segment on average; positive change indicates worsening of condition.
3. Training sustained in 16 of 19 patients.

Source: Based on data of T. Kavanagh & Shephard (1980).

Figure 9.1: An example of an 'exercise-log' for monitoring prescribed exercise.

Day	Type of exercise	Distance (km)	Time (min, s)	10-second pulse count (before exercise)	(after exercise)	Symptoms and comments
Sunday	Jogging	5.6	40.10	11	21	–
Monday	Jogging	5.6	40.15	12	22	Slight tightness in chest
Tuesday	Jogging	5.6	40.00	10	20	Had a good day
Wednesday	Jogging	5.6	40.04	11	21	–
Thursday	Rest day	–	–	–	–	–
Friday	Jogging	5.6	40.10	11	21	–
Saturday	Rest day	–	–	–	–	–

S.M. Fox (1979) has advocated a similar pattern of tapering supervision following infarction. His plan envisions twelve weeks at three sessions per week, twelve weeks at two sessions per week, twelve weeks at one session per week and twelve weeks at one session alternate weeks. The patient himself is encouraged to exercise at least three times per week throughout, either on his own or at some community facility. S.M. Fox has proposed that supervised training be terminated when the patient attains a reasonable level of physical working capacity, the required standard decreasing from 10 Mets in men and 8 Mets in women aged less than 49 years to 7 Mets in men and 6.5 Mets in women over 70 years of age.

Jogging technique

Although it is sometimes shrouded in mystery, the technique of jogging is simple. Basic needs are a good pair of shoes, clothes that are permeable to sweat, and (possibly) a cheap wallet-style-computer with timing and pacing options. The patient should run with short steps, landing in a flat-footed manner. The body is held erect, with the shoulders and neck relaxed. Running on the toes or an exaggerated heel roll are liable to cause various orthopaedic injuries. The shoes that are chosen should not be too light — the aim is comfort rather than a racing performance. The sole should be thick and resilient enough to absorb some of the shock of ground impact. Arch and ankle support should be provided, and the heel should not be too low. Padding around the instep and at the back of the heel will minimise chafing. Hard running surfaces (concrete or tiled floors and sidewalks) are best avoided. Natural turf should also be well-groomed, without pot-holes or obstacles.

Hot climates

Sustained jogging produces an increase in core temperature in 'post-coronary' patients, much as in normal individuals (R.J. Shephard & Kavanagh, 1975; T. Kavanagh & Shephard, 1975b; T. Kavanagh *et al.*, 1975a; T. Kavanagh *et al.*, 1977a; R.J. Shephard *et al.*, 1978a). Indeed, since the rise of core temperature is a function of the percentage of maximum oxygen intake that is exerted (B. Nielsen, 1969), a cardiac patient is more vulnerable to hyperthermia than a fit young man at any given speed of running. Limiting temperatures for the runner are summarised in Table 9.8. These values should be approached with caution if the patient is obese, or is not yet acclimatised to summer heat. The best remedy for a prolonged hot spell

Table 9.8: Limiting Environmental Temperatures for Outdoor Running and Jogging, as Specified by US National Road Running Club

	Temperature	Relative
Dry bulb (°C)	Wet bulb (°C)	humidity (%)
35.0		
29.4	24.3	60
26.7	23.3	75

Table 9.9: Some Changes Induced by Running over a Marathon Distance, Shown by Data for Post-coronary Patients Participating in 1975 Boston Marathon Run

Decrease in body mass	2.8 ± 0.5 kg	(4.1 ± 0.8%)
Sweat loss	3.6 ± 0.5 l	
Estimated dehydration*	0.7 ± 0.5 l	(1.8 ± 1.5%)
Rectal temperature	1.6 ± 0.5 °C	
Plasma		
Na^+	$+4 \pm 3 \quad mmol \cdot l^{-1}$	
K^+	$0 \pm 0.2 \ mmol \cdot l^{-1}$	
HCO'_3	$-1.5 \pm 0.8 \ mmol \cdot l^{-1}$	
urea	$+5.8 \pm 1.7 \ mg \cdot dg^{-1}$	

* Dehydration is less than sweat loss as a result of: (i) fluid ingestion; (ii) metabolic production of water; and (iii) (probably) liberation of water from glycogen.

Source: R.J. Shephard *et al.* (1978a).

may be a temporary replacement of jogging by swimming.

A group of post-coronary patients who ran the Boston marathon in 1975 averaged a 2.9 kg decrease in body mass and a 1.6°C increase in rectal temperature, despite copious use of fluids (Table 9.9). If the weather is warm, it is important to choose clothes that allow a ready evaporation of sweat, and to insist upon an adequate fluid intake. A jogger should be 'pre-loaded' with 500 ml of fluid a few minutes before running begins, and should ingest a further 150 ml every 15 minutes while he is running. During exercise, this type of intake is not easily achieved, since it is much larger than dictated by the sensation of thirst. During exercise, the sodium and potassium ion content of the plasma either rise or remain constant (R.J. Shephard & Kavanagh, 1975; R.J. Shephard *et al.*, 1978a; Table 9.9). There is thus little point in spending money on expensive replacement fluids — indeed, by causing an unnecessary rise in serum potassium, certain proprietary fluids may increase the danger of a dysrhythmia. The best drink for the runner is probably water or an isotonic solution of glucose. Following exercise, the potassium and sodium lost in the sweat should be replaced. Normally, this is accomplished by increased salting of food, but during a prolonged spell of hot weather, a cumulative mineral ion deficit can develop (C.H. Wyndham & Strydom, 1972). The affected patient becomes irritable and loses 'weight'. The blood volume and thus the stroke volume are reduced, so that a given rate of work induces a higher heart rate and a higher cardiac work rate. This may lead to a worsening of angina and/or an increased frequency of abnormal heart rhythms. The remedy is to maintain salt intake, and to moderate training temporarily if symptoms of mineral deficiency develop.

Cold weather

Very cold weather also restricts outdoor activity. Cold air causes cutaneous vasoconstriction, with an increase in central blood volume and a rise in systemic blood pressure. Inspiration of cold, dry air may also induce bronchospasm in an individual with sensitive airways (R.J. Shephard, 1977b), and it is reputed to provoke angina through a reflex narrowing of the coronary arteries. Substantial adaptation to cold is possible through an appropriate choice of clothing and the adoption of a brisk movement pattern. Cross-country skiing, for example, is an enjoyable sport on a sunny afternoon even when the temperature is as low as $-15°$C. Much depends on the wind chill factor (Table 9.10) and the extent of radiant heating from the sun; the comfort of a given environment may decrease rapidly once the sun sets, a point to be noted by those exercising in the evening. If inspiration of cold air is inducing symptoms, a patient may find it helpful to use a jogging mask (T. Kavanagh, 1970). This device allows the inspiration of air that has been warmed and humidified within the patient's own sweat suit.

It is important to note that the 'warm-up' must be extended if injuries are to be avoided in cold weather. Sudden chilling during the warm-down phase can be a danger if too much clothing has been worn, and garments have become saturated with sweat. Another danger, most marked in late February, is that of slipping on patches of ice. Freezing

Table 9.10: Thermal Comfort in Relation to Air Speed

Thermal comfort*	Air speed (m•sec^{-1})			
	0	5	10	20
Pleasant	10	26	27	28
Cool	0	19	21	21.5
Very cold	−14	11	14	16
Bitterly cold	−50	−11	−4	0

* All temperatures refer to dry air, and are expressed in degrees Celsius.

rain is an obvious hazard, but greater danger comes from small ice patches formed by alternate melting and freezing of the winter snows. Finally, the dirty windshields of the winter season put the night-time jogger at considerable danger from passing motorists.

Slowing of training

Many factors necessitate a temporary reduction of the training prescription for a 'post-coronary' patient. In place of pleasant tiredness, there may be persistent muscle soreness; if ignored, this could progress to a frank musculo-skeletal injury. The systemic blood pressure, both in rest and in exercise, may be increased by a period of domestic or business anxiety. Myocardial irritability may be augmented by a viral infection. Finally, the patient may complain of increased chest pain, an abnormal heart rhythm or a vague malaise suggesting an extension of the disease process. All of these items should be referred to the supervising physician as soon as possible; he will then decide whether a more formal reduction of prescription is necessary and, if so, for how long this should be enforced.

Recruitment and Compliance

The major challenges to exercise prescription are patient recruitment and compliance. The statistics are discouraging. Even if an exercise programme is established on company premises, the proportion of staff recruited to such a programme is unlikely to exceed 20 per cent (M. Collis, 1975; R.J. Shephard *et al.*, 1980a). Many participants will be people who were previously taking exercise in some other facility. Finally, as many as 50 per cent of 'high-risk' recruits may drop out of

Table 9.11: Drop-out Rate Observed in 'Post-coronary' Exercise Rehabilitation Programmes

Period of rehabilitation (months)	Drop-out rate (cumulative % of initial sample)	Drop-out rate plus poor attendance (cumulative % of initial sample)	Percentage of drop-outs due to medical problems	Authors
36	40	–	–	V. Gottheiner (1968)
36	25	–	–	H.K. Hellerstein (1968)
60	52	–	–	E.R. Nye & Poulsen (1974)
22	56	–	–	E.H. Bruce et al. (1976)
2–5	36	57	36.4	E. Kentala (1972)
6–12	52	78*	32.3	
12	40	61*	7.1	L. Wilhelmsen et al. (1975)
48	70	87*	–	
12	23	–	–	
24	38	–	–	
36	50	–	11.9	P. Rechnitzer et al. (in preparation)
36	4.4	17.2†	17.4	R.J. Shephard & Kavanagh (in preparation)

* Some of subjects reported exercising on their own.

† A further 12.7 per cent of subjects had moved to other cities, but were continuing to exercise three or more times per week.

Source: Based in part on data accumulated by N.R. Oldridge (1979).

an exercise class over a six-month period.

In patients who have already sustained a myocardial infarction, losses are not quite so severe (Table 9.11). The Southern Ontario multicentre exercise-heart trial lost about ten per cent of its residual sample every six months (R.J. Shephard, 1979b). The Toronto Rehabilitation Centre has fared even better, a total of 17.2 per cent of initial recruits having poor or zero attendance at the exercise class over an average of three years (R.J. Shephard, 1979b).

Recruitment

Factors influencing middle-aged adults to join a fitness programme differ from those that sustain their interest (Stiles, 1967; Heinzelman & Baggley, 1970). In a 'representative' group of US men, Stiles (1967) concluded that fear of incapacitation and a desire for buoyant health were frequent reasons for beginning to exercise. Less common initial motivations were a desire to compete and a history of family involvement in a specific sport. Heinzelmann & Baggley (1970) noted that workers joined their employee-fitness programme in order: (i) to feel healthier; (ii) to reduces chances of a heart attack; and (iii) to help research. The President's Council on Fitness (1973) cited as common reasons for regular physical activity: (i) a desire for good health (23 per cent); (ii) a belief that exercise was 'a good thing'; and (iii) a wish to lose 'weight' (13 per cent). Non-participants blamed their inactivity upon (i) lack of time (13 per cent); (ii) the amount of exercise taken at work (11 per cent); (iii) medical reasons (8 per cent); and (iv) age (5 per cent); they were the older, less well-educated and less affluent members of the sample, and were less likely to have participated in exercise programmes at school. D.V. Harris (1970) commented that middle-aged men who were physically active had a history of participation in athletic camps, school and university sports teams. Typically, they enjoyed both competition and the resultant fatigue, and their parents had encouraged them to participate in sports from an early age. B.C. Brunner (1969) also observed that middle-aged men joined a fitness programme to keep fit and develop a sense of well-being, while non-participants complained of lack of time.

Recruitment apparently occurs for similar reasons in other parts of the world. P. Teraslinna *et al.* (1970) listed improvement of health (63 per cent), improvement of fitness (19 per cent) and control of body 'weight' (7 per cent) as the perceived motives of Finnish executives who joined an exercise programme. The men recruited lived near the exercise facility, had an above average initial level of activity

Table 9.12: Reasons for Participation in an Industrial Fitness Programme

Variable	Always or frequently a motivation		Rarely or never a motivation	
	Men (%)	Women (%)	Men (%)	Women (%)
Health and fitness	83.2	91.2	16.8	8.9
Release of tension	58.5	57.5	41.5	42.5
Games and competition	70.0	38.3	30.0	61.7
Fun and enjoyment	90.4	92.5	9.6	7.5
Socialising, making friends	37.9	56.0	62.1	43.9
Self-discipline	50.0	52.5	50.0	46.5
Appearance	51.2	88.3	48.8	16.7

Source: Based on data of R.J. Shephard *et al.* (1980a).

and, contrary to many studies, were likely to be cigarette smokers.

R.J. Shephard *et al.* (1980a) studied US office staff who joined an employee fitness programme at the Westchester (NY) head offices of General Foods. They noted that male recruits had an above average maximum oxygen intake and muscle strength, but were also somewhat overweight and fat. Women participants were closer to the actuarial 'ideal' body mass, but had lower levels of cardio-respiratory and muscular fitness than the men. Factors of programme acceptability such as travelling time from the employee's home, hours worked in the office and the cost of an annual membership ($48) had little impact upon participation. Perceived attractions of the increased activity (Table 9.12) included health, fitness, competition (particularly in the men) and appearance (particularly in the women). General and specific health beliefs of employees were well developed, but contrary to the arguments advanced by Marshall Becker and his associates (M. Becker & Maiman, 1975; M. Fishbein & Ajzen, 1975; M. Becker *et al.*, 1977), the relationship between health beliefs, health practices and health outcomes was limited (Table 9.13). Our findings thus suggest that personal trial of an exercise programme may be a more effective technique of recruitment than a campaign intended to induce a more general change of attitudes and values.

In older adults (K.H. Sidney & Shephard, 1977a), findings are similar; reasons why men joined an experimental pre-retirement

Table 9.13: A Comparison of Health Beliefs between Participants in an Employee Fitness Programme and Control Workers from the Same Company (Scores Expressed in Arbitrary Units)

Variable	Men		Women	
	Members (n = 256)	Non-members (n = 217)	Members (n = 153)	Non-members (n = 151)
General health beliefs				
Current health	4.58	4.46†	4.59*	4.29
Possibility of improvement	1.41*	1.67	1.55	1.66
Heart-attack beliefs				
Smoking a risk factor	4.06	4.14	3.86*	4.16
Beliefs about exercise				
Prevents heart attacks	1.85*	2.21†	1.91*	2.19†
Spouse believes in it	1.57*	1.28	1.46	1.23
Friends believe in it	1.83*	1.46	1.71*	1.36
Reasons for exercise				
Health	1.92*	2.23†	1.63*	2.05†
Fun	1.84	1.81	1.66*	1.88
Socialising	2.69	2.83	2.48*	2.85
Self-discipline	2.50*	2.69†	2.49	2.67†
Personal appearance	2.51*	2.78†	1.85*	2.20†

* Significantly better score than corresponding sub-group ($P < 0.01$).
† Subjects in non-member sample exercising away from the facility show favourable scores relative to those not taking any exercise.

Source: Based on data of R.J. Shephard *et al.* (1980a).

exercise class included (in order of perceived importance) the improvement of health and/or fitness, opportunity for exercise instruction and testing, altruism ('to help science') and hedonistic ('fun', 'curiosity'). Women recruits again cited improvement of health and fitness, opportunities for instruction and testing, altruism and hedonism, but they also remarked upon anticipated gains of mental vigour and alertness, along with opportunities to socialise and pressure exerted by their friends. Other factors important to the motivation of this age group were the provision of appropriate facilities, instructions on how to exercise safely and opportunities for regular supervised activity. Not one of our elderly recruits had received any advice on the merits of increased physical activity from their personal physicians (R.J. Shephard, 1978b).

The situation is a little different after myocardial infarction. Many doctors have now accepted the value of progressive exercise in the treatment of younger 'post-coronary' patients, and recruits to such programmes are commonly received on the basis of medical referral. Given an incidence of three heart attacks per 1,000 men aged 35–65 years, and an average survival of ten years, the total patient base in a metropolitan area such as Toronto (population 2.5 million) is about 15,000. Relating these statistics to our actual enrolment of about 1,250, we would judge that one male patient in twelve is now being referred for exercise. Presumably, at least a proportion of such men have relatively small infarcts; this suggestion is strongly supported by: (i) the short average duration of ischaemic pain in the Toronto series (Table 9.14); and (ii) the low rates of recurrence and mortality seen in those patients recruited to a control programme of homeopathic exercise (1.5 and 0.4 events per 100 person-years respectively).

Compliance

Knowledge of factors influencing compliance with exercise programmes is in its infancy. Plainly, much depends upon the characteristics of the individual and our success in matching the prescribed programme to his temperament and abilities.

Drop-out rates among apparently healthy subjects depend greatly upon the basis of initial recruitment and screening, the type of programme that is offered and criteria of non-compliance. Thus, Teräslinna *et al.* (1969) had only one of 89 subjects defect over nine months of exercise. On the other hand, losses from a jogging programme amount to 35 per cent at ten weeks (J.H. Wilmore *et al.*, 1970), 41 per cent at six months (G.V. Mann *et al.*, 1969) and 53 per cent at seven months (J. Massie & Shephard, 1971; H.L. Taylor *et al.*, 1973). Typical figures for a gymnasium-based exercise programme are a 17 per cent sample attrition at three months (H.P. Elder, 1969) and an 18 per cent loss at seven months (J. Massie & Shephard, 1971). N. Oldridge (1977) noted that 50 per cent of his sample had defected at 18 months, 60 per cent at 48 months and 70 per cent at 84 months.

The gregarious middle-aged adult responds better to a group programme than to solitary jogging (J. Massie & Shephard, 1971), whereas the reverse is often true of the introvert. Among the Toronto

Table 9.14: Characteristics of Myocardial Infarction among Patients Referred to the Toronto Rehabilitation Centre

Duration of pain (min)	Proportion of sample (%)	Severity of pain	Proportion of sample (%)
Nil	4.2	Nil	4.1
0–2	11.7	Mild	29.6
2–10	22.3	Severe	29.6
10–20	3.2	Very severe*	25.5
20–30*	14.9	Unbearable*	11.2
30–60*	43.7		

* Typical of a classical myocardial infarction.

Source: Based on data of T. Kavanagh & Shephard (1973a).

sample of 'post-coronary' patients, a surprisingly large 45 per cent said that they were happiest when exercising on their own (R.J. Shephard & Kavanagh, 1978d). Possible attractions of solitary exercise for the cardiac patient are an absence of 'competition' and avoidance of comparisons with others who may be progressing faster in their prescribed activity.

Reactions to an industrial fitness programme depend upon the overall attitude of the employee (favourable or otherwise) towards his company (R.J. Shephard & Cox, 1980). In vigorous programmes, it is the heavy subjects with a large excess body mass, a high percentage of body fat and a low maximum oxygen intake who are the commonest defectors (Table 9.15). Presumably, the physical demands made upon them are excessive relative to either their physiological ability or their perceived needs. In some instances, a failure to fulfil the expectations of the instructor leads to a deterioration of self-image. In programmes where a more gradual progression of exercise intensity has been adopted, the interaction between initial fitness and compliance is less obvious (R.J. Shephard & Cox, 1980); however, a light, rhythmic gymnastics class selectively attracts the shorter members of an office population (mean height of participating men 173.5 ± 0.7 cm and of women, 160.3 ± 0.6 compared with values of 175.0 ± 1.5 and 162.3 ± 1.1 cm for 'drop-outs', and of 178.4 ± 0.9 and 161.9 ± 0.8 cm for non-participants). Other features of the 'drop-out' include extroversion, persistent cigarette smoking, a poor credit-rating (J. Massie & Shephard,

Table 9.15: Three Comparisons between Good Participants (P) and Drop-outs (D) from Exercise Programmes

Variable	Middle-aged volunteers Men		Middle-aged office workers				Elderly subjects Men and women	
			Men		Women			
	P	D	P	D	P	D	P	D
Body mass (kg)	76.9	84.8[2]	76.4	75.4	57.2	59.3	64.1	70.8
	±7.8	±11.6	±1.3	±2.7	±0.9	±1.8	±10.2	±12.2
Excess mass (kg)	9.6	16.1[2]	5.1	4.2	6.0	6.7	3.6	13.3[3]
	±6.9	±9.4					±6.0	±6.9
Body fat (%)	23.0	26.2[1]	21.1	19.9	27.9	28.5	22.2	28.6
	±4.0	±4.2	±0.7	±1.5	±0.7	±0.8	±5.6	±6.3
Maximum oxygen intake ($ml \cdot kg^{-1} \cdot min^{-1}$ STPD)	36.5	33.2	36.6	38.6	32.0	31.1	29.8	24.0[1]
	±10.2	±5.6	±0.8	±1.6	±0.5	±0.8	±1.4	±4.1
Percentage of smokers	25	55[1]						

1. $P < 0.05$.
2. $P < 0.01$.
3. $P < 0.001$.

Source: Data of J. Massie & Shephard (1971) for middle-aged volunteers, of R.J. Shephard & Cox (1980) for middle-aged office workers and of K.H. Sidney & Shephard (1978) for elderly subjects.

1971) and (at least in 'post-coronary' patients; Table 9.16) a 'Type A' personality, a 'blue-collar' job, light occupational activity and an inactive leisure (N. Oldridge, 1979b).

Among 'post-coronary' patients, some defections are attributed to severe disease (for example, worsening angina, or the onset of cardiac failure), but most authors agree that medical problems are a fairly infrequent cause of poor compliance (R.A. Bruce *et al.*, 1974b; T. Kavanagh *et al.*, 1979; R.J. Shephard *et al.*, 1979a). In the Southern Ontario multicentre exercise-heart trial, 22 percent of sample attrition was due to medical causes (13.2 per cent cardiac, 8.8 per cent non-cardiac; N. Oldridge & Andrew, 1979); 25 per cent of losses were regarded as unavoidable (factors such as a change of work shift or removal to another city) and 42 per cent were blamed on psycho-social causes. In Göteborg (L. Wilhelmsen *et al.*, 1975), drop-outs were

Table 9.16: Identification of the Exercise 'Drop-out', Based on a Multiple-regression Analysis

Characteristic	Cumulative likelihood of dropping out of programme in 2 years* (%)
Average patient	45
Cigarette smoker	58
Smoker + blue-collar worker	69
Smoker + blue-collar worker + inactive leisure	80
Smoker + blue-collar worker + inactive leisure + light activity at work	95

* For the purpose of the Southern Ontario multicentre exercise-heart trial, a 'drop-out' was defined as a person who failed to attend class sessions for eight consecutive weeks.

Source: Data from Southern Ontario multicentre trial, as reported by N. Oldridge (1979b).

Table 9.17: A Comparison of Drop-out Rates and Reinfarction Rates for the Southern Ontario Multicentre Exercise-heart Trial

	Cumulative drop-outs	Reinfarction rate (per 100 person-years)
Centres recruiting from hospitals (n = 367)	52.6%	5.1
Centres where physician referred (n = 384)	38.5%	2.7

Source: Based on preliminary analysis of data from Southern Ontario multicentre trial, as reported by R.J. Shephard (1979c).

blamed upon lack of transportation (34 per cent), poor motivation (24 per cent), cardiac problems (25 per cent) and other medical problems (17 per cent).

One striking feature of the Southern Ontario trial analysed to date has been a two-fold difference of compliance between cooperating centres. This reflects in part varying patterns of recruitment (physician referral versus the 'scouring' of intensive-care hospital wards; Table 9.17) — and in part differences in the personality of the individuals leading the exercise classes. The class leader must plainly be enthusiastic, but not to the point of making excessive demands upon his patients. There is a need for a regular feedback of test scores and interpretation of current symptoms, and in this connection the personal involvement of the medical director is very important. In such a setting, a relatively close linkage can be established between physical activity and health. Thus the perceived benefits reported by our 'post-coronary' patients (R.J. Shephard and Kavanagh, 1978d) have included advice on fitness, health and heart problems, regular testing, safe supervised exercise, encouragement and camaraderie. Many patients have also valued our associated programme of psychological rehabilitation, making a plea for its wider availability.

Some authors have found that the drop-out rate is highest in the first three months after recruitment (N.B. Oldridge, 1979). If this were generally true, it would have important implications for both the design of experiments and the use of scarce resources in the rehabilitation of 'post-coronary' patients. In fact, if the annual loss from the Southern Ontario multicentre exercise-heart trial is expressed as a percentage of the residual sample, overall defections amount to about 20 per cent in the fourth as in the first year of recruit-ment (R.J. Shephard, 1979c).

Techniques of sustaining exercise compliance become of particular importance one to two years after recruitment, when the average 'post-coronary' patient must be weaned from one supervised class per week to one class in eight weeks. As might be predicted, the transition is harder for extroverts than for introverts (R.J. Shephard & Kavanagh, 1978d). T. Kavanagh & Shephard (1979) noted that 67 per cent of patients who had reached a plateau of training and 63 per cent of patients who were still progressing found it 'no problem' or 'relatively easy' to continue with their prescribed activity while making only one visit to the Centre every eight weeks. The remainder of the sample missed the encouragement they had drawn from other members of the class and the discipline of regular observation, complaining that 'suitable' exercise facilities were lacking in their area of residence. Nevertheless, attendance at the eight-weekly classes was good. After allowing for an average of one legitimate absence per year (due to an acute infection, or a journey out of town), the attendance averaged more than 90 per cent of potential. It may be that the patient accepts the reduced class frequency as a practicable commitment, and is thus willing to reschedule conflicting engagements, avoiding the establish-ment of a pattern of chronic non-attendance.

Safety of Prescribed Exercise

The safe operation of an exercise class is essential not only in its own right, but also in terms of sustaining compliance and avoiding expensive litigation.

Cardiac problems

The cardiac problems that may arise from injudicious exercise have already been discussed in Chapter 3. Current estimates of risk run from one in 100,000 to one in 300,000 man-hours of exercise, figures varying with the precise status of the 'post-coronary' patients that are included in a class. A cardiac facility operating five one-hour classes per week, each with 50 members, might thus encounter one episode of ventricular fibrillation in eight years. This is a sufficiently likely event that staff should have the training to administer prompt and effective resuscitation.

Many patients experience some warning of impending reinfarction (symptoms such as increasing anginal pain, premature beats or general malaise). Prompt reporting of such problems prior to a class can allow a careful clinical and physiological re-evaluation of the individual, thereby minimising the chances of an emergency during the exercise session (H. Pyfer, 1979). Sometimes pride or worsening cerebral perfusion may cause a class member to ignore exercise-induced symptoms, and class members should thus learn to watch not only themselves but also their colleagues. The prescribed intensity of activity should be reduced for any adverse circumstance (environmental or personal) and should be halted for any acute infection. Subjects with deep exercise-induced ST segmental depression and/or dysrhythmias must be observed with particular care, the prescribed activity being kept to a cardiac frequency at least 10 beats$\cdot$min^{-1} below that causing symptoms and signs. Both the warm-up and the warm-down should be carefully carried out, and patients should sit when changing. Showers should be locked to prevent use of excessively hot or cold water, and ventilation should be adequate to prevent a build-up of humidity in the locker room.

The relatives of the patient and other class members should be taught the principles of cardiac resuscitation, and where possible exercise should be carried out in pairs.

Musculo-skeletal problems

In some exercise programmes for middle-aged adults, as many as a half of the group have had to stop exercising within six months due to musculo-skeletal problems (such as ankle and knee injuries, prolapsed intervertebral discs, stress fractures of the metatarsals and 'shin-splints'; Å. Kilbom *et al.*, 1969; G.V. Mann *et al.*, 1969). T. Kavanagh & Shephard (1977a) found that among participants in the 1975 World Masters' competition, 57.2 per cent had suffered an injury of sufficient severity to interrupt training during the previous year. Of those injured, 39.6 per cent had experienced at least one week of disability, 26.7 per cent had been incapacitated for between one and four weeks, and 33.7 per cent had been affected for more than four weeks.

This alarming toll of injuries is not necessary in a well-designed and carefully graded recreational or therapeutic programme. K.H. Sidney & Shephard (1977a) prescribed a regimen of increased activity for 42 men and women aged 60–83 years, encountering only one or two minor tendon pulls requiring no more than one or two weeks of reduced activity.

The risk of such problems apparently increases with age, as a result of: (i) greater muscle stiffness secondary to greater fatigue; (ii) less rapid relaxation of antagonist muscles; (iii) loss of elastic tissue, shortening of tendons and alterations in structure of the collagen molecule; (iv) loss of flexibility and degeneration of the joints; (v) a decreased blood supply to the tendons; (vi) loss of both organic matter and minerals from bone; (vii) clumsiness due to lack of recent exercise and impairment of special senses, balance and reflexes; and (viii) obesity.

Keys to the minimisation of musculo-skeletal problems include: (i) a thorough initial medical examination, with avoidance of stress upon vulnerable joints; (ii) adequate warm-up at each session of activity; (iii) gradual progression of the required training; (iv) the use of appropriate footwear and soft running surfaces such as well-groomed natural or artificial turf; (v) emphasis upon walking rather than jogging in the early phases of conditioning; (vi) a temporary reduction of the prescription if the pattern of activity is changed; and (vii) avoidance of violent calisthenics (especially rapid twisting movements and excessive stretching).

10 ADJUVANTS TO EXERCISE

It is not the purpose of this book to provide detailed instructions regarding such aspects of 'prudent living' as the reduction in body fat, adoption of special diets, cessation of smoking, relaxation and the use of various drugs.

Nevertheless, an exercise programme may involve several years of regular contact between class leader and participant, and many opportunities arise to offer advice on these issues. Furthermore, prudent living can itself have a beneficial effect upon prognosis. Indeed, some authors have gone so far as to claim that the benefits of regular exercise are brought about simply by reductions in body mass and systemic blood pressure (Chapter 8). A few comments will thus be made on possible adjuvants to exercise.

Reduction in Body Mass

Tables of 'ideal' body mass (Table 10.1) have been developed by the Society of Actuaries (1959). Their suggested classification of subjects by body frame (light, medium or heavy) is very subjective, and the present author has therefore proposed using as a reference criterion the average ideal mass for a given standing height, irrespective of body frame (R.J. Shephard, 1974d). The figures thus derived provide simple target 'weights' from the viewpoint of minimising cardiovascular mortality, but they must be interpreted with discretion. A very muscular individual may exceed the 'ideal' mass by 10 kg and yet have little body fat. At the other extreme, a woman may be 5 kg below the ideal mass, while combining an excess of fat with very poor muscular development. A low body mass was once linked to a poor prognosis, since it often heralded either tuberculosis or carcinoma. With current advances in medical treatment, there is no longer any obvious prognostic penalty in subjects who fall a little under the ideal mass; indeed, many people have a more pleasing appearance when their mass is a little less than the quoted figure.

The majority of sedentary, middle-aged North-Americans exceed the target figures. Typically, 5-10 kg of tissue is added between late adolescence and the age of 45 years (R.J. Shephard, 1977a).

Table 10.1: 'Ideal' Body Mass, Derived from Data of the Society of Actuaries (1959)

Standing height, for subjects wearing no shoes (cm)	Ideal mass,* for subjects wearing indoor clothing	
	Men (kg)	Women (kg)
147.3	—	48.5
149.9	—	49.9
152.4	—	51.2
155.0	—	52.6
157.5	57.6	54.2
160.0	58.9	55.8
162.6	60.3	57.8
165.1	61.9	60.0
167.6	63.7	61.7
170.2	65.7	63.5
172.7	67.6	65.3
175.3	69.4	66.8
177.8	71.4	68.5
180.3	73.5	—
182.9	75.5	—
185.4	77.5	—
188.0	79.8	—
190.5	82.1	—
193.0	84.3	—

* For discussion, see R.J. Shephard (1974d).

In older age groups, fat persists but some lean tissue is lost, so that the total body mass of a senior citizen gradually reverts towards the supposed target.

Since obesity is well recognised as a cardiovascular 'risk factor' (Table 10.2), one might anticipate substantial numbers of very heavy patients in a 'post-coronary' exercise programme. In practice, this does not seem to be the case. The number of very obese subjects reporting to a coronary rehabilitation class is quite small, and changes in body fat over the course of training are also quite limited (Table 10.3). One reason for this anomalous finding is that body fat has already been reduced during the hospital phase of treatment. It may also be that

Table 10.2: Mortality of Grossly Obese Men and Women from Selected Causes in Relation to Excess Body Mass for Subjects Aged 15–69 Years

Disease	Men*		Women*	
	+ 24 kg	+ 42 kg	+ 28 kg	+ 37 kg
Heart and circulation	131	185	175	178
Renal	146	298	93	122
Vascular diseases of brain	136	215	143	142
All causes	123	168	130	138

* Data expressed as a percentage of standard values for subjects of same sex. Excess mass associated with a given mortality ratio varies slightly with stature.

Source: Based on data of *Build and Blood Pressure Study*, Society of Actuaries (1959).

Table 10.3: Initial Body Composition of Patients Referred to a 'Post-coronary' Programme, and Changes Observed over One Year of either Vigorous or Homeopathic Exercise

	Vigorous exercise		Homeopathic exercise	
	Initial	One year	Initial	One year
Body mass (kg)	74.6	+0.1	75.6	+1.5
	±10.5	±1.8	±11.0	±3.4
Skinfold thicknesses:				
triceps (mm)	10.9	−0.1	10.1	+1.2
	±4.3	±2.5	±2.5	±1.6
subscapular (mm)	20.2	−1.1	19.6	+3.3
	±6.1	±5.4	±3.8	±6.9
suprailiac (mm)	18.3	−1.8	18.9	+0.2
	±8.7	±5.8	±8.2	±6.7
Estimated body fat (%)	27.3	−0.4	26.2	+1.2
	±5.7	±3.0	±3.8	±1.9

Source: Based on Toronto segment of Southern Ontario multicentre trial, to be reported by R.J. Shephard, Cox & Kavanagh.

those with persistent obesity seek some alternative form of treatment, or indeed reject medical advice concerning lifestyle.

Patients who are above the ideal mass often claim that they are carrying muscle rather than fat. Some bias towards a well-muscled

Table 10.4: The Average Thickness of Eight Skinfolds in Subjects
Approximating the 'Ideal' Body Mass of Table 10.1

Skinfold site	Skinfold thickness (mm)	
	Men	Women
Chin	5.8	7.1
Triceps	7.8	15.6
Chest	12.0	8.6
Subscapular	11.9	11.3
Suprailiac	12.7	14.6
Waist	14.3	15.3
Suprapubic	11.0	20.5
Knee (medial aspect)	8.6	11.8
Average, eight folds	10.4	13.9

Source: R.J. Shephard (1977a).

sample is indeed possible among recruits to an exercise class.
However, there are several simple methods of checking this potential
alibi. An increase in body mass after the age of 25 is more likely to
be fat than muscle. The amount of fat can be estimated by caliper
measurements of skinfold thickness (Table 10.4). More direct
assessments of the percentage body fat are also possible by such
techniques as water displacement, underwater weighing, isotopic
determinations of body water and determinations of lean body mass
from ^{40}K counts.

On a warm day, elimination of body heat is impeded in a fat person.
Heat energy can be transferred through the insulating layer of
subcutaneous adipose tissue only at the expense of an increased skin
blood flow. The associated increase in body mass boosts the oxygen
cost of most physical tasks (G. Godin & Shephard, 1973b). This in turn
throws a greater strain on both the heart and the musculo-skeletal
system. When planning a training programme for an obese subject,
gentle progression is thus important in avoidance of cardiac and
musculo-skeletal problems and an associated high drop-out rate.

The desired result of an activity programme is loss of fat rather than
a loss of 'weight'. In a woman who has taken too little activity and too
little food for many years, an increase in total body mass through
some muscular development may be a healthy development. The

method of reducing body fat is simply to create a negative energy balance. If the body consumes less food energy than the combined costs of lean tissue synthesis and external work, the body fat content must diminish (W. O'Hara *et al.*, 1979). Drastic or even complete starvation is sometimes proposed for the obese individual, but this is dangerous unless conducted in a hospital setting; risks are particularly grave in the coronary-prone patient, where potassium ions liberated by tissue breakdown could provoke a fatal dysrhythmia. Since the original gain in body mass in a middle-aged adult has typically occurred over a span of ten to 20 years, it is usually better to aim at a relatively slow correction of the problem, with the intention of creating a new lifestyle that will persist once the target body mass has been reached. Starvation diets occasionally achieve dramatic initial reductions in excess mass, but the fat is commonly replaced once dietary restrictions are lifted (E. Sohar & Sneh, 1973; J.A. Innes *et al.*, 1974).

Body mass can undoubtedly be reduced by a modest restriction of diet, even in the absence of deliberate physical activity, but this has the major disadvantage that tissue protein is sacrificed along with the unwanted fat. A combination of increased activity (500–1,000 $kJ \cdot day^{-1}$, as developed through a typical exercise prescription), and a normal or slightly reduced energy intake (e.g., 500 $kJ \cdot day^{-1}$ diminution of food supply) provides the most effective 'reducing' regimen. Regularly spaced meals help to avoid the peaks and troughs of blood sugar that favour overeating, but snacks, alcohol and sweetened soft drinks must be held to a minimum. A daily energy deficit of 1,000 kJ will reduce body mass by at least 1 kg per month, more if energy loss is accelerated by an increased protein turnover. This is a satisfactory regimen for the average 'coronary-prone' patient who is 10–15 kg overweight, although more drastic measures may be needed for the occasional individual who presents with 50–100 kg of excess fat.

Although the necessary increase in physical activity was once regarded as impracticable by some nutritionists, simple calculations show that the exercise prescription of Chapter 9 readily meets the requirements of fat loss. The prescribed energy expenditure (60 per cent of maximum oxygen intake) amounts to an added 20–2 $kJ \cdot min^{-1}$, or 600–60 kJ over a 30-minute exercise class. If two flights of stairs are also climbed only three times during the day, a further 100 kJ are added, for a total of 700–60 $kJ \cdot day^{-1}$. A negative energy balance may give rise to a rapid early decrease in body mass. This reflects a loss of tissue fluids, probably including water 'coupled' to food stores such as glycogen (R.J. Shephard, 1980c). Although the phenomenon is sometimes exploited by those marketing dubious methods of 'instantaneous weight reduction', any such fluid loss is replaced within a few days, to the great discouragement of the 'weight watcher'. The early loss of fluid is often accompanied by disturbances of mineral balance, and this problem must be carefully watched in an individual with ischaemic heart disease.

The response of the post-coronary patients to a year of exercise rehabilitation (Table 10.3) is a little disappointing in terms of further changes in body fat content. Nevertheless, if the required activity does no more than maintain the fat loss achieved in hospital, this is in itself a major accomplishment relative to the known failure rate of traditional 'weight-loss' programmes.

Special Diets

Saturated fat

A number of trials are currently evaluating the preventive and thera- peutic value of diets low in saturated (animal) fat (Chapter 5). In general, it seems that the patient with a risk of ischaemic heart disease gains a marginal advantage of prognosis if he switches to a vegetable-oil diet that has a low cholesterol content (Dayton *et al.*, 1969). However, dramatic benefits cannot be expected from a sudden change of feeding patterns in late life. A high proportion of the undesired serum cholesterol comes not from the diet (500–600 mg·day^{-1}), but rather from hepatic and intestinal synthesis (about 1,000 mg·day^{-1}). If energy intake is excessive relative to physical activity and other sources of energy expenditure, cholesterol formation will occur whether fat or sugar is ingested (K.J. Ho *et al.*, 1970). Since atherosclerotic changes begin in childhood (Chapter 1), dietary manipulations in adult life are unlikely to resolve existing vascular disease such as advanced plaque formation with thrombosis and calcification. While a high serum cholesterol remains a risk factor for the patient who has already sustained a myocardial infarction (Table 10.5), there is no guarantee that prognosis can be improved by dietary attempts (J. Stamler, 1971) to reduce serum cholesterol. Furthermore, critics of low-animal-fat diets have pointed to several risks of alternative eating patterns, including: (i) a build-up of the wax-like vegetable fat ceroid (which is not attacked by body enzymes; A.N. Howard, 1970); (ii) an accumula- tion of straight-chain (trans-) unsaturated fatty acids, with possible damage to cell membranes (M.G. Enig, 1979); and an increased intake of refined sugar (which may favour both cholesterol formation and

Table 10.5: Classification of Blood Lipid Abnormalities with Main Basis of Treatment

Type of abnormality	Characteristics	Treatment Drug	Diet and Exercise
I	Increased low-density lipoproteins, lack of enzymes to break down chylomicrons, xanthomata	Thyroid hormone	Medium-length tri-glycerides
II	Increased low-density lipoproteins, lack of serum bile acids — inherited	Clofibrate and/or cholestyr-amine	Unsaturated fat
III	Increased very-low-density lipoproteins, xanthomata	Clofibrate	Exercise, negative energy balance
IV	Increased very-low-density lipoproteins, reduced low-density, increased cholesterol synthesis		Exercise, negative energy balance
V	Increased high- and low-density lipoproteins	Thyroxine + clofibrate	Exercise, negative energy balance, high-protein diet

Source: D.S. Fredrickson (1974).

damage to the pancreatic islets).

The first practical step in the dietary treatment of a coronary-prone individual is to obtain a lipid profile. Certain specific abnormalities of cholesterol and triglyceride metabolism can be corrected by use of drugs and dietary modification (Table 10.5). Some post-coronary patients with less clear-cut lipid disorders may still seek possible prognostic gains from a restricted diet and a low fat intake, but others may decide that the purchase and preparation of special food for one member of the family would cause a domestic upheaval that is unwarranted by present scientific evidence.

Increased physical activity modifies serum cholesterol only if there is an associated negative energy balance. However, vigorous endurance exercise induces favourable changes in the ratio of high-density to low-density lipoproteins, with some reduction in serum triglyceride readings (Chapter 4).

Vitamins

While large quantities of vitamins are consumed by the public, there is little evidence that such materials are deficient in a normal well-balanced western diet. Indeed, in war-time experiments, volunteers survived for several months on a vitamin-free-diet before symptoms occurred.

Exercisers are particularly prone to ingest large quantities of vitamins and other dietary supplements (T. Kavanagh & Shephard, 1977a). There seem several reasons for this. Successful competitors from Eastern Europe follow this practice, partly because the food in many communist states is less varied than in North America and partly because Eastern physiologists argue that for optimum performance the body must be 'saturated' to the point that the excretion of a given vitamin exactly matches the amount ingested. In North America, the more active members of the total population are often 'health-conscious' individuals and this causes them to explore possible methods of improving physique, including the use of dietary supplements.

A number of vitamins, particularly members of the B complex, are involved in carbohydrate metabolism, and the need for such compounds may thus rise with an increase in daily energy expenditure. However, if the diet remains well balanced, the added demand for vitamins is balanced by the added intake of food. One possible minor exception is the small loss of water-soluble vitamins that occurs in an individual who sweats heavily (R.J. Shephard, 1980c). Massive doses of vitamin C are sometimes taken by athletes in an attempt to ward off upper respiratory infections, and speed recovery following musculo-skeletal injuries (T. Kavanagh & Shephard, 1977a), although there is little hard evidence that the supplement is of benefit in either situation. Among 'post-coronary' patients, there is also a vogue for ingestion of vitamin E, although there is no objective evidence that this affects prognosis (R.E. Olson, 1973; T.W. Anderson, 1974).

Smoking Withdrawal

Cigarette-smoking is a clearly-identified 'risk factor' for the development of clinically manifest ischaemic heart disease (Chapter 2).

Table 10.6: Some Adverse Effects of Smoking upon Oxygen Transport and the Cardiovascular System

---

Decreased maximum oxygen intake:
    combination of CO with haemoglobin
    displacement of oxygen dissociation curve for haemoglobin
    combination with myoglobin
    ? effects on tissue enzymes
Increased work of breathing:
    bronchospasm
    chronic bronchitis
Increased cardiac work rate:
    increase in heart rate
    increase in systemic blood pressure
    increased velocity of myocardial contraction
    increased stroke volume and cardiac output
Decreased coronary blood flow
Decreased flow to skeletal muscles
Increased risk of abnormal cardiac rhythm
Increased platelet adhesiveness
Increased serum free fatty acids

Source: A. Rode & Shephard (1971b); A. Rode *et al.* (1972); Wright & Shephard (1979).

Several constituents of cigarette smoke (including carbon monoxide and nicotine) have adverse effects upon oxygen transport and the cardiovascular system (Table 10.6). Among ostensibly healthy middle-aged adults who smoke, the reduction in 'coronary risk' associated with regular exercise habits is also less than that seen in non-smokers (Table 10.6). Further, continued smoking increases the risk of recurrent infarction for patients who are already enrolled in a rehabilitation programme. It is thus logical to commend smoking withdrawal as an important adjuvant to an increase of physical activity in both secondary and tertiary preventive programme.

It is not our intention to discuss here the various possible techniques of smoking withdrawal, although a few practical points deserve emphasis. Firstly, an initial exercise test and/or participation in a regular training programme may provide motivation to quit smoking, particularly if clinically significant findings are carefully interpreted to

Table 10.7: Effects of Smoking Habits and of Physical Activity upon Total Mortality (47 Per cent due to Ischaemic Heart Disease)

Habitual level of activity	Total mortality (relative to corresponding sedentary group)	
	Never smoked regularly	Smoked > 20 cigarettes·day^{-1}
Sedentary	1.00	1.00
Light	0.69	0.95
Moderate	0.58	0.75
Heavy	0.57	0.70

Source: Based on data of E.C. Hammond (1964).

Table 10.8: Smoking Status of Distance Runners by Age at Which They Began Running

Smoking status	Began running	
	Before age 21	After age 21
Never smoked (%)	56	36
Former smoker (%)	36	60
Current smoker (%)	8	4

Source: Based on data of P. Morgan *et al.* (1976).

the patient (Table 10.8). The cigarette habit leads to various respiratory symptoms such as cough, sputum and breathlessness, with a substantial associated increase in the work of breathing (A. Rode & Shephard, 1971b). However, the severity of the respiratory disorder does not become obvious to a sedentary middle-aged adult until he tries to exercise. Equally, the initial stress test may provide the first warning of myocardial ischaemia. Personal experience of a smoking-withdrawal clinic has shown that exercise-induced dyspnoea and ST segmental depression are both strong factors influencing the decision of an individual to stop smoking (R.J. Shephard *et al.*, 1972).

The percentage of continuing smokers among men attending the Toronto 'post-coronary' rehabilitation programme is about 35 per cent (T. Kavanagh *et al.*, 1977c). A large proportion of our group stopped smoking soon after infarction. There is little evidence that the remaining subjects followed this example with continued rehabilitation. Nevertheless, the combined effects of regular exercise and contact with Centre staff probably played a useful role in avoiding the recidivism that normally afflicts ex-smokers.

Relatively few middle-aged adults who engage in distance running are smokers. Some authors have argued that this reflects the attraction of health conscious non-smokers to active pursuits. P. Morgan *et al.* (1976) presented statistics for Masters' Athletes. The initial percentage of smokers was much the same as in the general population (64 per cent in men who began distance running after age 21 years), but at the time of examination (after many years of running) it was only four to eight per cent. In this group, it is thus likely that running caused smoking cessation. However, the required weekly mileage (40–50 km) falls outside the scope of most recreational programmes.

It is important to persuade patients to quit smoking and not merely to switch from cigarettes to a cigar or pipe. Although the latter two forms of tobacco usage are normally associated with a lower primary risk of ischaemic heart disease than cigarette smoking, this is mainly because the smoke is not inhaled, with a correspondingly smaller absorption of carbon monoxide. Unfortunately, many cigarette smokers continue to inhale the more pungent smoke if they switch to a cigar or a pipe, so that their final health status may actually be worsened by this change of behaviour (C.M. Castleden & Cole, 1973).

Any decision to stop smoking should be linked with a total appraisal of health attitudes; otherwise, the potential gain in life expectancy may be whittled away by adverse changes such as an increase in mental tension, or a large increase in body fat. The ideal goal is to change attitudes in at least four areas of health behaviour, smoking cessation being linked to an increase in physical activity, control of food intake and adoption of a more relaxed attitude to life. In many patients, the well-disciplined atmosphere of the regular exercise class provides a format that is helpful in realising these objectives. But even if the patient shows a transient period of tension, or a small gain in body mass following smoking withdrawal, this should not be regarded as an indication to resume the cigarette habit; the accumulation of one or two kilograms of additional body mass is a negligible risk factor relative to the continued inhalation of tobacco smoke.

Relaxation

In the view of many authors, typical coronary-prone individuals are tense, restless, time-oriented individuals, with what M. Friedman and Rosenman (1974) would class as 'Type A' behaviour (Chapter 11). Of the 751 patients referred to the Southern Ontario multicentre exercise heart trial, 489 cases (65.1 per cent) were placed in this category.

Participation in an exercise programme sometimes has a relaxing effect, with a reduction of state anxiety (W.P. Morgan, 1979), cardiac frequency (J.F. Patton *et al.*, 1977), blood pressure (H.J. Montoye, 1975), lactate production (J.O. Holloszy *et al.*, 1971), catecholamine output (L. Hartley *et al.*, 1972) and rating of perceived exertion (J.F. Patton *et al.*, 1977). However, the response depends very much upon the manner in which physical activity is pursued. Despite advice to the contrary, many patients with ischaemic heart disease choose to participate in a tense, competitive manner. They arrive at the rehabilitation class begrudging the time that must be devoted to physical activity, their minds seething with other plans and problems. The prescribed exercise is performed in a rigid, obsessional manner, with the hope not only of improving physical condition, but of out-performing other class members. If business or social commitments prevent the daily dose of exercise, such individuals may show a substantial increase in tension and anxiety.

In these circumstances, real benefit may be gained from various types of relaxation therapy — deep-breathing exercises, yoga and even hypnosis. At the Toronto Rehabilitation Centre, instruction in hypnosis is arranged for many of the 'post-coronary' patients. The rudiments of the necessary procedures are taught to individuals by a physician with special experience in this art, and then regular weekly practice classes are scheduled for groups of between eight and ten men. Over the course of a year or so, the majority of patients reach the point where they can induce deep relaxation on their own and, by daily practice of hypnosis, many of these individuals apparently develop a healthier attitude to life. While this is difficult to quantify, T. Kavanagh *et al.* (1973b) found that over the first year of rehabilitation, the improvements in exercise-test responses in patients receiving hypnosis almost matched the gains of those enrolled in the exercise class!

Drugs

Space does not permit a detailed discussion of the place of drugs in the treatment of ischaemic heart disease. However, comment will be made on interactions between physical activity and some of the more commonly used pharmaceutical agents.

Nitroglycerin

Patients with exercise-induced angina may find a need to take trinitrin, isosorbide dinitrate or a related drug immediately before or during prescribed activity. The implication is that in addition to the primary myocardial infarction, other areas of the heart muscle are becoming perilously short of oxygen. Such a patient is at a greater risk of recurrence than the individual with an uncomplicated infarct and, accordingly, training must proceed more cautiously. In particular, activity must be kept below an intensity that would provoke cardiac failure (J.O. Parker *et al.*, 1966), and a close watch must be kept for any worsening of angina that would herald a potential reinfarction.

Nitroglycerin substantially augments the amount of work that can be performed by symptom-limited patients (Table 10.9). Some (R.E. Goldstein *et al.*, 1971; J.P. Bronstet *et al.*, 1978) but not all (A.N. Goldbarg, 1973) authors have also found gains from the administration of longer-acting nitrates. Failure to respond to these compounds may reflect either a non-ischaemic cause for the supposed anginal pain, or advanced coronary disease (L.D . Horwitz *et al.*, 1972).

The nitrates as a class were originally thought to be coronary vasodilator agents, although it would be surprising if much dilatation could occur in the hardened vessels of a typical anginal patient. Such drugs may have some effect upon coronary collateral vessels (W. Ganz *et al.*, 1978). Amyl nitrate also causes a general arteriolar dilatation (D.T. Mason *et al.*, 1972), while nitroglycerin is reputed to have a positive inotropic action that shortens the duration of systole (B.E. Strauer, 1973). Nevertheless, it is now widely accepted that most nitrates act primarily through an increase in venous pooling (H. Westling, 1971). Cardiac filling pressure is reduced, with a reduction in the systemic blood pressure and thus the work rate of the heart (B.F. Robinson, 1968; R.E. Goldstein *et al.*, 1971; V. Kötter *et al.*, 1978). A small reduction in pressure can be beneficial to a heart that is failing from oxygen lack, but an excessive fall in diastolic filling pressure reduces cardiac output and thus physical performance. It is still hotly debated whether the response can be improved by using a

Table 10.9: Changes in Response to Progressive Cycle-ergometer Test with Sublingual Nitroglycerine, a Long-acting Nitrate (Nifedipine) and Placebo in Patients with Angina

Drug	Max. heart rate (beats·min^{-1})	Max. systolic blood pressure (mm Hg)	Max. work performed (kp-m)	Final ST depression (mV)
Control	122	170	3,015	0.38
Placebo (30 min)	125	168	3,220	0.39
(180 min)	127	174	3,313	0.39
Nitroglycerine (immediate)	140	183	4,861	0.33
Nifedipine (30 min)	143	164	4,254	0.40
(180 min)	146	171	4,947	0.34

Source: Based on data of J.P. Bronstet *et al.* (1978).

combination of nitrates with β-blocking drugs that counter coronary vascular spasm (H.I. Russek, 1968; W.S. Aronow & Kaplan, 1969; D.J. Battock *et al.*, 1969; J.P. Bronstet *et al.*, 1978; C. De Ponti *et al.*, 1978). Presumably, much depends upon the extent of coronary calcification. Some authors also advocate combining nitrates with calcium inhibitors; the latter modulate the breakdown of adenosine triphosphate and thus affect the development of tension by the myocardium (I.P. Clements *et al.*, 1978; B. Niehnes *et al.*, 1978).

Since nitroglycerin reduces cardiac stroke volume, the heart rate for a given power output is increased after administration of this drug. The assessment of responses to sub-maximal exercise then becomes complicated, particularly if reliance is placed upon heart-rate measurements at a given work load. However, to the extent that patients with angina take nitroglycerin as a normal prelude to exercise, it can be argued that the observed performance scores are realistic.

The response of anginal patients to regular, slow, long-distance exercise is often disappointing, and such individuals fare much better if transferred to a modified interval training programme (T. Kavanagh & Shephard, 1975a). The rest intervals apparently allow opportunity for re-oxygenation of poorly vascularised areas of the myocardium. The need for nitroglycerin can be reduced by a thorough warm-up and (in cold weather) the use of a jogging mask (T. Kavanagh, 1970).

Fortunately, the modification of the exercise/heart-rate relationship by nitroglycerin does not seem to prevent some training from occurring, provided that the patient is made sufficiently comfortable that he can increase his activity by a significant amount.

β-Blocking agents

Agents that block β-receptors of the sympathetic nervous system (for example, propranolol) are given to an ever-increasing proportion of 'post-coronary' patients. One common reason for such therapy is to decrease the frequency of premature ventricular contractions and other abnormal cardiac rhythms. Catecholamines provoke such disturbances by causing a patchy disturbance of ventricular function; there is an increase in calcium conductance across the cell membrane which increases contractility and shortens the refractory period, while at the same time an increase in potassium conductance accelerates repolarization (A.M. Katz, 1977). Both of these changes favour re-entry of the electrical signal into a part of the myocardium that has already undergone contraction. β-Blocking agents counter this trend by making the myocardial membrane less sensitive to catecholamines (P. Kühn, 1977).

Abnormalities of ventricular rhythm such as premature ventricular contractions and tachycardia are of particular importance as possible precursors of ventricular fibrillation. The need for β-blocking drugs is thus a warning that exercise testing and prescription must proceed with caution.

A.N. Goldbarg *et al.* (1971) found that after administration of propranolol the heart rate of healthy adults was reduced at rest (9 beats·min^{-1}), in light activity (17 beats·min^{-1}) and during maximal effort (36 beats·min^{-1}). However, there was considerable compensation for this bradycardia through an increase in the end-diastolic volume, with a resultant increase in stroke volume and a widening of arterio-venous oxygen difference. Maximum oxygen intake was unchanged, but the period for which maximum power output could be sustained was shortened by 25 per cent. Other suggested effects of propranolol have included a favourable distribution of coronary blood flow within the myocardium (L.C. Becker *et al.*, 1971) and an enhanced release of oxygen from the red cells (F.A. Oski *et al.*, 1972).

It is uncertain how far these various patterns of adaptation operate when β-blocking drugs are administered to patients with advanced coronary vascular disease. If a reduction in heart rate, systemic blood pressure and myocardial contractility occur, this should reduce the oxygen demand of the myocardium (C.R. Jorgensen *et al.*, 1977).

Propranolol is thus commended by most authors (H.I. Russek, 1968; D.J. Battock *et al.*, 1969; G.R. Dagenais *et al.*, 1971; A.N. Goldbarg, 1973) for the relief of pain in anginal patients. Most but not all (W.S. Aronow & Kaplan, 1969; A.N. Goldbarg, 1973) investigators find that the exercise tolerance of the anginal victim is improved by β-blockade. Much probably depends upon the cause of his disability. If the angina is arising from an excessive myocardial oxygen demand, then propranolol will help performance. However, if activity is limited by poor myo-cardial pumping, a further reduction in contractility will have a deleterious effect upon effort tolerance (D.T. Mason *et al.*, 1972); indeed, it may even precipitate cardiac failure. There may thus be advantages in the use of newer and more selective drugs such as practolol and oxprenolol, which produce cardiac β-blockade with less depression of myocardial contractility (E.A. Amsterdam *et al.*, 1971).

The slow heart rate of the patient treated by β-blockade complicates the normal process of stress testing and exercise prescription. The ideal arrangement would be to halt administration of the drug a few days prior to laboratory evaluation. However, withdrawal must be arranged with the concurrence of the supervising clinician, and a gradual tapering of dosage over a week or longer is necessary to avoid provoking a 'rebound' dysrhythmia. If, for any reason, the drug cannot be with-drawn, exercise tolerance cannot be judged from observations of heart rate; exercise prescription must be based on the power output as measured on a cycle ergometer, or the oxygen intake attained during treadmill walking. Any attempt to push such a patient to a normal target heart rate would of course be fraught with disaster.

A slowing of the heart-rate response to exercise is not necessarily an indication of improved physical condition in this class of person. It is equally conceivable that the clinical status has worsened, and the supervising physician has found it necessary to increase the dose of β-blocking agent. If the exercise prescription has previously been based upon heart rate, the first administration of β-blocking drugs is an urgent indication to re-evaluate the permitted work rate.

α-Blocking agents

α-Blocking agents such as phentolamine are occasionally administered to improve myocardial contractility. Such drugs are helpful to the patient whose performance is limited by function of the cardiac pump (H. Zebe *et al.*, 1978). α-Blockade leads to a substantial drop of end-diastolic pressure, with an increase in stroke volume and exercise tolerance.

Calcium antagonists

Drugs such as Verapamil and Nifedipine inhibit calcium transport. In consequence, myocardial-tension development is reduced, heart rate is slowed and blood pressure falls, all of these changes being helpful to the patient with exercise-induced angina (J.P. Bronstet *et al.*, 1978; I.P. Clements *et al.*, 1978; B. Niehnes *et al.*, 1978). The delay in calcium transport at the myocardial membrane also decreases the likelihood of developing a ventricular dysrhythmia (P. Kühn, 1977). Indications for the use of these compounds are much as for β-blocking agents; they should be avoided if there is any suspicion of cardiac failure.

Cardiac glycosides

Cardiac glycosides such as digoxin may be administered to treat residual heart failure following myocardial infarction, and/or to lower ventricular rate in the presence of an abnormal atrial rhythm. In either case, recovery of myocardial function is less than complete, and the exercise prescription must be correspondingly cautious.

Unfortunately, it is particular difficult to interpret behaviour of the exercise electrocardiogram after administration of digoxin, since this drug can of itself delay repolarisation, giving rise to ST segmental depression (L. Zwillinger, 1935; A.M. Katz, 1977). The slow resting heart rate of over-digitalisation must also be distinguished clearly from a training bradycardia.

Functional effects upon the myocardium are complex. Contractility and the velocity of cardiac contraction are increased (E.H. Sonnenblick *et al.*, 1965). At the same time, end-diastolic pressure and ventricular dimensions are diminished (J.O. Parker *et al.*, 1969; R.O. Malmborg, 1965). It is thus difficult to predict whether the cardiac glycosides will increase or decrease myocardial oxygen consumption, angina and symptom-limited effort tolerance.

Diuretics

Diuretics are commonly administered to 'post-coronary' patients who show a tendency to cardiac failure. They are an indicator of an adverse prognosis (T. Kavanagh *et al.*, 1977c).

Such drugs lower blood pressure, and thus the rate-pressure product. They also reduce ventricular volume and cardiac output, and thus have a beneficial effect upon those patients whose effort tolerance is impaired by angina. If there is depletion of body potassium stores, the ECG may show a falsely positive ST depression during exercise (A.J. Georgopoulos *et al.*, 1961).

Hypotensive agents

Hypotensive agents such as the Raowolfia alkaloids may be administered to patients with ischaemic heart disease in order to control an associated hypertension. Heart rate, cardiac output and myocardial contractility may all be reduced (R.L. Kahler *et al.*, 1962; S.I. Cohen *et al.*, 1968). However, the potential reduction in cardiac work rate is offset by an increase in ventricular volume.

Again, there is a likely implication of advanced atherosclerotic disease, with an impaired exercise response. In the early stages of therapy, control of blood pressure may be less than perfect, the patient swinging from hypertension to hypotension. Allowance must be made for this when monitoring the blood-pressure response to exercise. If the patient is in the hypotensive phase, particular care must be taken to ensure a slow warm-down, with avoidance of hot showers. Carelessness in this respect could cause hypotensive collapse or ventricular fibrillation.

Sedatives and relaxants

In view of the personality disorders encountered in many patients with ischaemic heart disease (Chapter 11), a case could be made for the prescription of sedative and/or relaxant drugs. However, the problem of impaired myocardial function can be life-long, and the danger of addiction to a 'remedy' such as Valium or Librium is then very real.

Endurance exercise has an immediate arousing effect, but if it is timed to take place two to three hours prior to the patient's bed-time, it has an effective secondary sedative action. The degree of relaxation that results from exercise depends upon the spirit in which it is pursued (see the comments on relaxation above).

Insulin

Maturity-onset diabetes is frequently associated with ischaemic heart disease. Before acceptance into an exercise programme, the blood sugar should be well controlled. Care should also be taken to have a sweetened drink before commencing an extended bout of exercise.

The long-term prognosis of the diabetic is improved by an increase in physical activity, and in many cases the need for insulin is diminished or abolished (J. Devlin, 1963; G.M. Grodsky & Benoit, 1967).

11 PSYCHO-SOCIAL CONSIDERATIONS

Although physicians place great emphasis upon statistics for mortality and recurrence rates in ischaemic heart disease, a more important aspect of therapy in many respects is the success of psycho-social readaptation. This chapter will look briefly at the issues of employment, resumption of normal sexual activity and adjustments of mood state.

Employment

We have already noted (Table 2.2) that premature death from ischaemic heart disease leads to a substantial economic loss. The typical cardiac victim is a successful, well-trained executive at the peak of his career. Sudden death robs society of a potential ten or 20 years of benefit from accumulated skills and experience. One estimate calculated the cost to the US economy at $19.4 billion per year (H.E. Klarman, 1964). The same author estimated the additional costs of caring for cardiac cripples at $3.0 billion per year. At the time of Klarman's report, the emphasis was upon work classification (L.H. Bronstein, 1959; R.J. Clark, 1959; D. Gelfand, 1959; T.V. Parran et al., 1959), with cardiologists making maximum use of residual function in the light of physiological, psycho-social and occupational evaluation (Table 11.1; N.K. Weaver, 1959; H.K. Hellerstein, 1979). It was soon found that the great majority of cardiac patients could return to gainful employment without risk to themselves or their employers (D.J. Turell & Hellerstein, 1958). More recently, the process of re-integration into society has been aided by active rehabilitation. S.R. Doehrman (1977) found that 60 per cent of one sample had resumed work after three to four months, 79 per cent at six months and 81 per cent at one year. N.K. Weaver (1959) had an even better experience (Table 11.2).

Those who remain unemployed after six months seem unlikely to change their status. Age is the main determinant of successful re-adaptation, the percentage returning to work being 88 per cent at 45–60 years, 85 per cent at 60–5 years, and 67 per cent in those over 65 years (E. Weinblatt et al., 1966; B.M. Groden, 1967; S. Fisher, 1970;

279

Table 11.1: Apparent Needs of Patients with Ischaemic Heart Disease Attending the Cleveland Work Classification Unit

Reassurance	73%
Intellectual interpretation	60
Vocational guidance	41
Emotional rehabilitation	28
More medical treatment	15
Vocational rehabilitation	8
Physical rehabilitation	6
Diagnosis	3
Avocational guidance	2

Source: T.V. Parran *et al*. (1959).

Table 11.2: Cumulative Percentage of Patients Resuming Work at an Oil Refinery

Number of months post-infarction	Percentage of patients returned to work
0	5.2
1	17.7
2	34.4
3	63.5
4	75.0
5	87.5
6	93.8

Source: Based on data of N.K. Weaver (1959).

S. Hinohara, 1970; R. Nagle *et al*., 1971). A second important variable is the severity of infarction. One year after the acute episode, E. Weinblatt *et al*. (1966) found 86 per cent employment in those who were not severely disabled, compared with 54 per cent in those who had severe disability. A history of vigorous physical activity prior to infarction doubles the chances of a return to full-time work (E. Weinblatt *et al*., 1966). Other important variables include motivation, skills and experience (R.J. Clark, 1959; D. Gelfand, 1959; A. Morgan Jones, 1959; T.V. Parran *et al*., 1959), financial status (R. Nagle *et al*., 1971), the attitude of relatives (R. Mulcahy *et al.*, 1972), the physical demands of the job (B.M. Groden, 1967; N.K. Wenger *et al.*, 1973) and the presence of associated diseases such as diabetes (B.M. Groden, 1967; S. Hinohara, 1970; N.K. Wenger *et al.*, 1973).

The anxiety that follows infarction (T. Hackett & Cassem, 1973) may delay a return to work (S. Hinohara, 1970), but it does not seem to be a major determinant of ultimate employability. S. Fisher (1970a) found no greater anxiety levels among the unemployed than in those who resumed their job, while H.A. Wishnie *et al.* (1971) and N.K. Wenger *et al.* (1973) considered anxiety and depression were limiting factors in no more than a quarter of chronically unemployed cardiac patients.

A proportion of more severely disabled patients benefit from coronary by-pass surgery (Chapter 12). G.K. Barnes *et al.* (1977) found that after such treatment 19 per cent of those previously unemployed returned to full-time work, and a further 35 per cent accepted part-time employment.

Given that most patients do resume regular work, should any restriction be placed on such activity? If the job involves occasional heavy tasks such as lifting, these should be simulated in the laboratory under telemetric control. If severe ST depression or dysrhythmias develop during this testing, the two possible options are: (i) to proscribe those duties that provoke undesirable signs; or (ii) to prescribe local muscular training until the heaviest physical demands are better tolerated. Attention must also be directed to the psychological demands of the job; while argument continues over 'stress' and infarction (L.E. Hinckle, 1972), a surprisingly large percentage of patients note business problems in the period immediately preceding a coronary attack (Chapter 3). The typical history is of a man who is spending long hours at each of two jobs. It is thus discouraging to find that after their 'heart attack' many patients remain fiercely competitive, still working 44–72 hours per week (D.E. Sharland, 1964). A. Jezer & Warshaw (1960) suggested that before returning to work employees should undergo a 'stress interview', with simultaneous recording of the electrocardiogram and blood pressure. L. Zohman & Tobis (1970) added a galvanic skin response measurement to the protocol in order to quantify the stress imposed.

Some employers have feared the legal implications of employing 'post-coronary' patients (L. Price, 1959; Ungerleider & Gubner, 1959). The number of cases where employment has been judged a primary or a contributing cause of myocardial infarction has increased dramatically in recent years. An early study from New York State set the annual total of Compensation Board payments for heart disease at $2 million (L.J. Goldwater & Weiss, 1951). In contrast, the US Disability Insurance Program received 43,979 claims for arteriosclerotic and degenerative heart disease between July 1955 and August 1956; furthermore, 64.2 per cent of these claims were allowed (A.B. Price, 1959). A cause-and-effect relationship may be postulated if the 'heart attack' begins less than six hours following performance of some unusual task; the case for compensation is naturally strengthened if there is a history of bridging symptoms (M. Texon, 1959).

The employment record of the cardiac patient is usually well up to average. W.E.R. Greer (1959) examined the experience of the Gillette razor company. Some 23.5 per cent of employees with ischaemic heart disease were premium workers (expected figure 20 per cent), while 8.8 per cent were base or unsatisfactory employees (expected figure 8 per cent). Absenteeism averaged 13.3 days per year (expected figure 11.3 days per year), and there were no major accidents among the cardiac group (expected figure 2.6 per cent of employees losing two or more weeks' work per year from major accidents). We may conclude that, given adequate rehabilitation and proper placement, the 'post-coronary' patient can become a safe and effective member of the labour force.

Resumption of Sexual Activity

Relatively little is known about the sexual behaviour of the older person (A.C. Kinsey, 1948; W.R. Stokes, 1951; A.L. Finkle, 1959; G. Newman & Nichols, 1960; R.J. Shephard, 1978b), and information regarding the 'post-coronary' patient is even more sketchy. A major textbook on ischaemic heart disease (T.R. Harrison & Reeves, 1968) makes no mention of sexual activity, while an otherwise excellent monograph from the International Society of Cardiology (T. Semple, 1973) contents itself with the delicate comment: 'family relationships may so deteriorate that resumption of normal married life becomes very difficult'. Nevertheless, sexual relations are an important aspect of healthy living at all ages, and the physician who is guiding a patient's recovery from myocardial infarction should be able to offer competent advice on the resumption of normal sexual activity.

There is both subjective and physiological evidence that exercise helps the process of readaptation (H.K. Hellerstein, 1970; R.A. Stein,

1977). Certainly, the physical demands of sexual activity can be substantial in a young person. There are reports of heart rates rising to 170 beats·min^{-1} and systemic blood pressures reaching levels as high as 250/120 mm Hg (G. Klumbies & Kleinsorge, 1930; E.P. Boas & Goldschmidt, 1932; R.G. Bartlett & Bohr, 1956). Such figures would place an undesirable load upon the heart after infarction, particularly if due account is taken of: (i) the absence of a steady state; (ii) the contraction of small muscles; (iii) the combination of isometric and isotonic work, often with a need for postural support; and (iv) associated autonomic reactions (J.S. Skinner, 1979). However, the typical 'post-coronary' patient has been married for many years, and his response to normal intercourse is much less dramatic than that of a young student. A peak pulse rate averaging 117 beats·min^{-1} (range 90-144 beats·min^{-1}) is sustained for only ten to 15 seconds, and the resultant cardiac stress can be compared with the ascent of a couple of flights of stairs (an oxygen consumption of 4.5 Mets; L. Zohman & Tobis, 1970; H.K. Hellerstein & Friedman, 1973).

Many patients harbour the myth that repeat infarctions tend to occur at orgasm, so that sexual intercourse should never again be attempted (T.P. Hackett & Cassem, 1973). A number of authors have documented the decreased frequency of intercourse following infarction, although a part of this change could be a normal con-comitant of aging (R.J. Shephard, 1978b). H.K. Hellerstein & Friedman (1970) noted a drop from 2.1 to 1.6 orgasms per week in 49-year-old men, and A. Bloch *et al.* (1975) a decrease from 1.2 to 0.6 per week. Others (W.B. Tuttle *et al.*, 1964; R.F. Klein *et al.*, 1965; D. Dorossiev *et al.*, 1976) report similar findings. The altered behaviour apparently bears more relationship to pscyhological factors including the sexual drive prior to infarction (Table 11.3) than to age, working capacity or disease severity.

A study from the Toronto Rehabilitation Centre (T. Kavanagh & Shephard, 1977b) noted that while 80 of 161 patients showed either no change or an increase in sexual activity, in the remaining 81 patients the frequency of intercourse was reduced. Reasons cited for the diminished frequency included the patient's apprehension (21 per cent), the wife's apprehension (23 per cent), loss of desire (37 per cent) and a combination of these factors (19 per cent). Of the patients with reduced frequency, 20 were encountering anginal pain and six were developing premature ventricular beats during intercourse. These 26 individuals noted that sexual activity was less enjoyable than before infarction. Eight of their number feared that intercourse would provoke

Table 11.3: Cited Reasons for Reduction in Sexual Activity

Reason	Author
Loss of desire	A. Bloch *et al.* (1975)
	H.K. Hellerstein & Friedman (1970)
	T. Kavanagh & Shephard (1977b)
Depression	A. Bloch *et al.* (1975)
Apprehension	A. Bloch *et al.* (1975)
	H.K. Hellerstein & Friedman (1970)
	T. Kavanagh & Shephard (1977b)
Wife's apprehension	A. Bloch *et al.* (1975)
	H.K. Hellerstein & Friedman (1970)
	T. Kavanagh & Shephard (1977b)
Symptoms and fatigue	A. Bloch *et al.* (1975)
	H.K. Hellerstein & Friedman (1970)
Impotence*	A. Bloch *et al.* (1975)
	H.K. Hellerstein & Friedman (1970)
	E. Weiss & English (1957)
	W.B. Tuttle *et al.* (1964)

* Many North American patients appear to deny impotence (J.S. Skinner, 1979).

Source: Based in part on reports collected by J.S. Skinner (1979).

another infarct, and in a further eight cases their wives had similar fears. The remainder of the 26 men were apathetic because of symptoms that arose during intercourse.

Formal tests of personality disclosed no clear relationship between reduced sexual activity and post-infarct depression. However, discussion with the wives revealed certain differences of behaviour relative to those with normal or increased sexual activity (Table 9.6). The gain in maximum oxygen intake with training (19.1 versus 11.6 per cent) also favoured the group who resumed normal sexual activity, an observation confirmed by R.A. Stein (1977). It is less clear whether the difference in training response is the cause or an effect of sexual problems. Certainly, self-esteem is important to successful completion of an exercise rehabilitation programme. T.H. Hackett & Cassem (1973) have commented on the decreased ego strength and sense of emasculation that exacerbate feelings of fatigue and weakness in the 'post-coronary' patient, and it is highly probable that the resumption of normal sexual activity plays an important role in restoring self-esteem.

Some authors (for example, M. Brenton, 1968; J.F. Briggs, 1972) have suggested that the cardiac patients should adopt a physically less demanding position such as side-lying when sexual activity is resumed. In the Toronto study, only 18 per cent of patients elected a more passive position and, whether cause or effect, all 18 per cent showed a decline in sexual activity. L. Zohman & Tobis (1970) also found that a change of technique hampered a return of normal sexual response. Passive positions are now largely discredited, since E.D. Nemec *et al.* (1964) have found that such changes yield no advantage in terms of lowering the heart rate or blood pressure at orgasm.

The relative risks of intercourse and normal rhythmic exercise can be judged from the respective incidence of symptoms; 12.4 per cent of the Toronto patients developed angina during intercourse, compared with 36.0 per cent during a standard laboratory stress test to 75 per cent of maximum oxygen intake (T. Kavanagh & Shephard, 1977b). Likewise, the percentage of patients experiencing ventricular premature beats was 3.7 per cent, compared with 4.6 per cent during the stress test. Nevertheless, in one series of just over 200 primary non-fatal infarctions, two patients admitted that their cardiac episodes had arisen during normal sexual activity (R.J. Shephard, 1974b). M. Ueno (1963) found 34 of 5,559 sudden deaths (0.6 per cent) were related to coitus, 0.3 per cent being attributable to cardiovascular disease, while H.K. Hellerstein & Friedman (1970) estimated sexually related cardiac fatalities at 0.6 per cent of deaths in the Cleveland area. Some 80 per cent of the Japanese incidents occurred during extra-marital affairs, many being associated with overeating and overdrinking. Given that the average frequency of intercourse in a coronary-prone man is about once in five days (H.K. Hellerstein & Friedman, 1970; A. Bloch *et al.*, 1975; T. Kavanagh & Shephard, 1977b), and allowing between ten and 15 minutes for the discharge of marital responsibilities (R.G. Bartlett, 1956; H.K. Hellerstein & Friedman, 1970; W.A. Littler *et al.*, 1974), it can be estimated that the risk of a first heart attack is increased at least two- to three-fold during the period of sexual activity (E. Massie, 1969; R.J. Shephard, 1974b).

It has been recommended that patients who are liable to angina take nitroglycerin, standard cardiac drugs and possibly tranquillisers prior to the sex act (J.F. Briggs, 1972; Q.R. Regestein & Horn, 1978; W.S. Aronow, 1979). Unfortunately, many of the medications commonly prescribed for the cardiac patient (digoxin, β-blockers, antidepressants, alcohol and tranquillisers, anti-hypertensive drugs) are liable to reduce libido, impair ejaculation and cause impotence (F.O. Simpson, 1974; R.S. Eliot & Miles, 1975). Because of the greater heart rate and blood pressure response evoked in such circumstances, there are strong medical arguments against marital adventures with an unfamiliar partner (L.D. Scheingold & Wagner, 1974). Coitus should also be avoided after a heavy meal, particularly if the subject is fatigued, anxious or emotionally upset. Reassurance may be necessary if the first few attempts at intercourse are unsuccessful following a prolonged period of abstinence; in this regard, advice from a general practitioner who is familiar with both the topic and the patient may be as effective as more specialised sexual counselling (B. Kushnir *et al.*, 1976).

In women who have sustained infarction, sexual frigidity and dissatisfaction are common, although such problems are almost always blamed upon the male partner rather than the disease process (L. Abramov, 1976). It may be wise to recommend some method of contraception other than the 'pill' to female cardiac patients (Chapter 12).

Adjustment of Mood State

Patients participating in a 'post-coronary' exercise rehabilitation programme often show serious disturbances of mood (J. Bendien & Groen, 1963; D.L. Keegan, 1973; T. Kavanagh *et al.*, 1977a), but it is less clear how far such disturbances are a reflection of the original personality (C.D. Jenkins, 1971; M.J. Segers & Mertens, 1974; B. Lebovits *et al.*, 1975; P. Siltanen *et al.*, 1975), and how far they reflect a reaction to the loss of financial, social and emotional security that accompanies a heart attack. The Napoleonic physician Corvisart (1806) wrote: 'repeated depressing emotions . . . may be the origin of refractory disorders of the heart'. More recently, M. Friedman & Rosenman (1974) described an association between a specific personality ('Type A') and heart disease, but others (E.H. Friedman, 1974; J.L. Marx, 1977; H. Selye, 1978) have argued that this thesis has been exaggerated, thereby causing unnecessary anxiety to patients fitting the 'Type A' description. D. Eden *et al.* (1977) went further, finding in a group of kibbutzim workers a negative correlation of overload, conflict and social pressure with conventional cardiac risk factors such as serum cholesterol. They concluded that the managers under study thrived in stressful situations.

Nevertheless, it seems likely that problems of personality and attitude can not only contribute to the critical 'coronary' incident (R.A. Keith, 1966; J.R.P. French & Caplan, 1970; M. Friedman & Rosenman, 1974), but also can influence the timing of the decision to call a physician, and the subsequent response to rehabilitation (D. Gelfand, 1959; B.D. McPherson *et al.*, 1967; M. Dobson *et al.*, 1971; T. Kavanagh *et al.*, 1973b). Clinicians also have the impression that there is an increased incidence of depression in the months immediately following myocardial infarction (A. Verwoerdt & Dovenmuehle, 1964; C.K. Miller, 1965; H.P. Klein & Parsons, 1968; D.L. Keegan, 1973). The question thus arises whether 'post-infarction' patients are individuals with a particular liability to depression (J. Brozek *et al.*, 1966), the 'heart attack' merely serving as a trigger that reveals an underlying personality defect.

T. Kavanagh *et al.* (1975b) applied the Minnesota Multiphasic Personality Inventory (MMPI) to a sample of 96 patients after between twelve and 15 months of rehabilitation. Almost all patients exceeded the theoretical D (depression) score of 50 (Figure 11.1), which may reflect in part the normal effect of age upon D scores, but about a third of the sample (34/96) had very high D scores (> 70 units, two standard deviations greater than normal). Individuals with the pathological increase in D score also showed high values for the 'neurotic triad' (hysteria, hypochrondriasis and psychasthenia; Table 11.4). Other authors (H.D. Ruskin *et al.*, 1970) have reported similar findings. It is popularly held that the MMPI is a measure of 'trait' rather than 'state', and in support of this view J. Brozek *et al.* (1966) found pre-existing high hypochondriasis scores in men who later sustained a 'heart attack'. On the other hand, A.M. Ostfeld *et al.* (1964) found no initial difference in MMPI scores between normal subjects and those individuals who subsequently developed myocardial infarction. A further possible complication is that individuals with an unusual personality tend to volunteer for physiological and psychological testing (R.J. Shephard & Kemp, unpublished data). Thus J. Naughton *et al.* (1968) recorded high D, Hy and Hs scores for a group of sedentary control subjects who agreed to complete the MMPI. However, depression inhibits physical activity (particularly in a post-coronary patient; D. Gelfand, 1959), and it is thus unlikely that a rehabilitation programme will selectively attract patients with a high D score. It could be argued that depression is a side-effect of the medication used to treat hypertension (rauwolfia and guanethidine) and dysrhythmia (β-blockers). Some 30 per cent of the depressed patients in the Toronto series were receiving propranolol, but scores

Figure 11.1: Distribution of depression (D) scores on the Minnesota Multiphasic Personality Inventory (MMPI). The solid line shows the anticipated distribution of normalised D scores and the broken line the distribution for a unimodal sample of patients with mild depression. The shaded area indicates the proportion of the sample with gross depression.

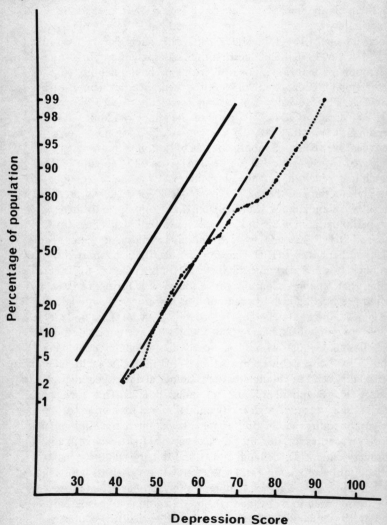

Source: T. Kavanagh *et al.* (1975b).

Table 11.4: Normalised Scores from Minnesota Multiphasic Personality Inventory Data for Post-coronary Patients, a Score of 50 on Each Measure Being Expected for a Normal Healthy Subject

Psychological characteristic	H.D. Ruskin *et al.* (1970)	T. Kavanagh *et al.* (1975b)	
		Entire sample (*n* = 96)	Grossly depressed patients (*n* = 34)
Depression	70.1	63.3	79.2
Hysteria	63.1	54.2	66.3
Hypochondriasis	63.7	55.4	64.2
Psychasthenia	59.2	55.5	65.2

for this sub-group did not differ from those for patients who were not receiving drugs. Possibly, the direct mood-depressing effect of β-blocking agents is outweighed by the resultant relief of symptoms.

We may conclude that a proportion of patients became severely depressed as a reaction to their infarction. T.H. Hackett & Cassem (1973) estimated that during the acute episode, 75 of 100 patients admitted to the coronary care unit became depressed. The peak effect was seen on the third day post-infarction. The abnormality of mood persists with the return home, as the patient senses the threat of invalidism, loss of autonomy and independence. Contributory factors include weakness resulting from the heart attack and subsequent bed rest, sexual problems (T.H. Hackett & Cassem, 1973), inappropriate and inadequate explanation from the attending physician (S. Hinohara, 1970), interaction with an over-anxious wife (H.D. Ruskin *et al.*, 1970; M. Dobson *et al.*, 1971; M. Skelton & Dominian, 1973), frequent hospital admissions (A. Verwoerdt & Dovenmuehle, 1964) and the patient's own anxiety, lack of confidence and fear of sudden death (V.B.O. Hammett, 1963; S. Fisher, 1970). In the Toronto series (T. Kavanagh *et al.*, 1975b), the depressed group were older than those with normal D scores (average age 51 as opposed to 45 years). A higher proportion of the depressed group also suffered from angina and hypertension. Prior to infarction, a higher percentage reported facing major worries, both in business (74.1 per cent of sample versus 60.6 per cent) and at home (32.2 versus 20.0 per cent). However, the information was collected retrospectively, and it could thus reflect either a true difference in exogenous pressure (C.M. Parkes *et al.*, 1969; C.D. Jenkins, 1971), or a magnified perception of difficulties secondary to depression. As previously noted by M. Dobson *et al.* (1971), the depression was also related to physical disability, affecting subjects that showed a poorer than average training response. It could be argued that depression weakened motivation, leading to exaggeration of symptoms and inadequate training (R.R.H. Lovell & Verghese, 1967). On the other hand, in the Toronto experiments, depressed and non-depressed subjects attained an almost equal walking distance and speed. Despite equal effort, the training response was poorer in the depressed subjects. The most reasonable explanation of our findings is thus that difficulties encountered in training contributed to their depression, and indeed it is arguable that some cases might have responded more favourably to a less vigorous programme.

Many patients deny their depression (A.D. Weisman & Hackett, 1961), to the point where it may be overlooked (J.G. Bruhn, 1973; T. Kavanagh *et al.*, 1975b; M. Dobson *et al.*, 1971). However, the psychological profile has important implications when planning a rehabilitation programme. The non-depressed hypomanic patient is a driving, ambitious individual, eager to excel in his prescribed exercise, and he must be cautioned against training in too aggressive and competitive a manner. Such an individual may use the mechanism of denying symptoms to enable him to cope with heavy business commitments or strenuous physical exertion in the face of niggling pains. To a point, this is a useful mechanism, and it accounts for his favourable progress after infarction. On the other hand, it can lead to a dangerous delay in seeking medical advice when symptoms warn that a recurrence of the infarction is imminent (V.B.O. Hammett, 1963).

The depressed patient, in contrast, may need much encouragement in order to undertake the rehabilitation needed for a return to work (D. Gelfand, 1959). Nevertheless, the Toronto Rehabilitation Centre team ultimately persuaded 95 per cent of their depressed patients to resume full-time employment. Depressed patients are likely to benefit from psychotherapy (C.A. Adsett & Bruhn, 1968), hypnosis (T. Kavanagh *et al.*, 1974a) or a combination of these two types of treatment. Small-group sessions allow covert problems to be revealed and discussed, with substantial therapeutic benefit. Some psychiatrists have regarded depression as a functionally useful withdrawal from a noxious situation, but in the context of ischaemic heart disease there is a good deal of evidence that hope and optimism are necessary to a favourable prognosis (W.A. Greene, 1954; B.Z. Lebovits *et al.*, 1967;

A.H. Schmale & Engel, 1967; J.G. Bruhn *et al.*, 1971).

Patients frequently comment on the improvement of mood that follows participation in a regular exercise programme (W.P. Morgan *et al.*, 1970, 1971). This thus seems an important reason for recommending an increase in physical activity. Amidst a list of medical prohibitions (food, cigarettes, alcohol, sex, . . .) exercise stands out as both a positive recommendation and a means of reducing the dependency of the cardiac victim. Nevertheless, it is not easy to document large changes of mood by objective tests. In one group of 'post-coronary' patients who progressed to marathon running (T. Kavanagh *et al.*, 1977a), D scores were lower than in the average cardiac patients, but were still substantially greater than for the general population. T. Kavanagh *et al.* (1977b) carried out a longitudinal 'follow-up' on 44 patients with high initial scores for depression and the 'neurotic triad'. Four years later, there was a substantial reversion towards normal scores (Table 11.5). Likewise, J.G. Bruhn (1973) found that relative to an inactive group, post-coronary patients who increased their physical activity had lower scores for depression and hypochrondriasis, with higher scores for ego strength. H.K. Hellerstein (1965) also showed decreases in depression and psychasthenia scores among patients enrolled in his cardiac reconditioning programme. It is arguable that at least a part of these various changes reflects an inevitable adaptation of the patient and his spouse to the problems created by the infarct (A. Verwoerdt & Dovenmuehle, 1964; M. Skelton & Dominian, 1973). Furthermore, in the Toronto study, the sample was initially selected on the basis of a high D score, thus increasing the likelihood that scores would revert towards the mean (B.D. McPherson *et al.*, 1967; C.O. Dotson, 1973). Several other groups of investigators have described a reduction in depression coincident with exercise participation (A. Verwoerdt & Dovenmuehle, 1964; J. Naughton *et al.*, 1968; B.M. Groden & Brown, 1970; W.P. Morgan *et al.*, 1970; J.G. Bruhn, 1973; E.H. Friedman & Hellerstein, 1973) but, in the one controlled trial (J. Naughton *et al.*, 1968), the decrease in depression was not significantly enhanced by training. B.D. McPherson *et al.* (1967) suggested that much of the observed improvement might be a result of group support rather than exercise *per se*, since some changes occurred when patients carried out homoeopathic doses of exercise. Certainly, in the Toronto series, gains of aerobic power were as great in those who did not improve their D score as in those who did; however, persistently high D scores were linked to a lability of resting systemic blood pressure and a worsening

Table 11.5: Changes of Minnesota Multiphasic Personality Inventory Score over Four Years of Exercise Rehabilitation for Subjects with High Initial D

Variable	Initial score	Final score	Δ	P	Normal score
Depression (D)	29.0	25.9	−3.1 ± 6.0	< 0.05	16.7
Hysteria (Hy)	25.1	22.5	−2.6 ± 4.9	< 0.05	16.5
Hypochondriasis (Hs)	18.2	16.0	−2.2 ± 4.9	< 0.05	11.3
Psychasthenia (Pt)	30.6	28.6	−2.1 ± 5.7	< 0.05	23.0

* Data are here presented as 'raw' scores.

Source: T. Kavanagh *et al*. (1977b).

of exercise-induced ST segmental depression (T. Kavanagh *et al.*, 1977b).

W.P. Morgan (1979) has emphasised that excessive training can have an adverse effect upon mood, with associated physiological disturbances (heart rate, blood pressure, catecholamine output and — in women — menstrual disorders). This picture of 'overtraining' is well recognised among athletes, but it can also develop in a post-coronary patient who is exercising too hard.

One last personality characteristic that deserves comment is the MF (masculinity/femininity) scale of the MMPI. 'Post-coronary' patients have a high score on this variable (T. Kavanagh *et al.*, 1977b). One may link this observation to the feminine characteristics of heavy smokers (A. Rode *et al.*, 1972). It is conceivable that stress may arise because of a conflict between the individual's personality and the perceived demands of a traditional male sex role (H.I. Russek, 1966), with both recourse to cigarettes and development of a heart attack. Alternatively, the MF score could be increased as a consequence of emasculating changes forced upon the patient by his heart attack. The lack of change in MF scores over four years of rehabilitation seems rather against the latter explanation. Finally, since most of the Toronto sample were well-educated 'white-collar' workers, it is possible that a high level of education affected the choice of cultural vocational and avocational attitudes (ballet, poetry, art, . . .) in a manner leading to a 'feminine' score.

12 MISCELLANEOUS TOPICS

This chapter will examine briefly a miscellany of topics relating to exercise and ischaemic heart disease, including problems of the female patient, anginal pain, by-pass operations and peripheral vascular disease.

The Female Patient

Until recently, the loss of productive years from ischaemic heart disease in women amounted to only a small fraction of the male total. In a classical study of 100 coronary heart disease patients under the age of 40 years, only four cases were women (R.E. Glendy et al., 1937). More recent Canadian statistics (Table 2.2) put female deaths between one quarter and one fifth of the male total. Since the relative immunity of women to heart attacks is particularly noticeable in the younger age groups, it has been argued that women gain an advantage from their characteristic pattern of hormone secretions. In support of this view, animals gain some protection from oestrogen-feeding, and men who have undergone bilateral orchidectomy in early life are also less liable to heart attacks (J.B. Hamilton, 1948; M.M. Gertler & White, 1976). On the other hand, several recent observations have tended to discredit the hormonal hypothesis, as follows:

(1)   Men suffering myocardial infarctions have a personality that is rated as feminine rather than masculine on traditional assessments such as the Terman-Miles test (Chapter 11); they are less aggressive, less adventurous, less enterprising and less self-assertive than controls, being 'actively sympathetic and concerned with domestic affairs, art and literature' (M.M. Gertler & White, 1976).

(2)   'Post-coronary' men have above average serum levels of oestradiol, with possible adverse effects upon the metabolism of sugar and fat.

(3)   Women taking female sex hormones for purposes of contraception apparently have an increased risk of 'heart attacks' (W.H.W. Inman & Vessey, 1968; J.E. Wood, 1972; L.D. Ostrander & Lamphiear, 1978), with a reduction in hepatic triglyceride lipase

(D. Applebaum-Bowden & Hazzard, 1979).
(4) Finally, the incidence of 'heart attacks' in women has increased progressively as they have adopted a more 'masculine' lifestyle.

Current thinking is thus that women gained a substantial part of their historic immunity to myocardial infarction through such characteristics as a low average consumption of cigarettes. Furthermore, this advantage is now being dissipated through heavy smoking and the adoption of aggressive 'Type A' behaviour in occupational and leisure activity.

Relatively few authors have compared the circumstances of heart attacks in men and women (B. Wikland, 1971; M. Romo, 1972; G. Bentsson, 1973). M. Romo (1972) found that 15 per cent of men were physically active during or immediately prior to infarction, whereas only one per cent of women were active at the time of attack (Chapter 3). This may reflect a lack of heavy physical activity among middle-aged European women prior to 1970. If so, the statistics that are now being collected will probably show a higher proportion of incidents in women who are exercising.

The paradoxical behaviour of the ST segment in women has already been discussed (G. Cumming *et al.*, 1973b; K.H. Sidney & Shephard, 1977b; Chapter 7). 'Abnormal' electrocardiograms are as frequent in elderly women as in men. However, female subjects show less evidence of coronary atherosclerosis at angiography, and they sustain less heart attacks than the men. One possible explanation of the paradox (K.H. Sidney & Shephard, 1977b) is that the ventricular wall has a lesser cross section in women than in men. Attempts to develop a similar systemic pressure thus place the myocardial fibres under greater tension, and ischaemia occurs during vigorous exercise, even if the coronary vasculature is relatively normal. If this explanation is correct, it is then necessary to explain why ischaemia does not provoke fibrillation in the women. Possibly, the intensity of effort needed to reveal ischaemia (75–100 per cent of maximum oxygen intake) is not normally attained by a middle-aged lady.

There have been several comparisons of prognosis between men and women. One early report found that the five-year survival after myocardial infarction was only 39 per cent in women, compared with 60 per cent in men (J.L. Juergens *et al.*, 1960). However, a part of this difference was due to the greater average age of the females (67.5 as opposed to 60.0 years). More recent studies have found either no difference in prognosis (G.E. Honey & Truelove, 1957), or a slight advantage to female patients compatible with the normal difference of

Table 12.1: Probability of Death within First 4.5 Years of Diagnosis of
Angina or Myocardial Infarction — a Comparison of Statistics for
Women and Men, Based on Abnormality of Four Variables

Variable	Probability of cardiac death			
	Women		Men	
	Normal	Abnormal	Normal	Abnormal
Electrocardiogram	0.047	0.149	0.062	0.190
Systemic blood pressure	0.102	0.093	0.101	0.227
Serum cholesterol	0.048	0.163	0.137	0.122
Blood-sugar regulation	0.071	0.278	0.133	0.197

Source: E. Weinblatt *et al.* (1973).

Table 12.2: Perceived Reasons for Joining a Physical-activity
Programme — a Comparison of Ranked Data for Elderly Men and
Women

Men	Women
1. Physical health	1. Physical health
2. Programme and facilities	2. Programme and facilities
3. Altruism	3. Psychological well-being
4. Recreational/hedonistic	4. Altruism
	5. Recreational/hedonistic
	6. Socialising

Source: K.H. Sidney & Shephard (1977a).

longevity between older men and women (E. Weinblatt *et al.*, 1973;
A. Vedin *et al.*, 1975). Diabetes has a greater adverse effect on post-
infarction prognosis in women, while angina has less impact in a woman
than in a man. The last finding may reflect the fact that a larger proportion of women have vague symptoms that prove not to be true
angina (E. Weinblatt *et al.*, 1973). Likewise, a much higher proportion
of women than men are diagnosed as hypertensive, but many have
labile hypertension. The recorded pressure therefore has less influence
on prognosis in women than in men. On the other hand, a high serum
cholesterol has a greater adverse effect in women (Table 12.1).

Attitudes to an increase in physical activity differ substantially

Table 12.3: Attitudes towards Physical Activity as Assessed by the Kenyon Inventory – a Comparison of Data for Elderly Men and Women

Concept of physical activity	Arbitrary score	
	Men	Women
Aesthetic experience	49.2	51.0
Health and fitness	48.2	49.2
Catharsis of tension	45.9	48.0
Social experience	46.9	46.1
Ascetic experience	34.2	33.8
Pursuit of vertigo	38.6	30.9
Game of chance	29.7	29.7

Source: K.H. Sidney & Shephard (1977a).

between men and women (M. Dosch *et al.*, 1975). Women are less attracted to physical development than men, but are more interested in psychological well-being and a reduction in body fat, with improvements of posture and carriage (R.J. Shephard, 1977a). Appealing items of programme content for the female include health and fitness, relief of tension, plus the social and aesthetic aspects of activity; however, there is less appreciation of the vertiginous component than in men (Tables 12.2 and 12.3).

Track events are well accepted by young women, but older females still resist a programme that places a heavy emphasis upon jogging, particularly if they are somewhat obese. At the Toronto Rehabilitation Centre, a battery of cycle ergometers has provided a satisfactory basis for regular exercise. These machines allow the women to undertake a graded activity programme while conversing with their friends. Swimming and aquabatics (underwater gymnastics) are other forms of exercise suitable for an older woman who is somewhat obese; during such activities, excess body fat provides a useful bonus of both buoyancy and insulation against cool water.

Anginal Pain

Anginal pain arises from myocardial ischaemia (L. Katz & Landt, 1935; Chapter 1). The chain of events leading to this symptom often includes a rise in peripheral venous tone and thus in cardiac work-load (H. Westling, 1971). The tissue malfunction is reversible, in contrast with infarction (where the myocardial cells die and are replaced by scar tissue). It might therefore be inferred that angina is an earlier manifestation of ischaemic heart disease than is an infarct. However, in practice, this is not the case. Angiograms often show extensive disease in the patient with angina. The cumulative likelihood of death in the first five years after diagnosis is very similar for angina and for myocardial infarction (E. Weinblatt *et al.*, 1973), while disability prior to death is typically greater among those with angina. Furthermore, the prognosis of the post-infarction patient is substantially worsened by concurrent angina (R.J. Shephard, 1979a), while the development of an infarct may cure angina, at least temporarily.

Angina usually has a precipitating cause (such as exposure to cold, physical activity or emotional excitement), and recovery is relatively rapid as soon as the provoking agent is withdrawn. A proportion of patients can 'walk through' an exercise-induced anginal attack. Possibly, continued exercise leads to dilatation of either the normal or the collateral blood supply to the affected segment of myocardium, or possibly a progressive increase in systemic blood pressure improves myocardial flow. In any event, 'walking through' an attack is not a technique to recommend to angina patients. Careful measurements usually show impaired cardiac contractility (decrease of $\dot{V}_{max}$, dP/dt and circumferential fibre shortening; M.H. Ellestad, 1975) with a stiff-ening of the ventricular wall (A.M. Fogelman *et al.*, 1972) during an attack. If affected individuals persist with physical activity in the face of anginal pain, they can precipitate a situation where stroke output diminishes, end-diastolic volume increases and cardiac failure develops (J.O. Parker *et al.*, 1966; T.W. Moir & Debra, 1967). The astute clinician will infer impairment of myocardial function from an atrial or ventricular 'gallop' rhythm, heard immediately following an exercise bout.

There is a general relationship between exercise-induced ST-segmental depression and angina, but many patients can develop several millimetres of ST displacement and a rise in end-diastolic pressure without symptoms (M. Ellestad, 1975). Again, some women show both retrosternal discomfort and ST changes without angio-graphically demonstrable narrowing of the coronary vessels (R. Gorlin, 1967; T.N. James, 1970; W. Likoff, 1972). Despite these anomalies, ECG telemetry during exercise provides an objective basis for distinguishing angina from musculo-skeletal pains and symptom-claiming associated with a secondary cardiac neurosis.

Patients who show a deep ST-segmental depression or true angina following infarction have an adverse prognosis. Training is contra-indicated for the individual who develops angina or cardiac failure at rest. In other anginal patients, activity must be prescribed with caution. If there is ECG evidence of exercise-induced ischaemia, the maximum permissible level of training should be defined by a laboratory stress test (R.E. Goldstein & Epstein, 1973; L.T. Sheffield & Roitman, 1973), and the individual should be taught the symptom pattern of angina as a further safeguard in regulating his habitual activity. Some authors (for example, J.J. Kellermann *et al.*, 1977) have observed a substantial improvement in effort tolerance when anginal patients undertake regular bouts of vigorous continuous training. Others have found a poor response to continuous activity, possibly because the patients were unable to reach a training threshold (T. Kavanagh & Shephard, 1975a); nevertheless, when the individuals concerned were transferred to a modified interval training plan, gains in maximum oxygen intake were almost as large as those seen in asymptomatic 'post-coronary' patients.

The optimum regimen for the person with angina seems to be about a minute of exercise, followed by a slow-walking recovery interval of sufficient duration to allow oxidation of accumulated metabolites (typically 1–1½ minutes). Sudden bursts of activity without a warm-up must be avoided, as must sustained isometric contractions. Exercise is also contraindicated for this class of patient if there has been recent emotional excitement, a heavy meal or exposure to extreme heat or cold.

If a patient is severely disabled by chest pain, preliminary medication with trinitrin and/or the administration of oxygen may help to raise confidence sufficiently so that a significant volume of training can be undertaken. Trinitrin affords relief to about 90 per cent of anginal victims, usually within five minutes of sub-lingual administration. If relief is not obtained, one must suspect either a loss of potency in the drug or a non-anginal explanation of the discomfort. Other drugs used in the relief of angina are discussed in Chapter 11. The angina threshold is lowered by exposure to carbon monoxide, whether from cigarette smoking (W.S. Aronow, 1976) or freeway travel (W.S. Aronow *et al.*, 1972). Regular ingestion of alcohol may also have an adverse effect (J. Orlando *et al.*, 1976).

The frequency of exercise-induced ST segmental depression and angina diminishes with conditioning (A. Kattus, 1970; J. Detry &

Bruce, 1971; D.R. Redwood *et al.*, 1972; T. Kavanagh *et al.*, 1973b).
Possible explanations include: (i) a lesser emotional reaction to a given
exercise task; (ii) a decrease in cardiac work rate for a given intensity of
exercise (D.R. Redwood *et al.*, 1972; D.N. Sim & Neill, 1974; C.K.
Kennedy *et al.*, 1976); and (iii) a true increase in myocardial blood
supply. Often, the first of these mechanisms is the most important.
Angina arises because a patient fears he will be unable to complete a
task or senses that he is being hurried (W.A. Aronow, 1979).
Substantial benefit is then derived from reassurance, judicious use of
tranquillisers and sedatives and simple psychotherapy. L. Zohman &
Tobis (1967) provided an interesting demonstration of the importance
of psychological factors in an experiment where patients were
supplied with compressed air via a mask; this led to a 50 per cent
increase in effort tolerance and a 20 per cent decrease in ECG changes
at a given work rate, changes comparable with those observed after a
short period of training. With regard to the third mechanism, A.A.
Kattus & Grollman (1972) found little relationship between development of the coronary collateral circulation and relief of angina.
However, more recent observations (G. Kober *et al.*, 1978) have noted
a better recovery of left ventricular function in patients with well-
developed collateral vessels.

By-pass Operations

There remain substantial differences of opinion concerning the indications for and the benefit to be anticipated from coronary by-pass
operations in ischaemic heart disease. The goals of surgery are similar
to those of exercise rehabilitation — extension of longevity,
restoration of function and an improvement in the quality of life.
There is good evidence that a by-pass may provide six to twelve
months of relief from disabling angina (W.C. Sheldon *et al.*, 1969;
E.L. Alderman *et al.*, 1973). In some instances, this may reflect an
increase in blood flow to ischaemic areas of the myocardium (J.A.
Walker *et al.*, 1971; D.G. Greene *et al.*, 1972; P. Lichtlen *et al.*, 1973).
However, in other patients, the mechanism of pain relief seems to be
the provocation of a perioperational infarct (H.I. Russek, 1970; R.E
Goldstein & Epstein, 1973; R.S. Ross, 1975; G.A. Guinn & Mathur,
1976; G.M. Lawrie *et al.*, 1977; H.D. McIntosh & Garcia, 1978).

There are reports that surgery has improved longevity in patients
with significant disease of the left main coronary artery (T. Takaro

et al., 1976; R.C. Read *et al.*, 1978), isolated disease of the anterior descending artery (W.C. Sheldon *et al.*, 1975), two-vessel disease (K.E. Hammermeister *et al.*, 1977), severe three-vessel disease (J.F. McNeer *et al.*, 1974; R.C. Read *et al.*, 1978) and anginal pain with minimal laboratory exercise (J.R. Margolis, 1975). Proponents of medical treatment suggest that there is no sound theoretical reason for such claims, since the majority of coronary veins grafts do not remain patent for more than one to two years (M.L. Murphy *et al.*, 1979). They argue that surgeons have generally compared their data with inappropriate controls — a medically treated group reported by the Cleveland Clinic (A.V.G. Bruschke *et al.*, 1973), or other non-concurrent data drawn from the literature (A. Oberman *et al.*, 1972; J.O. Humphries *et al.*, 1974). Randomised controlled trials fail to support the claims made for surgical treatment (V.S. Mathur & Guinn, 1975; M.L. Murphy *et al.*, 1979). Some surgeons have in turn retorted that this reflects the unexpectedly poor experience of the surgically treated patients. If the controlled series had received the best possible standard of surgery, benefit would have been observed. Thus W.D. Johnson (1979) claimed that in patients without significant irreversible myocardial damage, surgery should yield a 95 per cent five-year survival rate, irrespective of the number of diseased vessels, 90 per cent of patients getting partial relief and up to 70 per cent total relief from angina (Table 12.4). However, cynics have replied that part of the apparent improvement in surgical statistics reflects the extension of operative treatment to patients with less severe disease. The debate continues, but for the present we must conclude that the superiority of surgical treatment has only been established for patients with left main coronary artery disease (F. Kloster *et al.*, 1975; M.H. Frick *et al.*, 1976; T. Takaro *et al.*, 1976; Table 12.5).

Functional tests have shown little difference in the incidence of dysrhythmia during normal daily activity between surgically and medically treated patients (N. de Soyza *et al.*, 1976). There have been reports of augmented tolerance to exercise, with a higher limiting rate-pressure product (W.D. Johnson *et al.*, 1970; E.A. Amsterdam *et al.*, 1973), a decrease in left-ventricular end-diastolic pressure (W.D. Johnson *et al.*, 1970; K. Chatterjee *et al.*, 1972), a gain in cardiac index (K. Chatterjee *et al.*, 1972) and an increased ventricular ejection fraction after surgery (G. Rees *et al.*, 1971; M.G. Bourassa *et al.*, 1972), but other investigators have found no greater improvements than would be expected during conservative treatment (A.G. Tilkian *et al.*, 1976). The quantitation of left-ventricular function after a by-pass operation

Table 12.4: Relief of Angina with Coronary By-pass Surgery, Based on Data for 1,150 Unselected Patients

Angina status	Ventricular function		
	Normal (47% of sample) (%)	Mild impairment (34% of sample) (%)	Severe impairment (19% of sample) (%)
Total relief*	66	66	63
Improved	25	23	24
No change	6	7	6
Worsened	3	4	7

* Figures for 1975–6 show 68.5 per cent of patients with total relief of angina.

Source: W.D. Johnson (1979).

Table 12.5: Long-term Results of Coronary By-pass Surgery

Type of vessel	Post-operative period (yr)	Progression of stenosis (%)
Vessels with patent grafts	1	57
	6	66
Vessels with occluded grafts	1	53
	6	57
Non-grafted vessels	1	9.5
	6	46

Source: Based on data of M.G. Bourassa *et al.* (1978).

is complicated by changes in both ventricular volume and compliance (J.H. Caldwell *et al.*, 1975; U. Sigwart *et al.*, 1975; B. Sharma *et al.*, 1976). Nevertheless, a disappointingly small percentage of subjects show improved left-ventricular performance (R. Balcon & Rickards, 1973; K.E. Hammermeister *et al.*, 1974; P. Steele *et al.*, 1977).

J.C. Manley (1979) has suggested that the response to surgery depends on both pre-operative left-ventricular impairment (which reflects the size of the scar) and the patency of the graft (Table 12.6). If initial function is relatively normal, substantial gains in performance

Table 12.6: Improvement of Left-ventricular Function in Relation to Extent of Scarring and Success of Revascularisation

Extent of myocardial scar	Improvement of left-ventricular function	
	Good revascularisation (%)	Poor revascularisation (%)
Small	94	73
Moderate	75	56
Large	20	25

Source: Based on data of J.C. Manley (1979).

appear soon after surgery, and persist as long as the graft remains patent. However, gains are less likely if there is initially a moderate or a severe impairment of function and, in patients who have suffered a post-operative infarction, a deterioration in ventricular performance is likely. While revascularisation can improve the function of a hypo-kinetic segment of the ventricular wall, it is unlikely to restore the contraction of akinetic tissue (J.C. Manley & Johnson, 1972; W.P. Geis *et al.*, 1975). A combination of persistent angina, a low resting cardiac index, a poor ejection fraction and an elevated left-ventricular end-diastolic pressure points to a large infarct and a poor response to surgery (P.E. Cohn *et al.*, 1975). On the other hand, the patient who has normal resting function but develops angina and a rising left-ventricular end-diastolic pressure during exercise may well benefit from a by-pass operation. If there is a clear-cut aneurysm with paradoxical motion of the ventricular wall, function may be improved by excision of the affected segment (D.E. Harken, 1972; W. Delius *et al.*, 1973; R.W. Hacker, 1973; M. Rothlin *et al.*, 1973).

Peripheral Vascular Disease

Many patients with ischaemic heart disease also have atherosclerotic lesions in their peripheral vasculature (L.K. Widmer *et al.*, 1969). Such lesions worsen prognosis for several reasons, as follows:

(1)   They generally lead to an increase in systolic blood pressure and thus in cardiac work-load.
(2)   They hamper peripheral perfusion, compounding problems that

arise from poor maintenance of the cardiac stroke volume during vigorous exercise.

(3) Peripheral ischaemia may limit participation in a training programme (as a result of the development of intermittent claudicant pain when the patient walks a short distance).

(4) A combination of diabetes and peripheral ischaemia may progress to gangrene, with a need to amputate one or both lower limbs. The diseased heart must then sustain the heavy demands of locomotion in a wheel chair, on crutches or on a prosthesis (T. Kavanagh *et al.*, 1973a).

The pain of intermittent claudication is typically felt in the calf muscles (J.A. Gillespie, 1960). It is brought about by moderate exercise (such as walking 200 metres) and is relieved by rest. S.O. Isacsson (1972) observed symptoms of this type in 2.8 per cent of a random sample of 55-year-old men living in Malmo, Sweden. While the main risk factor is cigarette smoking, Isacsson also noted a significant correlation between calf blood flow and reported leisure activity.

The traditional treatment of claudicant pain has been surgical (excision of the thrombus, vascular graft or lumbar sympathectomy). However, A. Singer & Rob (1960) commented that the condition of 20 out of 22 patients receiving conservative treatment remained unchanged or improved, and a more recent review estimated that surgery was necessary in only 20 per cent of patients (British Medical Journal, 1976).

The walking distance to the onset of claudicant pain can be extended by a programme of regular exercise (S. Hedlund & Porjé, 1964; O.A. Larsen & Lassen, 1968; B. Ericsson *et al.*, 1971; Table 12.7), although the mechanism leading to the improvement of function remains unclear. H. Sanne & Sivertsson (1968) noted a development of collateral vessels in the cat when experimental occlusion of the femoral artery was followed by five weeks of treadmill training. On the other hand, O.A. Larsen & Lassen (1968) did not see any increase in limb flow when men with peripheral vascular disease underwent a training programme. Other possible mechanisms for improvement of peripheral oxygen supply include: (i) a recanalisation of existing vessels; (ii) a strengthening of the active muscles; and (iii) an increased peripheral oxygen extraction related to a redistribution of blood flow between skin and muscle, a redistribution of flow between active and inactive fibres and possibly an increased oxygen extraction within a given fibre through an increase in enzyme activity

Table 12.7: The Influence of Endurance Training upon Patients with Intermittent Claudication, Based on Data for Eleven Months of Training

Variable	Exercise group (n = 7)		Control group (n = 6)	
	Initial status	Change (%)	Initial status	Change (%)
Walking distance	273 m	+ 95	298 m	+ 17
Painless distance	186 m	+ 104	184 m	− 22
Maximum flow	15.7 ml/dl	+ 41	17.5 ml/dl	+ 6

Source: B. Ericsson *et al.* (1971).

(S. Zetterquist, 1971). It is also conceivable that psychological support allows a patient to perform more work before activity is halted by symptoms.

Practical suggestions for the claudicant subject include: (i) the wearing of well-insulated footwear in cold weather; (ii) correction of any anaemia; (iii) cessation of smoking; and (iv) the taking of a peripheral vasodilator drug prior to vigorous exercise. The traditional Buerger's exercises involve elevating the legs at 45-90° for three minutes, three or four times per day. Such therapy is supposed to improve collateral flow by inducing a reactive vasodilatation. However, if the exercises have more than a psychological effect, it is likely that this arises through a strengthening of the leg muscles, with a resultant facilitation of perfusion of the active fibres (J.P. Clausen & Larsen, 1971; M. Hirai, 1974).

13 EPILOGUE: THE BOTTOM LINE

While commercial organisations increasingly keep their focus upon the 'bottom line', there remains resistance to a cost-benefit analysis of health care. Somehow, it seems distasteful to set a dollar value on an individual human life. Nevertheless, how available health care resources should be deployed is becoming an important ethical decision. For example, is it appropriate to spend money on the primary and secondary prevention of heart disease, or should it be diverted to modern marvels of treatment such as by-pass surgery and cardiac transplants? Accordingly, this final chapter will attempt a brief review of cost-benefit issues from the standpoint of the patient, the physician and the community as a whole.

Cost-benefit Considerations for the Patient

Heart disease and health insurance costs

Strident argument continues between the proponents and antagonists of 'socialised' medicine, but prepaid health care by government and/or private insurance carriers is becoming a fact of life in almost all nations. Even in New York, the last bastion of free-enterprise medicine, L.R. Zohman (1973) found that a third of patients attending her exercise test and rehabilitation facility received 50 per cent or more reimbursement from Health Insurance carriers. Furthermore, social provision for the disabled and their dependants has become a responsibility of the state. Thus, fatal and non-fatal episodes of ischaemic heart disease impose a substantial financial burden upon the community (Table 13.1). Measured in current (1981) dollars, this amounts to at least $900 per wage-earner (R.J. Shephard, 1977a).

Since many of the causes of ischaemic heart disease reflect personal lifestyle (including items such as cigarette consumption, physical inactivity, overeating, and 'Type-A' behaviour, it becomes an important question of public policy how firm a government should be in moulding individual behaviour patterns.

One possible way of encouraging a favourable lifestyle is to develop a system of differential health-insurance premiums, based upon the risk-taking behaviour of the insured person. This approach has been adopted successfully with automobile insurance (reduced premiums for teetotallers), fire insurance (reduced premiums for non-smokers) and some forms of life assurance (increased premiums if overweight, reduced premiums for non-smokers). The concept would be more difficult to apply and to police if a total allowance were to be made for 'diseases of choice' when calculating annual insurance premiums. For example, it could be argued that a small proportion of those who are obese have an intractable metabolic disorder; this is not their choice, and it would be unfair to penalise such individuals. Nevertheless, a potential instrument for measuring overall risk-taking behaviour has now been developed by the Canadian Federal Government — a health-hazard-appraisal questionnaire. A simple computer programme calculates the difference between the individual's calendar age and an appraised age based upon personal lifestyle (cigarette smoking habits, physical inactivity, excessive consumption of alcohol, failure to use a seat belt, etc.). At present, the score from this instrument is being used as a motivational tool, and there is now evidence that a favourable change of appraised age can result from participation in an employee fitness programme (Table 13.2).

A second possible tactic for discouraging poor health behaviour is to charge the resultant health cost at source, imposing a heavy tax on items such as cigarettes and alcohol. For some reason, this expedient is politically more acceptable than the use of differential health-insurance premiums. Nevertheless, it remains difficult to attribute an appropriate cost to any given risk factor and, to avoid the wrath of powerful lobbies maintained by the industries concerned, the tax that is levied rarely covers the full health cost of the adverse behaviour. Furthermore, there is a danger that a government may perceive the tax as a source of revenue rather than as a partial payment of health costs already incurred. It is then but a short step to accept and even tacitly to encourage the risk-taking behaviour. Physical inactivity is particularly difficult to tax, except indirectly through such items as petrol for cars and electricity for power appliances. A possible alternative is to offer tax relief to corporations that introduce low-cost employee-fitness programmes. The self-employed could receive similar encouragement through tax deductions for membership in approved health clubs.

A third method of health promotion is a massive advertising campaign. There seems sufficient evidence to warrant persuading people to become physically more active. In the past, it has been argued that advertising is singularly ineffective in changing personal habits. While commercial Fitness Spas often spend a substantial proportion of their

Table 13.1: Estimated Impact of Cardiovascular Disease upon the US Economy, Measured in 1962 Dollars

	Annual cost (billion dollars)
Direct costs:	
personal services and supplies (hospital care, services of physicians and nurses, provision of drugs)	2.6
non-personal items (research, training, public-health services, capital construction and insurance schemes)	0.5
Indirect costs:	
premature death (see Table 2.2)	19.4
loss of output from illness	3.0
intangibles (e.g. pain, suffering, orphanhood)	5.2
Total	30.7

Source: H.E. Klarman (1964).

Table 13.2: Appraised Age, as Determined by the Canadian Health Hazard Appraisal, Showing the Change of Score among Men and Women Participating Regularly in an Industrial Fitness Programme

Nature of participation	Change of appraised age over 6 months	
	Men	Women
Control subject	−0.42	1.37
Non-participant	0.25	1.87
Drop-out	−0.24	−0.27
Low adherent	−0.44	0.53
High adherent	−1.91	0.39

Source: R.J. Shephard, Corey & Cox (in preparation).

income on recruitment, it is possible that the individuals thus attracted have already been active elsewhere. Again, the short-term results of massive 'lifestyle' documents such as the US Surgeon General's reports on 'Smoking and Health' have been disappointing. On the other hand, the funds allocated to smoking-withdrawal programmes have remained only a small fraction of those expended by cigarette manufacturers in promoting their sales. More encouragement can be drawn from long-term changes in the cardiac epidemic (Chapter 2). The most reasonable explanation of the downturn in cardiac deaths is that there has been a slow but progressive improvement in lifestyle in response to 15 years of well-coordinated health education.

Techniques of mass stress-testing

Some authors have advocated mass stress-testing, both as a means of detecting individuals who are vulnerable to a 'heart attack' and as a prelude to an increase in physical activity. In the United States, it is current wisdom that an exercise ECG should be obtained prior to the prescription of physical activity for any patient over 35 years of age (K.H. Cooper, 1970; American College of Sports Medicine, 1975). This is largely an example of the practice of 'defensive medicine'. Physicians fear to use less than the maximum available diagnostic aids in case a cardiac emergency should occur, with a subsequent claim of professional negligence (G.H. Siegel, 1973). However, we have already seen that an exercise stress-test is a relatively ineffective screening procedure when dealing with apparently healthy 35-year-old subjects. In Canada, the option of universal physician-supervised stress-tests was reviewed at a National Conference on Fitness and Health (W.R. Orban, 1974); delegates concluded that such a policy would generate unwarranted expense. A simple, three-tiered test structure was proposed as a workable alternative. At the lowest level of sophistication would be a self-administered test, the Canadian Home Fitness Test (R.J. Shephard, 1980a). This would cost from $5-7, the charge being borne by the individual himself. The relative safety of the procedure would be assured by details of test design (R.J. Shephard, 1980a), and by completion of an initial health questionnaire (PAR-Q, the physical activity readiness questionnaire; D. Chisholm *et al.*, 1975). The score from the Home Fitness Test was intended to motivate patients to an increase in physical activity, while providing them with an approximate guide to a suitable exercise prescription.

At the second level of sophistication, the Canadian National Conference proposed a more comprehensive fitness test, supervised by paramedical personnel, and costing about $15. In some instances, this cost might be borne by the individual, and in other instances it might be arranged as an employee benefit. A prototype of this system can be seen in seven 'fitness vans' currently operated by the Province of Ontario. These are staffed by five paramedical workers, and they offer simple assessments of lung function, muscle strength, body fat and flexibility in addition to an ECG-monitored version of the Canadian Home Fitness Test. The ECG is used primarily to obtain an accurate heart-rate count, although the paramedical staff of the vans have had instruction in ECG interpretation, and are thus able to refer suspicious-looking records to a physician for expert appraisal. At the third level of investigation is a full physician-supervised laboratory stress-test. Many clinics in the United States charge $150–200 (L.R. Zohman, 1973) for this service.

It is obviously much cheaper to leave the great mass of routine exercise testing to paramedical personnel, but questions may be asked concerning the safety of such an approach. In practice, the risks are remarkably small. The Canadian Home Fitness Test has now been carried out by upwards of 500,000 people, with no serious complications (R.J. Shephard, 1980a). A typical experience from a series of 15,000 supervised tests is a transient loss of consciousness in three subjects and one minor ankle strain (R.J. Shephard, 1980a). Many would maintain that the involvement of a physician helps to avoid a heart attack during testing or subsequent prescribed exercise. However, we found that different physicians advised anywhere from 0.7 to 15.0 per cent of ostensibly healthy patients against performance of the Canadian Home Fitness Test. Furthermore, the proportion of ECG abnormalities observed during testing was unrelated to the proportion of subjects that had been excluded. On the basis that prolonged exercise such as a marathon ski event increased the risk of a heart attack by a factor of only three or four (R.J. Shephard, 1976), we calculated that if five million middle-aged Canadian men and women performed the Canadian Home Fitness Test once every year, 16 to 33 years would elapse before there was a single fatality attributable to the test. On the reasonable assumption that the PAR-Q test would exclude at least a half of the 'high-risk' patients, the time to a cardiac emergency would increase to 33–66 years. The advantage of having a physician present to administer resuscitation during the 66th year seems indisputable. However, if his cardiac resuscitation had a success rate of 80 per cent, the cost would exceed $25 billion dollars per resuscitation measured in 1981 currency. While the physician might be successful in his treatment of the emergency, it is further quite unlikely that he would have averted the incident, since there are few clear guidelines as to precipitating factors. Permissible test limits for the three most promising indicators (excessive ST depression, excessive dysrhythmias and excessive rise in systemic blood pressure) are all hotly debated between different laboratories. Plainly, there are more economic strategies than physician supervision for combating one emergency in 330 million man-years; one obvious possibility is the training of the general population in techniques of cardiac resuscitation (L.A. Cobb *et al.*, 1975).

If tests are conducted in their entirety by paramedical workers, the disposition of the exercise electrocardiogram becomes an important consideration. Some physicians have argued that paramedical personnel should be required to use a device other than an ECG for accurate heart-rate counting. The main basis for this suggestion is that patients may believe they have received ECG clearance for exercise, when in fact they have not. There are two simple remedies: (i) the patient can be given a written statement that the ECG is used only to count the heart rate; or (ii) the paramedical worker can be taught to interpret the ECG. The latter approach seems the more sensible, and indeed H. Blackburn (1968) has shown that a competent technician can provide more accurate routine screening than a physician (Chapter 7). Test records that appear to be abnormal can be referred to a resident cardiologist for evaluation, and where necessary the patient can then be referred for a full medically supervised stress-test. If a large population is to be screened, another possible option is to group subjects by age, sex and fitness level, carrying out the stress-tests 16 at a time. A bank of 16 ECGs can then be monitored by an intensive-care nurse and a cardiology resident on a highly cost-effective basis; indeed, with careful scheduling, two individuals can carry out at least 100 stress tests per hour (R.J. Shephard, 1980a).

Value of screening

Using this last approach, the cost of a medically supervised ECG stress-test can be brought under $2.50 per individual (Table 13.3). The examination takes a little over the optimal time for a screening procedure, but nevertheless it is well accepted by most patients. The main argument against its general application is a low effectiveness in detecting ischaemic heart disease (Table 7.1; Chapter 7). Furthermore, there are inevitably many false positive diagnoses, a situation that creates both cardiac cripples and an unnecessary demand for the potentially dangerous procedure of coronary angiography. Taking account of the costs of angiography, the total expense involved in bringing ten of 1,000 screened individuals to by-pass sugery and a further ten patients to a test-reinforced improvement in lifestyle exceeds $60,000, more than $3,000 for every individual that is helped (Table 7.3). Moreover, the value of such help is doubtful. The usefulness of coronary by-pass

Table 13.3: Cost of Mass Stress-testing with Medically Supervised
ECG Recording

Test time =	10 min	
Staff	one salaried physician at $42•h^{-1}	= $ 7.00
	one coronary care nurse at $21•h^{-1}	= $ 3.50
	ten junior assistants at $6•h^{-1}	= $10.00
Equipment	depreciation at $20,000•yr^{-1}	= $ 2.38
Supplies		= $16.00
Total for 16 patients		= $38.00
	Cost per patient = $2.43	

Source: Based on calculations of R.J. Shephard (1980a).

surgery in the absence of cardiac symptoms remains highly debatable
(Chapter 12), and there are cheaper and possibly more certain means of
reinforcing behavioural change than mass screening.

Cost-effectiveness is substantially improved (Table 7.3) if exercise
testing is limited to candidates identified as having a high risk of
ischaemic heart disease on the basis of simple clinical questioning
(family history, smoking habits, excess body mass, etc.).

Medical supervision of exercise programmes

Similar questions of cost-effectiveness may be posed concerning the
medical supervision of exercise programmes. To reach informed and
ethical decisions, it is necessary to set a dollar value upon the life that
is being protected. For example, an apparently healthy 40-year-old
man has the potential to earn for 25 years and collect a pension for a
further ten years. Given a current annual income of $30,000, his total
financial worth is thus $900,000, measured in 1981 dollars. In
contrast, a post-coronary patient aged 50 may have the prospect of
survival for only ten years. Assuming the same annual salary, his total
worth would be about $300,000. How do these figures compare with
the cost of providing a medically supervised exercise programme?

Let us suppose that a middle-aged population of five million adults
are each performing five hours of exercise per week. The total number
of exercise-related cardiac emergencies will then be about 910 per
year (R.J. Shephard, 1976). This estimate is admittedly based on many
assumptions, but it is partially corroborated by an alternative figure of

1,900 incidents per year, derived from the experience of *males* with an above-average cardiac risk (individuals who have already survived a non-fatal heart attack). Grouping the population of five million adults into 100,000 exercise classes, each with 50 members, the risk that an emergency will arise in any given class is about one in 110 per year. By using a simple self-administered health questionnaire, the risk is reduced, probably to one in 220 class-years or lower. Let us assume that medical cover is to be provided, and that 100,000 physicians are persuaded to undertake regular supervisory duties for an honorarium of $50 per class. The cost of such supervision is $12,500 per class-year, $2,750,000 per emergency or about $3.5 million per successful resuscitation; unfortunately, this cost is almost four times the worth of the person whose life has been saved.

The risk of a cardiac emergency is greater when dealing with 'post-coronary' patients. W. Haskell (1978) has estimated that in recently designed 'cardiac' rehabilitation programmes there is one cardiac emergency in 1,000 man-years. Given a class size of 50 patients, the risk is one in 20 class-years, $250,000 per emergency or about $300,000 per successful resuscitation. Although the financial worth of the 'post-coronary' patient is lower than that of his healthy counterpart, there is plainly more economic justification for medical supervision of a 'cardiac' exercise programme.

Assuming a class size of 40–50 patients, and allowing one hour of physician time, one hour of gym time and 2½ hours of physical activity supervisor time per session, H. Pyfer & Doane (1973) calculated a total operating cost of $4.50 per person-session over the first three months of post-coronary rehabilitation, $4.00 per person-session for the remainder of the first year, and $25 per person-month (three sessions per week) thereafter. L.R. Zohman cited a similar figure ($5 per session for supervised cycle-ergometer exercise). In Toronto, we have used one physician and four supervisors for a group of 50 'cardiac' patients (R.J. Shephard, 1976); the cost is about $90 per session, excluding gymnasium rental (R.J. Shephard, 1976).

It is also instructive to calculate the economic cost of insuring against a cardiac emergency. One recent discussion recommended a minimum personal protection of $500,000 per incident (R.B. Parr & Kerr, 1975), with additional coverage for the responsible hospital or university. Let us suppose an apparently healthy 40-year-old man with a net worth of $900,000, and a risk of one in 220 class-years. Simple calculation suggests that an appropriate charge for insurance would be $82 per person-year. A class of 50 members could thus be insured for an annual premium of $4,100; if resuscitation were 80 per cent successful, the cost would drop further to $820 per class-year. Parallel calculations can be carried out for 50-year-old post-coronary patients with a worth of $300,000 and a risk of one cardiac emergency in 20 class-years. An appropriate insurance cost is then $300 per participant-year, or $15,000 per class-year ($3,000 per class-year, given 80 per cent success of resuscitation). However, these relatively low figures are based on well-designed medically supervised programmes. A cost at least ten times greater would be anticipated for less satisfactory classes (W. Haskell, 1978).

Few people would seriously argue against medical supervision of exercise in the early stages of post-coronary rehabilitation (B. Erb, 1969; J.K. Cooper & Willig, 1971). On the other hand, the possibility of arranging long-term medically supervised rehabilitation may be limited by the willingness of physicians to undertake this type of duty. The annual incidence of non-fatal infarcts is about 250 per 100,000 population, and about a half of these are suitable candidates for exercise rehabilitation (L.L. Brock, 1974). Thus, the total number of recruits to a Canada-wide cardiac rehabilitation programme might be 30,000 patients per year. Assuming an average survival of ten years, the size of the post-coronary exercise class would soon grow to 300,000 members. Maintaining a 1:50 physician/patient ratio there would be a need for 6,000 suitably trained physicians (cost $75 million per year) and 6,000 gymnasia equipped for cardiac resuscitation.

It is hardly surprising that both Canadian and US experts have recommended a progressive 'tapering' of medically supervised exercise programmes (Chapter 9) over a period of between one and two years following infarction. There is pragmatic justification for such a plan, since the mortality of patients who remain enrolled in an exercise programme drops progressively in the second and subsequent years of activity (Chapter 6).

Cost-benefit Considerations for the Physician

Traditionally, the Hippocratic oath has kept physicians from crass cost-benefit analyses in the operation of their practices. Such a view of medicine was appropriate when the main diagnostic tool was a $2 stethoscope, office costs were limited to the occasional re-upholstering of a living-room chair and secretarial help could be obtained by buying an occasional bouquet for one's wife. However, current patterns of practice demand the use of expensive diagnostic equipment, salaried paramedical assistants and costly office suites, and in this situation a careful cost-benefit analysis is necessary to economic survival (H. Pyfer & Doane, 1973).

Primary and secondary prevention

Many physicians believe that lifestyle counselling is too expensive to be undertaken within the fee schedules offered by insurance carriers. If such a viewpoint were correct, this would present a major obstacle to the development of practical programmes for the prevention of ischaemic heart disease. However, there has been a rapid growth in commercial lifestyle counselling services such as 'weight-watchers' and 'smoke-enders', suggesting that the medical community has a false perception of the economics of health promotion.

There is some virtue in offering incidental counsel on exercise, obesity and smoking habits during the course of a general medical examination, but the keys to a successful preventive programme include: (i) automation; (ii) gathering of a sufficient audience; and (iii) delegation of attitude changing to well-trained professionals. Many patients spend at least 15 minutes in the doctor's waiting room, and a good tape/slide presentation on a healthy lifestyle could be offered at this time for a capital investment of perhaps $1,000. The cost could be reduced proportionately if several doctors shared a common waiting room.

One-to-one lifestyle counselling is uneconomic, but an instructor with appropriate group skills can sustain the effective involvement of up to 30 patients. The role of the physician should be to supervise such programmes, monitoring the medical information that is transmitted, but leaving to behavioural experts the detailed organisation of a given class-session. Often, a meeting place such as a church hall can be reserved for a nominal fee, so that a nightly payment of $2-3 per patient is enough to meet the costs of therapy. Pre-paid insurance does not always cover charges for lifestyle counselling. Nevertheless small payments often serve a useful function, encouraging the patient to adhere to the proposed lifestyle.

Exercise testing and prescription

Many practices are sorely underequipped for purposes of exercise testing and prescription. Other physicians are dazzled by promotional literature, and make excessive purchases of electronic gadgetry that are hard to justify. The most economical arrangement is to ensure that

Table 13.4: Costs of Maintaining a Simple Exercise Test Facility

		$	Per year $
Office space, 20 square metres			2,000
Paramedical professional			20,000
Equipment:	defibrillator	1,000	
	electrocardiogram	500	
	cycle ergometer	200	
	sphygmomanometer	200	
	skinfold calipers	200	
	handgrip dynamometer	200	
	flexibility test	200	
	spirometer	400	
	timing device	25	
	oxygen and medical supplies	200	
		$4,125	
	amortized over five years:		825
Supplies and repairs			1,000
	Total:		$23,825

Capacity 20 patients per day, 4,600 patients per year

Cost per patient: $ 5.20*

---

* This estimate does not include allowance for medical consultation, initial training costs, delays in response to billings or administration. In the first year of operation, these factors could increase costs by up to 50 per cent (H. Pyfer & Doane, 1973). H. Pyfer & Doane have calculated the much higher cost of $ 48 per maximum exercise-tolerance test. However, this is based on a much smaller-scale operation (40 cardiac patients), with incomplete usage of facilities. They also make the generous allowance of half an hour of physician time and one hour of paramedical time for each stress test. L.R. Zohman (1973) presents calculations based upon $ 155 per stress test; again this higher figure reflects underutilisation of the facility (50 patients per month) and a generous allowance for medical consultation.

one set of equipment is shared by a group of at least three to four physicians. Given a case load of 20 patients per day, the approximate cost per patient (exclusive of medical consultation and billing charges) can be as low as $ 5.20 (Table 13.4). The main expense is the salary of a well-trained paramedical professional. Given an adequate case load, a simple facility such as that outlined in Table 13.4 should not impose a severe financial burden upon a group medical practice.

Malpractice insurance

Theoretically, the physician who performs or supervises an exercise test at a level of care commensurate with his training should be immune from malpractice suits. Unfortunately, much effort has been expended by personal-injury lawyers in recent years, and in some cases substantial damages have been awarded against physicians on account of problems arising from exercise testing, exercise prescription and authorisation of a return to normal employment (E.L. Sagall, 1979). Successful suits have been based on professional negligence (harm resulting from acts of commision or omission), failure to obtain 'informed consent' for the test or exercise programme, and a combination of these factors. The present author has personal recollection of one patient, an apparently healthy middle-aged shop assistant, who performed a brief sub-maximal step test on company premises. She had been given a careful preliminary medical examination, and the step test was performed under medical supervision, without apparent mishap. Nevertheless, the following day, she complained of a swollen, painful ankle, and was unable to stand at work for about three months. She presented a claim for damages, although it was difficult to determine whether her tendonitis had been provoked by the step test or had arisen elsewhere. Certainly, there was no evidence that the condition was caused directly by a deviation from normal standards of care, and the patient could not prove that her own actions in the 24 hours following the test had not contributed to her condition. On the advice of her lawyer, she was thus persuaded to accept normal occupational-disability payments for the period that she was absent from work.

The appropriate level of medical care for exercise testing and prescription is now clearly documented in numerous publications. Defence against malpractice must thus be based on testimony and records showing that such norms of clinical expertise were met.

E.L. Sagall (1979) noted common basis for legal claims as follows:

(1)   Failure to detect pre-existing medical abnormalities contra-indicating a proposed stress test or conditioning programme;

(2)   Failure to monitor the patient adequately before, during and after exercise;

(3)   Lack of skill or delay in the handling of an emergency;

(4)   Lack of equipment, drugs and trained personnel necessary for effective resuscitation;

(5)   Lack of informed consent;

(6)   Inadequate documentation of the procedures followed;

(7) Inappropriate clearance for return to work with subsequent reinfarction.

E.L. Sagall suggested that the consent form should list specifically all hazards of exercise, including death, myocardial infarction, acute congestive heart failure and cerebrovascular accident. It should also explain appropriate alternative procedures with their risks. He commented that the signing of a printed consent form (G.H. Siegel, 1973; American College of Sports Medicine, 1975) might not be enough to establish informed consent. The physician should therefore note in his records at the time of testing that a verbal explanation had been fully understood by the patient.

Given that fatalities occur almost exclusively among 'cardiac' patients, and that resuscitation is about 80 per cent successful, the risk of death is approximately one in 50,000 patients. Assuming the net worth of a 'post-coronary' patient is $ 300,000, an appropriate insurance allowance would be $ 6 per test, more than 100 per cent of the basic cost of the examination.

In contrast, when a sub-maximal test is performed on a 'normal' adult, the risk of a cardiac emergency is about one in 80 million; assuming an 80 per cent chance of successful resuscitation, the cost of providing $ 1,000,000 insurance would then be no more than 0.25 ¢ per test. Given the total annual test population of 4,600 patients postulated in Table 13.4, insurance against possible fatalities in healthy subjects would not add more than five per cent to operating costs.

Cost-benefit Considerations for the Community

Physical activity has potential benefits for the community in terms of the prevention of ischaemic heart disease, plus a more general impact on other health problems (smoking, obesity, diabetes, etc.), productivity and the costs of self-care during old age (Table 13.5). Against these possible gains must be set the costs of promoting physical activity and of providing the necessary facilities.

Costs of ischaemic heart disease

In discussing cost-benefit considerations for the patient, we estimated the probable cost of ischaemic heart disease at $ 900 per wage-earner per year. The community would not recover all of this money if there were a mass increase in physical activity. The most optimistic forecasts

Table 13.5: Potential Annual Savings from an Increase in Physical Activity, Calculated per Wage-earner, Assuming 20 Per cent Participation in the Exercise Programme

	$ per annum
Ischaemic heart disease	90
Chronic chest disease	?
Improved lifestyle	150
Absenteeism	37
Employee turnover	216
Geriatric care	17
	510*

*   In estimating this figure, note that: (1) not all savings are necessarily mutually exclusive; (2) ischaemic heart disease patients may live to collect longer pensions; (3) geriatric savings have been adjusted downwards by 25 per cent to allow for the cost of specific exercise classes for the elderly.

(Chapter 5) point to an immediate halving of cardiac deaths ($900/5 × 2 = $90 p.a.). However, cynics have suggested that the resultant survivors might live to collect a substantial old-age pension, eventually requiring several years of expensive geriatric care that would have been avoided by a heart attack. From the purely economic point of view, savings to the community are most likely if exercise postpones death from 40 to no later than 65 years of age.

Costs of other health problems

A stronger economic case can be made for the savings that result from avoidance of other health problems, particularly the chronic chest disease that is linked to cigarette smoking (C.M. Fletcher, 1959). It is uncertain how far physical activity checks the cigarette habit, but there is some evidence that the commencement of long-distance running can have this type of effect (P. Morgan *et al.*, 1976).

In our employee fitness programme, 'high adherents' showed a gain of 1.5-2 years appraised age relative to 'non-participants' and 'drop-outs' over a six-month study (R.J. Shephard & Cox, in preparation). Assuming an income of $30,000 per year, this is equivalent to a total of between $45,000 and $60,000 per individual, or $650-850 per participant per year of life. At present, sustained participation in employee fitness programmes does not exceed 20 per cent of company staff, so the community saving is the smaller sum of $130-70 per individual per year.

Industrial productivity

Important practical effects of an employee fitness programme are a decrease of absenteeism and a reduced employee turnover (M. Cox & Shephard, 1979). In our study, 'high adherents' showed a drop in in absenteeism relative to other employees. The resultant saving averaged 1.4 days per employee per year. Assuming 230 days were spent earning $30,000, the annual saving per employee would average $183, or 0.61 per cent of salary. Given a company of 1,400 employees, with 20 per cent of high adherents, the total payroll saving would be a useful $51,000 per annum (0.12 per cent).

An even bigger cost factor is the employee turnover rate. In the company that we examined (M. Cox & Shephard, 1979) there was an average turnover rate of 20 per cent per annum. The cost was $6,000 per individual, $1,200 per employee per year (or four per cent of payroll). However, 'high adherents' to the industrial fitness programme had a turnover rate of only two per cent per annum (some 0.4 per cent of payroll). Given 20 per cent participation in the employee fitness programme, the overall turnover should thus drop from 20 to 16.4 per cent, with a payroll saving of 0.72 per cent. In a company of 1,400 employees, this could yield a total dividend of just over $300,000 per annum.

Costs of geriatric care

In 1975, the annual cost of institutional care for the elderly citizens of Canada amounted to $1,897 million, about $82 per citizen and $200 per wage-earner (R.J. Shephard, 1978b). Measured in 1981 dollars, the cost would be at least $250 per wage-earner.

Much of this expense is incurred simply because senior citizens become too weak to look after themselves. If increased physical activity were to push back the age of dependency by eight or nine years without altering the age at death, this would reduce the number of dependent patients by a factor of two thirds. Given also some impact on acute and chronic care (particularly for cardiorespiratory diseases) and a small reduction in mental illness, 1975 geriatric costs for Canada would have shown a 44 per cent reduction, as follows:

Active and chronic care $= \$ 1,169 \text{ M} \times 1/3 = \$ 386 \text{ M}$
Mental care $= \$ \quad 60 \text{ M} \times 1/10 = \$ \quad 6 \text{ M}$
Extended care $= \$ \quad 668 \text{ M} \times 2/3 = \$ 445 \text{ M}$

    Total saving $= \$ 837 \text{ M}$

Against this saving, it would be necessary to set the costs of suitable exercise classes for the elderly. The true financial benefit to the community would thus be about $633 million per year, or 34 per cent of geriatric-care costs. Assuming a participation rate of 20 per cent, the annual savings from a geriatric exercise programme would be $17 per wage-earner per year ($250 × 34% × 20%).

Costs of promoting physical activity

There are few reliable guides to the costs of promoting physical activity. One may presume that at one extreme there is a potentially active minority of adults who are easily persuaded to undertake regular exercise, but at the other extreme there are very inactive individuals who would be recruited only with extreme difficulty.

One possible indicator of the expenditure needed to influence life-style is the budget for advertising cigarettes (about $300 M per year in the US). Much of this money maintains the cigarette habit rather than recruits new smokers. Nevertheless, the annual cost is approximately $3 per wage-earner, with a 40–50 per cent adult participation rate.

A second statistic is the advertising budget for commercial health spas. One popular chain of health clubs in Southern Ontario boasts about 130,000 members, and it is reputed to spend $1,500,000 per year on advertising. Since the majority of those recruited sign an initial three-year contract, and some subsequently renew their membership, it costs this company about $50 for every contract that is completed. The club membership accounts for less than five per cent of the adults in Ontario, and it is thus difficult to be certain that the advertising programme has achieved any large-scale conversion to the habit of regular exercise. Many of the people who join both private and industrial fitness clubs have previously been active elsewhere (R.J. Shephard *et al.*, 1980a).

In Canada, governmental expenditures on the promotion of fitness are made through agencies such as the Canadian crown corporation 'Participaction', the Federal Department of Health and Welfare, and corresponding Provincial and municipal departments. The overall Federal expenditure on 'lifestyle' programmes was estimated at $45 million for the fiscal year 1973/4 (M. Lalonde, 1974). However, this total covered a wide range of public-health programmes, and even in 1981 it is unlikely that governmental allocations for the promotion of physical activity exceed $10 million per year (about 80 ¢ per wage-earner). Some ten years of expenditure at this rate has undoubtedly increased Canadian awareness of a need for voluntary activity, but changes in behaviour have been quite small. Particular effort has been concentrated on Saskatoon, and in that city as many as 50 per cent of adults have been persuaded to participate in specific projects such as a communal 'walk around the block'.

Costs of facilities

Many forms of physical activity involve substantial expense in terms of equipment, facilities and land usage (R.J. Shephard, 1977a; Tables 13.6 and 13.7). Indeed, at a first glance, the potential health savings seem eclipsed by the costs of the increased activity. However, if due allowance is made for economies from careful scheduling and incomplete participation, the cost-benefit ratio becomes more favourable.

Jogging is often regarded as the 'poor-man's sport', but a realistic appraisal of costs would amount to $200-300 per individual per year, at least $100 of this being attributable to clothing and equipment. Cross-country skiing (minimal equipment about $20 per year, amortized over five years) appears to be cheaper than jogging, although account must also be taken of the short 'season' (typically, two months of the year). While these costs do not deter an executive, many blue-collar workers perceive fitness as an expensive luxury. Thus, when a Hamilton hospital arranged 'post-coronary' exercise classes for employees at a steel mill, they found that in order to ensure regular attendance it was necessary to offer not only a free programme but free parking facilities.

Capital costs of physical facilities include construction and the land that is used by both the playing area and parked vehicles. The total expense would be much lower if the provision of recreational lands became a firmer condition of permission for residential developments. The costs cited in Table 13.7 exceed the basic fees charged by many commercial fitness clubs; for instance, a new and lavishly equipped YMCA in North Toronto is offering membership for $500 per year. This discrepancy arises partly because the costs of Table 13.7 are calculated per wage-earner rather than per participant, and partly because the space allocated is sufficient to allow all of the population

Table 13.6: Costs of One-year Jogging Programme

	$
Two pairs of good-quality running shoes	80
Two pairs of socks	10
Sweat suit (five-year depreciation)	5
Rain gear (five-year depreciation)	5
Stop watch (five-year depreciation)	5
Shorts (five-year depreciation)	2
Winter track admission ($ 1 per night)	90
Total*	197

* No allowance has been made for added food consumption. Depending on the distance covered and the type of food eaten, this could range from $ 25 to $ 100 per year.

Table 13.7: Estimated Capital Cost of Providing Facilities for Selected Types of Exercise in a Metropolitan Population of 2.4 Million, Measured in 1981 Dollars

Sport	Construction ($ billion)	Costs[2] Land ($ billion)	Total ($ billion)	Annual cost per wage-earner if loan at 15% interest ($)	Ratio to health savings of Table 13.5[3]
Football/soccer	1.4	14.0	15.4	2,310	0.076
Tennis (doubles, three shifts)[1]	2.0	1.8	3.8	570	0.057
Conservation park (swimming)	—	0.45	0.45	68	0.023[4]
Urban swimming (360 per pool):					
indoor	5.2	8.4	13.6	2,040	0.067
outdoor	1.7	8.4	10.1	1,515	0.050
Urban skating (1,000 per rink):					
indoor	2.1	4.2	6.3	945	0.031
outdoor	1.1	4.2	6.3	795	0.026

1. It is assumed that the tennis courts are distributed on a neighbourhood basis, with no specific need for parking facilities.
2. Costs are calculated on the basis that all of the 2.4-million population will wish to use the facilities at peak hours. The values cited would drop proportionately if: (a) usage could be scheduled in one hour segments of a 12-hour day; and (b) participation rates were only 20 per cent of the total population.
3. Assuming usage scheduled over twelve-hour day with 20 per cent participation, at 1 hour per participant; eg. (2310/12)/5 × 510.
4. Assuming occupancy by 20 per cent of population throughout twelve-hour day.

to participate at peak hours. Commercial fitness organisations are profitable because: (i) scheduling allows distribution of member usage over at least twelve hours per day; (ii) only a small segment (commonly less than ten per cent of members) make full use of their privileges; and (iii) supplements are usually charged for popular activities such as tennis and squash.

Even a humble walk to the station is surprisingly expensive if careful accounting is made. Let us suppose than an 8-km walk is introduced into the normal working day. Although there is no charge for facilities (since sidewalks are probably available), a good pair of shoes may cost $50 per year, and a further expense arises from the food energy consumed — about 1.3 MJ per day, equal to four or five slices of bread per day, or about $25 of bakery products per year. On the credit side, we may note that maintenance costs are lower for a sidewalk than for a road, and the non-pedestrian will use gasoline ($270 \, \text{l} \cdot \text{yr}^{-1}$, $65 at 24 ¢ per litre) and parking facilities or will pay bus fares ($230 per year). The calculation is interesting in showing the problem of present-day society. Given the fact of universal car ownership, the cost of operating a vehicle over a short-haul journey that can and should be walked is remarkably low — indeed, for a family of four it is only about 22 per cent of self-propulsion! Plainly, it is desirable to modify our economic structure to correct this situation, conserving both our health and non-renewable resources such as gasoline in the process.

The next decade will undoubtedly see a trend towards demechanisation. Rising energy costs will encourage use of our muscles for performing more everyday activities. It may become economically advantageous to walk to the station and to use a handmower to cut the lawn. But even if this change is not realised, it would be wrong to conceive our cost-benefit analysis rigidly in terms of dollars and cents. Good health and an ability to live life to the full are priceless commodities. Those who have personal experience of a healthy life-style do not need strong economic incentives to persist in an active way of life — indeed, many are prepared to make considerable financial investments to enhance their newly discovered happiness.

BIBLIOGRAPHY

Abramov, L. Sexual life and sexual frigidity among women developing acute myocardial infarction. *Psychosom. Med., 38*, 418–25 (1976)

Acker, J. Early activity after myocardial infarction. In: *Exercise Testing and Exercise Training in Coronary Heart Disease*, ed. J.P. Naughton, H.K. Hellerstein & I.C. Mohler (Academic Press, New York, 1973) pp. 311–14

Adams, G.E., Bonner, E.A., Ribisl, P.M. & Miller, H.S. Blood pressure during heavy work on the treadmill and bicycle ergometer. *Med. Sci. Sports, 10*, 50 (1978)

Adelson, L. Sudden death from coronary disease — the cardiac conundrum. *Postgrad. Med., 30*, 139–47 (1961)

Adsett, C.A. & Bruhn, J.G. Short-term group psychotherapy for post-myocardial infarction patients and their wives. *Canad. Med. Assoc. J., 99*, 577–84 (1968)

Alderman, E.L., Matlof, H.J., Wexler, L., Shunway, N.E. & Harrison, D.C. Results of direct coronary artery surgery for treatment of angina pectoris. *New Engl. J. Med., 288*, 535–9 (1973)

Aldinger, E.E. & Sohal, R.S. Effects of digitoxin on the ultrastructural myocardial changes in the rat subjected to chronic exercise. *Amer. J. Cardiol., 26*, 369–74 (1970)

Allan, T.M. & Dawson, A.A. ABO blood groups and ischaemic heart disease in man. *Br. Heart J., 30*, 377-82 (1968)

Allen, J.G. Aerobic capacity and physiological fitness of Australian men. *Ergonomics, 9*, 485–94 (1966)

Altekruse, E.B. & Wilmore, J.H. Changes in blood chemistry following a controlled exercise program. *J. Occup. Med., 15*, 110–13 (1973)

American College of Sports Medicine. Guidelines for graded exercise testing and exercise prescription and behavioural objectives for physicians, program directors, exercise leaders and exercise technicians (Amer. Coll. Sports Med., Madison, Wisc., 1975)

American Heart Association. Report of committee on electro-cardiography (Chairman C.E. Kossmann). Recommendations for standardization of leads and specifications for instruments in electrocardiography and vectorcardiography. *Circulation 35*, 583–602 (1967)

American Heart Association, Committee on Exercise. *Exercise Testing and Training of Apparently Healthy Individuals. A Handbook for Physicians* (American Heart Association, New York, 1972)

Amery, A., Billiet, L., Conway, J. & Reybrouck, T. Comparison of cardiac output determined by a CO_2 rebreathing method at rest and during graded sub-maximal exercise. *J. Physiol., 267*, 34–5p (1977)

Amery, A., Julius, S., Whitlock, L.S. & Conway, J. Influence of hypertension on the hemodynamic response to exercise. *Circulation 36*, 231–7 (1967)

Amsterdam, E.A. Function of the hypoxic myocardium. In: *Congestive Heart Failure*, ed. D.T. Mason (Yorke Medical Books, New York, 1976) pp. 147–58

Amsterdam, E.A., Hughes, J.L., Mansour, E., Salel, A.F., Bonnano, J.A., Zelis, R. & Mason, D.T. Circulatory effects of practolol: selective cardiac beta adrenergic blockade in arrythmias and angina pectoris. *Clin. Res., 19*, 109 (abstr.) (1971)

Amsterdam, E.A., Hughes, J.L., Miller, R.R., Massumi, R.A., Zelis, R. & Mason, D.T. Physiologic approach to the medical and surgical treatment of angina pectoris. In: *Exercise Testing and Exercise Training in Coronary Heart Disease*, ed. J.P. Naughton, H.K. Hellerstein & I.C. Mohler (Academic Press, New York, 1973) pp. 103–17

Amsterdam, E.A. & Mason, D.T. Exercise testing and indirect assessment of myocardial oxygen consumption in evaluation of angina pectoris. *Cardiology 62*, 174–89 (1977)

Andersen, K.L., Shephard, R.J., Denolin, H., Varnauskas, E. & Masironi, R. *Fundamentals of Exercise Testing* (World Health Organization, Geneva, 1971)

Anderson, T.W. Double blind trial of vitamin E in angina pectoris. *Amer. J. Chem. Nutr., 27*, 1174–8 (1974)

Anderson, T.W. The myocardium in coronary heart disease. In: *Proceedings of International Symposium on Exercise and Coronary Artery Disease*, ed. T. Kavanagh (Toronto Rehabilitation Centre, Toronto, 1976) pp. 32–44

Anderson, T.W. A new view of heart disease. *New Scientist 77*,

374–6 (1978a)

Anderson, T.W. *Comments to Conference on Decline in CHD Mortality* (National Institutes of Health, Bethesda, Md., 1978b)

Anderson, T.W, & Halliday, M.L. The male epidemic: 50 years of ischaemic heart disease. *Publ. Hlth. (Lond.), 93*, 163–72 (1979)

Anderson, T.W. & Le Riche, W.H. Ischaemic heart disease and sudden death, 1901–1961. *Brit. J. Prev. Soc. Med., 24*, 1–9 (1970)

Applebaum-Bowden, D. & Hazzard, W.R. Ethinyl estradiol lowers liver levels of triglyceride lipase. *Circulation 59/60*, Suppl. II–186 (abstr.) (1979)

Arcos, J.C., Sohal, R.S., Sun, S.C. & Burch, G.E. Changes in ultra structure and respiratory control in mitochondria of rat heart hypertrophied by exercise. *Exp. Molec. Pathol., 8*, 49–65 (1968)

Arlow, J.A. Identification mechanisms in coronary occlusion. *Psychosom. Med., 7*, 195–209 (1945)

Armstrong, A., Duncan, B., Oliver, M.F., Julian, D.G., Donald, K.W., Fulton, M., Lutz, W. & Morrison, S.L. Natural history of acute coronary heart attacks. A community study. *Brit. Heart J., 34*, 67–80 (1972)

Armstrong, B.W., Workman, J.M., Hurt, H.H. & Roemich, W.R. Clinico-physiologic evaluation of physical working capacity in persons with pulmonary disease; rationale and application of a method based on estimating maximal oxygen consuming capacity from MBC and O_2V_e. *Amer. Rev. Resp. Dis., 93*, 223–33 (1967)

Armstrong, M.L. Regression of atherosclerosis. *Atheroscler. Rev., 1*, 137–82 (1976)

Aronow, W.S. Effect of cigarette smoking and of carbon monoxide on coronary heart disease. *Chest 70*, 514–18 (1976)

Aronow, W.S. Medical management of stable angina pectoris. In: *Heart Disease and Rehabilitation*, ed. M.L. Pollock & D.H. Schmidt (Houghton Mifflin, Boston, 1979) pp. 212–27

Aronow, W.S. & Cassidy, J. Five years follow-up of double Master's Test, maximal treadmill stress test and resting and post-exercise apexcardiogram in asymptomatic persons. *Circulation 52*, 616–18 (1975)

Aronow, W.S., Harris, C.N., Isbell, M.W. *et al.* Effect of freeway travel on angina pectoris. *Ann. Intern. Med., 77*, 669–76 (1972)

Aronow, W.S. & Kaplan, M.A. Propranolol combined with isosorbide dinitrate versus placebo in angina pectoris. *New Engl.*

J. Med., 280, 847–50 (1969)

Aronow, W.S., Kaplan, M.A. & Jacob, D. Tobacco: a precipitating factor in angina pectoris. *Ann. Intern. Med., 69*, 529–36 (1968)

Asano, K., Ogawa, S. & Furuta, T. Aerobic work capacity in middle- and old-aged runners. In: *Exercise Physiology*, ed. F. Landry & W.A.R. Orban (Symposia Specialists, Miami, Fla., 1978) pp. 465–71

Ascoop, C.A. What is an abnormal ischemic ECG response to exercise? In: *Coronary Heart Disease, Exercise Testing and Cardiac Rehabilitation*, ed. W.E. James & E.A. Amsterdam (Symposia Specialists, Miami, 1977) pp. 145–54

Ashley, F.W., & Kannel, W.B. Relation of weight change to changes in atherogenic traits: the Framingham study. *J. Chr. Dis., 27*, 103–4 (1974)

Asmussen, E. & Molbech, S.V. Methods and standards for evaluation of the physiological working capacity of patients. *Comm. Test. Obs. Inst.*, No. 4 (Hellerup, Denmark, 1959)

Åstrand, I. Aerobic work capacity in men and women with special reference to age. *Acta Physiol. Scand., 49*, suppl. 169, 1–92 (1960)

Åstrand, I. Blood pressure during physical work in a group of 221 women and men 48–63 years old. *Acta Med. Scand., 178*, 41–6 (1965)

Åstrand, I. The Scandinavian Committee on ECG classification. The 'Minnesota Code' for ECG classification. Adaptation to CR leads and modification of the code for ECGs recorded during and after exercise. *Acta Med. Scand.*, suppl. 481 (1967)

Åstrand, I. Electrocardiographic changes in relation to the type of exercise, the work load, age and sex. In: *Measurement in Exercise Electrocardiography*, ed. H. Blackburn (C.C. Thomas, Springfield, Ill., 1969) pp. 309–21

Åstrand, I. Circulatory responses to arm exercise in different work positions. *Scand. J. Clin. Lab. Invest.*, 27, 293–7 (1971)

Astrand, I., Åstrand, P.O. & Rodahl, K. Maximal heart rate during work in older men. *J. Appl. Physiol., 14*, 562–6 (1959)

Åstrand, P.O. Concluding remarks. *Canad. Med. Assoc. J., 96*, 907–11 (1967)

Åstrand, P.O., Cuddy, T.E., Saltin, B. & Stenberg, J. Cardiac output during submaximal and maximal work. *J. Appl. Physiol., 19*, 268–74 (1964)

Åstrand, P.O., Ekblom, B., Messin, R., Saltin, B. & Stenberg, J. Intra-arterial blood pressure during exercise with different muscle groups. *J. Appl. Physiol., 20*, 253–6 (1965)

Åstrand, P.O., Engström, L., Eriksson, B., Karlberg, P., Nylander, I., Saltin, B. & Thorén, C. Girl swimmers. *Acta Paed. Scand., 147*, supp., 1–75 (1963)

Åstrand, P.O. & Rodahl, K. *Textbook of Work Physiology* (McGraw Hill, New York, 1977)

Åstrup, P. Atherogenic compounds of tobacco smoke. In: *Atherosclerosis IV*, ed. G. Schettler, Y. Goto, Y. Hata & G. Close (Springer Verlag, Berlin, 1977) pp. 156–61

Åstrup, P., Hellung-Larsen, P., Kjeldsen, K. & Mellemgaard, K. The effect of tobacco smoking on the dissociation curve of oxhaemoglobin. *Scand. J. Clin. Lab. Invest., 18*, 450–7 (1966)

Åstrup, T. The effects of physical activity on blood coagulation and fibrinolysis. In: *Exercise Testing and Exercise Training in Coronary Heart Disease*, ed. J.P. Naughton, H.K. Hellerstein & I.C. Mohler (Academic Press, New York, 1973) pp. 169–92

Atkins, J.M., Matthews, O.A., Blomqvist, C.G. & Mullins, C.B. Incidence of arrhythmias induced by isometric and dynamic exercise. *Brit. Heart J., 38*, 465–71 (1976)

Auchincloss, J.H., Gilbert, R.G. & Bowman, J.L. Response of oxygen uptake to exercise in coronary artery disease. *Chest 65*, 500–6 (1974)

Avon, G., Ferguson, R.J., Chaniotis, L., Choquette, G. & Gauthier, P. *Estimation du Débit Cardiaque par 'CO$_2$ Rebreathing' avant et après l'Entrainement Physique chez le Coronarien. Anstract* (First Canadian Congress of Sport and Physical Activity, Montreal, 1973)

Ayotte, B., Seymour, J. & McIlroy, M. A new method for measurement of cardiac output with nitrous oxide. *J. Appl. Physiol., 28*, 863–6 (1970)

Bailey, D.A. & Mirwald, R.L. *A Children's Test of Fitness* (Action British Columbia, June, 1975)

Bailey, D.A., Shephard, R.J., Mirwald, R.L. & McBride, G.A. Current levels of Canadian cardio-respiratory fitness. *Canad. Med. Assoc. J., 111*, 25–30 (1974)

Balcon, R., Jewitt, D.E., Davies, J.P.H. & Oram, S. A controlled trial of propranolol in acute myocardial infarction. *Lancet* (ii), 917–20 (1966)

Balcon, R. & Rickards, A. Evaluation of results after aortocoronary bypass. In: *Coronary Heart Disease*, ed. M. Kaltenbach, P. Lichten & G.C. Friesinger (G. Thieme, Stuttgart, 1973) pp. 296–300

Ball, R.M., Bache, R.J., Cobb, F.R. & Greenfield, J.C. Regional myocardial blood flow during graded treadmill exercise in the dog. *J. Clin. Invest., 55*, 43–9 (1975)

Bang, H.O., Dyerberg, J. & Hjørne, N. Investigations of blood lipids and food composition of Greenlandic Eskimos. In: *Circumpolar Health*, ed. R.J. Shephard & S. Itoh (University of Toronto Press, Toronto, 1976) pp. 141–5

Banister, E.W. & Griffiths, J. Blood levels of adrenergic amines during exercise. *J. Appl. Physiol., 33*, 674–6 (1972)

Banister, E.W. & Taunton, J.E. A rehabilitation program after myocardial infarction. *Brit. Col. Med. J.*, 1–4 (October, 1971)

Banister, E.W., Tomanek, R.J. & Cvorkov, N. Ultrastructural modifications in rat heart-responses to exercise and training. *Amer. J. Physiol., 220*, 1935–40 (1971)

Barnard, R.J. Long-term effects of exercise on cardiac function. *Exercise Sports Sci. Rev., 3*, 113–33 (1975)

Barnard, R.J., MacAlpin, R.N., Kattus, A.A. & Buckberg, G.D. Ischemic response to sudden strenuous exercise in healthy men. *Circulation 48*, 936–42 (1973)

Barnes, G.K., Ray, M.J., Oberman, A., *et al*. Changes in working status of patients following coronary bypass surgery. *J. Amer. Med. Assoc., 238*, 1259–62 (1977)

Barry, A.J., Daly, J.W., Pruett, E.D.R., Steinmetz, J.R., Birkhead, N.C. & Rodahl, K. Effects of physical training in patients who have had myocardial infarction. *Amer. J. Cardiol., 17*, 1–7 (1966)

Bartle, S.H. & Sanmarco, M.E. Comparison of angiographic and thermal washout techniques for left ventricular volume measurement. *Amer. J. Cardiol., 18*, 235–52 (1966)

Bartlett, R.G. Physiologic responses during coitus. *J. Appl. Physiol., 9*, 469–72 (1956)

Bartlett, R.G. & Bohr, V.C. Physiologic responses during coitus in the human. *Fed. Proc., 15*, 10 (abstr.) (1956)

Bassett, D.R., Rosenblatt, G., Moellering, R.C. & Hartwell, A.S. Cardiovascular disease, diabetes mellitus and anthropometric evaluation in Polynesian males on the Island of Nichau, 1963. *Circulation 34*, 1088–97 (1966)

Bassler, T.J. Marathon running and immunity to atherosclerosis.

Ann. N.Y. Acad. Sci., 301, 579–92 (1977)

Battock, D.J., Alvarez, H. & Chidsey, C.A. Effects of propranolol and isosorbide dinitrate on exercise performance and adrenergic activity in patients with angina pectoris. *Circulation 39*, 157–69 (1969)

Bauss, R. & Roth, K. *Motorisch Entwicklung. Probleme und Ergebnisse von Längsschnittuntersuchungen* (Institut für Sportwissenschaft, Darmstadt, 1977)

Beard, O.W., Hipp, H.R., Robins, M., Taylor, J.S., Ebert, R.V & Bevan, L.G. Initial myocardial infarction among 503 veterans — 5 year survival. *Amer. J. Med., 28*, 871–83 (1960)

Beard, E.F. & Owen, C.A. Cardiac arrhythmias during exercise testing in healthy men. *Aerospace Med., 44*, 286–9 (1973)

Becker, L.C., Fortuin, N.J. & Pitt, B. Effect of ischemia and antianginal drugs on the distribution of radioactive microspheres in the canine left ventricle. *Circ. Res., 28*, 263–9 (1971)

Becker, M., Haefner, D.P., Kasl, S.V., Kirscht, J.P., Maiman, L.A. & Rosenstock, I.M. Selected psychosocial models and correlates of individual health-related behaviours. *Medical Care 15* (5) (suppl.), 27–46 (1977)

Becker, M. & Maiman, L.A. Socio-behavioural determinants of compliance with health and medical care recommendations. *Medical Care 13* 10–24 (1975)

Becklake, M.R., Frank, H., Dagenais, G.R., Ostiguy, G.L. & Guzman, G.A. Influence of age and sex on exercise cardiac output. *J. Appl. Physiol., 20*, 938–47 (1965)

Becklake, M., Varvis, C.J., Pengelly, L.D., Kenning, S., McGregor, M. & Bates, D.V. Measurement of pulmonary blood flow during exercise using nitrous oxide. *J. Appl. Physiol., 17*, 579–86 (1962)

Beiser, G.D., Epstein, S.E. & Goldstein, R.E. Impaired heart rate response to sympathetic nerve stimulation in patients with cardiac decompensation. *Circulation 37*, Suppl VI, 40 (1968)

Bendien, J. & Groen, J. A psychological statistical study of neuroticism and extroversion in patients with myocardial infarction. *J. Psychosomat. Res., 7*, 11–14 (1963)

Benditt, E.P. The origin of atherosclerosis. *Sci. Amer., 236* (2), 74–85 (1977)

Benestad, A.M. Determination of PWC and exercise tolerance in cardiac patients. *Acta Med. Scand., 183*, 521–9 (1968)

Benestad, A.M. The deteriorative effect of myocardial infarction upon physiological indices of work capacity. *Acta Med. Scand.*, *191*, 67–75 (1972)

Benfari, R.C. Lifestyle alteration and the primary prevention of CHD: the Multiple Risk Factor Intervention Trial (MRFIT). In: *Heart Disease and Rehabilitation*, ed. M.L. Pollock & D.H. Schmidt (Houghton Mifflin, Boston, Mass., 1979) pp. 341–51

Bengtsson, C. Ischaemic heart disease in women. *Acta Med. Scand.*, *549*, suppl., 1–128 (1973)

Bennett, D.H. & Evans, D.W. Correlation of left ventricular mass determined by echocardiography with vectorcardiographic and electrocardiographic voltage measurements. *Brit. Heart J.*, *36*, 981–7 (1974)

Berenson, G.S. & Burch, G.E. The response of patients with congestive heart failure to a rapid elevation in atmospheric temperature and humidity. *Amer. J. Med. Sci.*, *223*, 45–53 (1952)

Bergman, H. & Varnauskas, E. The haemodynamic effects of physical training in coronary patients. *Medicine and Sport 4*, 138–47 (Karger, Basel, 1970)

Bergström, K., Bjernulf, A. & Erikson, U. Work capacity, heart and blood volume, before and after physical training in male patients after myocardial infarction. *Scand. J. Rehabil. Med.*, *6*, 51–64 (1974)

Berkada, B., Akokan, G. & Derman, V. Fibrinolytic response to physical exercise in males. *Atherosclerosis 13*, 85–91 (1971)

Bevegard, S., Freyschuss, H. & Strandell, T. Circulatory adaptations to arm and leg exercise in supine and sitting positions. *J. Appl. Physiol.*, *21*, 37–46 (1966)

Bing, R.J., Hellems, H.K. & Regan, T.J. Measurement of coronary blood flow in man. *Circulation 22*, 1–3 (1960)

Biorck, G., Blomqvist, G. & Sievers, J. Studies on myocardial infarction in Malmo, 1935 to 1954. 1. Morbidity and mortality in hospital material. *Acta Med. Scand.*, *159*, 253–74 (1957)

Biss, K., Ho, K.J., Mikkelson, B., Lewis, L. & Taylor, C.B. Some unique biologic characteristics of the Masai of East Africa. *New Engl. J. Med.*, *284*, 694–9 (1971)

Bjernulf, A. Haemodynamic aspects of physical training after myocardial infarction. *Acta Med. Scand.*, *548*, suppl., 1–50 (1973)

Björntrop, B.P., Fahlen, M., Grimby, G., Gustafson, A., Holm, J., Renström, P. & Schersten, T. Carbohydrate and lipid metabolism in middle-aged physically well-trained men. *Metabolism 21*, 1037–44 (1972)

Blackburn, H. The exercise electrocardiogram. Technological, procedural and conceptual developments. In: *Measurement in Exercise Electrocardiography. The Ernst Simonsen Conference*, ed. H. Blackburn (C.C. Thomas, Springfield, Ill., 1968), pp. 220–58

Blackburn, H. Multifactor preventive trials in coronary heart disease. In: *Trends in Epidemiology*, ed. G.T. Stewart (C.C. Thomas, Springfield, Ill., 1972)

Blackburn, H. Disadvantages of intensive exercise therapy after myocardial infarction. In: *Controversy in Internal Medicine*, ed. F. Ingelfinger (W.B. Saunders, Philadelphia, 1974) p. 162

Blackburn, H. Preventive cardiology in practice: Minnesota studies on risk factor reduction. In: *Heart Disease and Rehabilitation*, ed. M.L. Pollock & D.H. Schmidt (Houghton Mifflin, Boston, Mass., 1979) pp. 245–75

Blackburn, H., Blomqvist, G., Freiman, A., Freisinger, G.C., *et al.* The exercise electrocardiogram: differences in interpretation. *Amer. J. Cardiol., 21*, 871–80 (1968)

Blackburn, H., Debacker, G. & Crow, R. Epidemiology and prevention of ventricular ectopic rhythms. *Adv. Cardiol., 18*, 208–16 (1976)

Blackburn, H., Taylor, H.L., Hamrell, B., Buskirk, E., Nicholas, W.C. & Thorsen, R.D. Premature ventricular complexes induced by stress testing, their frequency and response to physical conditioning. *Amer. J. Cardiol., 31*, 441–9 (1973)

Blake, H.A., Manion, W.C., Mattingly, T.W., *et al.* Coronary artery anomalies. *Circulation 30*, 927–40 (1964)

Blick, E.F. & Stein, P.D. *Work of the Heart: a General Thermodynamic Analysis* (Pergamon Press, New York, 1977)

Bloch, A., Maeder, J.P. & Haissly, J.C. Sexual problems after myocardial infarction. *Amer. Heart J., 90*, 536–7 (1975)

Blomqvist, C.G., Gaffney, F.A., Atkins, J.M. *et al.* The exercise ECG and related physiological data as markers of critical coronary artery lesions. *Acta Med. Scand., 615*, suppl., 51–62 (1978)

Blomqvist, C.G. & Mitchell, J.H. Exercise testing and electrocardiographic interpretation. In: *Heart Disease and Rehabilitation*, ed. M.L. Pollock & D.H. Schmidt (Houghton-Mifflin, Boston, 1979)

Blomqvist, G. Exercise physiology related to diagnosis of coronary artery disease. In: *Coronary Heart Disease: Prevention, Detection, Rehabilitation with Emphasis on Exercise Testing*, ed. S.M. Fox (Internationl Medical Corporation, Denver, Colorado, 1974) pp. (2-1)–(2-26)

Bloom, D.S. & Vecht, R.H. Circulatory changes during isometric exercise measured by transcutaneous aortovelography. *J. Physiol., 281*, 21–2p (1978)

Boas, E.P. & Goldschmidt, E.F. *The Heart Rate* (C.C. Thomas, Springfield, Ill., 1932)

Bonen, A., Gardner, J., Primrose, J., Quigley, R. & Smith, D. An evaluation of the Canadian Home Fitness Test. *Canad. J. Appl. Sports. Sci., 2*, 133–6 (1977)

Borer, J.S., Bacharach, S.L., Green, M.V., *et al.* Real-time radionuclide cineangiography in the non-invasive evaluation of global and regional left ventricular function at rest and during exercise in patients with coronary artery disease. *New Engl. J. Med., 296*, 839–44 (1977)

Boshoff, W.H. Ergonomic aspects of traditional and modern cultivation tasks in Uganda. In: *Proceedings of the Fourth International Congress on Rural Medicine* (Usada, Japan, 1965)

Bouchard, C., Hollmann, W., Venrath, H., Herkenrath, G. & Schlüssel, H. Minimalbelastungen zur Prävention kardiovaskularer Erkrankungen. *Sportarzt und Sportmedizin 7*, 348–57 (1966)

Bourassa, M.G. Corbara, F., Lésperance, J. & Campeau, L. Progression of coronary disease five to seven years after aortocoronary bypass surgery. In: *Coronary Heart Disease*, ed. M. Kaltenbach, P. Lichtlen, R. Balcon & W.D. Bussmann (G. Thieme, Stuttgart, 1978) pp. 139–44

Bourassa, M.G., Lésperance, J., Campeau, L. & Saltiel, J. Fate of left ventricular contraction following aortocoronary venous grafts. *Ciculation 46*, 724–30 (1972)

Bourne, G. An attempt at the clinical classification of premature ventricular beats. *Quart. J. Med., 20*, 219–43 (1927)

Braunwald, E., Ross, J. & Sonnenblick, E.H. *Mechanisms of Contraction of the Normal and Failing Heart*, 2nd edn (Little, Brown, Boston, Mass., 1976)

Brenton, M. *Sex and Your Heart* (Coward, New York, 1968)

Briggs, J.F. The role of emotions in the rehabilitation of the cardiac patient. In: *Changing Concepts in Cardiovascular Disease*, ed. H.I. Russek & B.L. Zohman (Williams & Wilkins, Baltimore,

1972) pp. 393–7

British Medical Journal. Intermittent claudication. *Brit. Med. J.*, *6019*, 1165–6 (1976)

Brock, L.L. Stress testing in work evaluation units. In: *Work Evaluation Units Sub-committee Newsletter* (American Heart Association, New York, 1967)

Brock, L. Early reconditioning for post-myocardial infarction patients: Spalding Rehabilitation Center. In: *Exercise Testing and Exercise Training in Coronary Heart Disease*, ed. J.P. Naughton, H.K. Hellerstein and I.C. Mohler (Academic Press, New York, 1973) pp. 315–23

Brock, L.L. Administrative considerations. In: *Coronary Disease, Exercise Testing, Rehabilitation Therapy*, ed. S. Fox (International Medical Corporation, Denver, Col., 1974) pp. (10-1)–(10-8)

Brodsky, M., Wu, D., Denes, P., Kanakis, C. & Rosen, K.M. Arrhythmias documented by 24 hour continuous electrocardiographic monitoring in 50 male medical students without apparent heart disease. *Amer. J. Cardiol., 39*, 390–5 (1977)

Brody, A.J. Master two-step test in clinically unselected patients. *J. Amer. Med. Assoc., 171*, 1195–8 (1959)

Bronstein, L.H. Experience of the work classification unit at BelleVue Hospital. In: *Work and the Heart*, ed. F.F. Rosenbaum & E.L. Belknap (P.B. Hoeber, New York, 1959)

Bronstet, J.P., Series, E., Guern, P., Vallot, F. & Pic, A. Matching Nifedipine and Nitroglycerine in the prevention of exercise-induced angina. In: *Coronary Heart Disease*, ed. M. Kaltenbach, P. Lichtlen, R. Balcon & W.D. Bussmann (G. Thieme, Stuttgart, 1978) pp. 309–16

Brown, B.G., Gundel, W.D., Gott, V.L. & Covell, J.W. Hemodynamic determinants of retrograde arterial coronary flow following acute coronary occlusion. *Circulation 46*, suppl. 2, 100 (Abstr.) (1972)

Brown, J.R. & Shephard, R.J. Some measurements of fitness in older female employees of a Toronto department store. *Canad. Med. Assoc. J., 97*, 1208–13 (1967)

Brozek, J., Keys, A. & Blackburn, H. Personality differences between potential coronary and non-coronary subjects. *Ann. N.Y. Acad. Sci., 134*, 1056–64 (1966)

Bruce, E.H., Frederick, R., Bruce, R.A. *et al.* Comparison of active participants and drop-outs in CAPRI cardiopulmonary rehabilitation programs. *Amer. J. Cardiol, 37*, 53–60 (1976)

Bruce, R.A. Atherosclerosis. In: *Coronary Heart Disease: Prevention, Detection, Rehabilitation with Emphasis on Exercise Testing*, ed. S.M. Fox (International Medical Corp., Denver, Col., 1974) chap. 1, pp. 1–16

Bruce, R.A, Alexander, E.R., Li, Y.B., Chiang, B.N., Ting, N. & Hornsten, T.R. Electrocardiographic responses to maximal exercise in American and Chinese population samples. In: *Measurement in Exercise Electrocardiography*, ed. H. Blackburn (C.C. Thomas, Springfield, Ill., 1969) pp. 413–44

Bruce, R.A., Blackmon, J.R., Jones, J.W. & Strait, G. Exercise testing in adult normal subjects and cardiac patients. *Pediatrics 32*, suppl., 742–56 (1963)

Bruce, R.A., Fisher, L.D., Cooper, M.N. & Gey, G.O. Separation of effects of cardiovascular disease and age on ventricular function with maximal exercise. *Amer. J. Cardiol., 34*, 757–63 (1974a)

Bruce, R.A., Hornsten, T.R. & Blackmon, J.R. Myocardial infarction after normal responses to maximal exercise. *Circulation 38*, 552–8 (1968)

Bruce, R.A., Kusumi, F., Culver, B.H. & Butler, J. Cardiac limitation to maximal oxygen transport and changes in components after jogging across the U.S. *J. Appl. Physiol., 39*, 958–64 (1975)

Bruce, R.A., Kusumi, F. & Hosmer, D. Maximal oxygen intake and nomographic assessment of functional aerobic impairment in cardiovascular disease. *Amer. Heart J., 85*, 546–62 (1973)

Bruce, R.A., Kusumi, F., Niederberger, M. & Peterson, J.L. Cardiovascular mechanisms of functional aerobic impairment in patients with coronary heart disease. *Circulation 49*, 696–702 (1974b)

Bruhn, J.G. Obtaining and interpreting psychosocial data in studies of coronary heart disease. In: *Exercise Testing and Exercise Training in Coronary Heart Disease*, ed. J.P. Naughton & H.K. Hellerstein (Academic Press, New York, 1973)

Bruhn, J.G., Wolf, S. & Philips, B.V. Depression and death in myocardial infarction: a psychosocial study of screening male coronary patients over nine years. *Psychosom. Res., 15*, 305–13 (1971)

Brunner, B.C. Personality and motivating factors influencing adult participation in vigorous physical activity. *Res. Quart.*, *40*, 464–8 (1969)

Brunner, D. Active exercise for coronary patients. *Rehab. Rec.*, *9*, 29–31 (1968)

Brunner, D. *Studies in Preventive Cardiology. Coronary Heart Disease — Epidemiology and Rehabilitation* (Government Hospital, Donolo, Jaffa, 1973)

Brunner, D. & Manelis, G. Physical activity at work and ischemic heart disease. In: *Coronary Heart Disease and Physical Fitness*, ed. O.A. Larsen and R.O. Malmborg (University Park Press, Baltimore, Md., 1971)

Brunton, T.L. On the action of nitrite of amyl on the circulation. *J. Anat. Physiol.*, *5*, 92–101 (1871)

Bruschke, A.V.G. Management of the patient with severe symptoms of coronary artery disease. In: *Coronary Heart Disease, Exercise Testing and Cardiac Rehabilitation*, ed. W.E. James & E.A. Amsterdam (Symposia Specialists, Miami, Fla., 1977) pp. 37–45

Bruschke, A.V.G., Proudfit, W.L. & Sones, F.M. Progress study of 590 consecutive nonsurgical cases of coronary disease followed 5–9 years. I. Arteriographic correlations. *Circulation* *47*, 1147–53 (1973)

Bruschke, A.V.G., Proudfit, W.L. & Sones, F.M. Progress study of 590 consecutive nonsurgical cases of coronary disease followed 5–9 years. II. Ventriculographic and other correlations. *Circulation 47*, 1154–63 (1973)

Brusis, O.A. Guidelines for supervised and non-supervised cardiac rehabilitation programs. In: *Coronary Heart Disease, Exercise Testing and Cardiac Rehabilitation*, ed. W.E. James and E.A. Amsterdam (Symposia Specialists, Miami, Fla., 1977) pp. 233–45

Bubenheimer, P., Samek, L., Schmeisser, H.J. & Roskamm, H. Echocardiographic evaluation of left ventricular function during exercise in untrained young men and athletes. In: *International Conference on Sports Cardiology*, ed. T. Lubich & A. Venerando (1980) pp. 787–92

Burch, G.E. & De Pasquale, N.P. Sudden, unexpected natural death. *Amer. J. Med. Sci.*, *249*, 86–97 (1965)

Burrow, R.D., Strauss, H.W., Singleton, R., *et al.* Analysis of left ventricular function from multiple gated acquisition cardiac blood pool imaging: comparison to contrast angiography.

Circulation 56, 1024–8 (1977)

Burt, J.J. & Jackson, R. The effects of physical exercise on the coronary collateral circulation of dogs. *J. Sports Med. Phys. Fitness 5*, 203–6 (1965)

Burton, A.C. *Physiology and Biophysics of the Circulation* (Year Book Publishers, Chicago, Ill., 1965)

Buskirk, E.R., Kollias, J., Piconreatigue, E., Akers, R., Prokop, E. & Baker, P. In: *International Symposium on the Effects of Altitude on Physical Performance*, ed. R. Goddard (Athletic Institute, Chicago, 1967)

Cadlwell, J.H., Stewart, D.K., Frimer, M., *et al.* Left ventricular volume during maximal supine exercise. *Circulation 51/52*, suppl. II, 140 (1975)

Cander, L. & Forster, R.E. Determination of pulmonary parenchymal tissue volume and pulmonary capillary blood flow in man. *J. Appl. Physiol., 14*, 541–51 (1959)

Cantwell, J.D., Walter, J.B., Watt, E.W. & Fletcher, G.F. Dynamic exercise training in post-myocardial infarction patients. *Med. Sci. Sports 5*, 66–7 (1973)

Cardus, D., Fluentes, F. & Srinivasan, R. Cardiac evaluation of a physical rehabilitation program for patients with ischemic heart disease. *Arch. Phys. Med. Rehabil., 56*, 419–25 (1975)

Carlson, L.A. Plasma lipids and lipoproteins and tissue lipids during exercise. In: *Nutrition and Physical Activity*, ed. G. Blix (Almqvist & Wiksell, Uppsala, 1967) p. 16

Carrier, R., Landry, F., Potvin, R., *et al.* Comparisons between athletes, normal and Eskimo subjects from the view of selected biochemical parameters. In: *Training: Scientific Basis and Application*, ed. A.W. Taylor (C.C. Thomas, Springfield, Ill., 1972)

Carrow, R.E., Brown, R.E. & Van Huss, W.D. Fiber sizes and capillary to fiber ratios in skeletal muscle of exercised rats. *Anat. Record 159*, 33–40 (1967)

Cash, J.D. & McGill, R.C. Fibrinolytic response to moderate exercise in young male diabetics and non-diabetics. *J. Clin. Pathol., 22*, 32–5 (1969)

Casssel, J., Heyden, S., Bartel, A.G., Kaplan, B.H., Tyroler, H.A, Cornoni, J.C. & Hames, C.G. Occupation and physical activity and coronary heart disease. *Arch. Int. Med., 128*, 920–8 (1971)

Castelli, W.P., Doyle, J.T., Gordon, T., Hames, C.G., Hjortland,

M.C., Hulley, S.B., Kagan, A. & Zukel, W.J. HDL cholesterol and other lipids in coronary heart disease — the cooperative lipoprotein phenotyping study. *Circulation 55*, 767–72 (1977)

Castleden, C.M. & Cole, P.V. Inhalation of tobacco smoke by pipe and cigar smokers. *Lancet* (2), 21–2 (July, 1973)

Cederlöf, R., Friberg, L. & Jonsson, E. Hereditary factors and 'angina pectoris'. A study of 5,877 twin-pairs with the aid of mailed questionnaires. *Arch. Env. Health 14*, 397–400 (1967)

Cermak, J. Changes of the heart volume and of the basic somatometric indices in 12–15 years old boys with an intense exercise regime. A long term study. *Brit. J. Sports Med., 7*, 241–4 (1973)

Chamberlain, D.A. Role of coronary ambulances in reduction of sudden coronary death. In: *Sudden Coronary Death*, ed. V. Manninen & P.I. Halonen (Karger, Basel, 1978a) pp. 191–2

Chamberlain, D.A. Beta-adrenergic blocking agents in prevention of sudden death. In: *Sudden Coronary Death*, ed. V. Manninen & P.I. Halonen (Karger, Basel, 1978b) pp. 196–205

Chapman, C.B. & Fraser, R.S. Studies on the effect of exercise on cardio-vascular function. III. Cardiovascular response to exercise in patients with healed myocardial infarction. *Circulation 9*, 347–51 (1954)

Chapman, J.M. & Massey, F.J. The interrelationship of serum cholesterol, hypertension, body weight, and risk of coronary disease. Results of the first ten years' follow up in the Los Angeles Heart Study. *J. Chron. Dis., 17*, 933–49 (1964)

Chatterjee, K., Swan, H.J.C., Parmley, W.W., Sustaita, H., Marcus, H. & Matloff, J. Depression of left ventricular function due to acute myocardial ischemia and its reversal after aortocoronary saphenous-vein bypass. *New Engl. J. Med., 286*, 1117–22 (1972)

Chiang, B., Perlman, L.V., Ostrander, L.D., *et al.* Relationship of premature systoles to coronary heart disease and sudden death in the Tecumseh epidemiological study. *Ann. Intern. Med., 70*, 1159–66 (1969)

Chidsey, C.A, Braunwald, E. & Morrow, A.G. Catecholamine excretion and cardiac stores of norepinephrine in congestive heart failure. *Amer. J. Med., 39*, 442–51 (1965)

Chisholm, D.M., Collis, M.L., Kulak, L.L., Davenport, W. & Gruber, N. Physical activity readiness. *Brit. Col. Med. J., 17*, 375–8 (1975)

Choquette, G. & Ferguson, R. Blood pressure reduction in 'borderline' hypertensives following physical training. *Canad. Med. Assoc. J., 108*, 699–703 (1973)

Chrastek, J. & Adimirova, J. Höher Blütdruck und körperliche Übungen. *Sportarzt und Sportmedizin 21* (3), 61–6 (1970)

Clark, R.J. Experience of the cardiac work classification unit in Boston, Massachusetts. In: *Work and the Heart*, ed. F.F. Rosenbaum & E.L. Belknap (P.B. Hoeber, New York, 1959) pp. 311–21

Clarke, H.H. *Physical and Motor Tests in the Medford Boy's Growth Study* (Prentice Hall, Englewood Cliffs, N.J., 1971)

Clarke, H.J. Physical activity and coronary heart disease. Washington, D.C. — President's Council on Physical Fitness and Sports. *Physical Fitness Research Digest 2* (2), 1–13 (1972)

Clarke, H.H. Update: physical activity and coronary heart disease. *Physical Fitness Research Digest 9* (2), 1–25 (1979)

Clarke, J.M., Shelton, J.R., Hamer, J., Taylor, S. & Venning, G.R. The rhythm of the normal human heart. *Lancet* (ii), 508–12 (1976)

Clausen, J.P. Circulatory adjustments to dynamic exercise and effect of physical training in normal subjects and patients with coronary artery disease. *Progr. Cardiovasc. Dis., 18*, 459–95 (1976)

Clausen, J., Felsby, M., Schønau-Jørgensen, F., Lyager-Nielsen, B., Roin, J. & Strange, B. Absence of prophylactic effect of propranolol in myocardial infarction. *Lancet* (ii) 920–4 (1966)

Clausen, J.P., Klausen, K., Rasmussen, B. & Trap-Jensen, J. Central and peripheral circulatory changes after training of the arms and legs. *Amer. J. Physiol., 225*, 675–82 (1973)

Clausen, J.P. & Larsen, N.A. Muscle blood flow during exercise in normal men studied by the Xe^{133} clearance method. *Cardiovasc. Res., *, 245–54 (1971)

Clausen, J.P., Larsen, O.A. & Trap-Jensen, J. Physical training in the management of coronary artery disease. *Circulation 40*, 143–54 (1969)

Clausen, J.P. & Trap-Jensen, J. Effects of training on the distribution of cardiac output in patients with coronary artery disease. *Circulation 42*, 611–24 (1970)

Clausen, J.P., Trap-Jensen, J. & Lassen, N.A. The effects of training on the heart rate during arm and leg exercise. *Scand. J. Clin. Lab. Invest., 26*, 295–301 (1970)

Clausen, J.P., Trap-Jensen, J. & Lassen, N.A. Evidence that the relative exercise-bradycardia induced by training can be caused by extra-cardiac factors. In: *Coronary Heart Disease and Physical Fitness*, ed. O.A. Larsen & R.O. Malmborg (University Park Press, Baltimore, Md., 1971) pp. 27–8

Clements, I.P., Vliestra, R.E., Dewey, J.D. & Harrison, C.E. Protective effect of verpamil infusion on mitochondrial respiratory function in ischemic myocardium. In: *Coronary Heart Disease*, ed. M. Kaltenbach, P. Lichtlen, R. Balcon & W.D. Bussman (G. Thieme, Stuttgart, 1978) pp. 284–96

Cobb, F.R., Ruby, R.L. & Fariss, B.L. Effects of exercise on acute coronary occlusion in dogs with prior partial occlusion (abstr.) *Circulation 37/38*, 104 (1968)

Cobb, L.A., Baum, R.S., Alvarez, H. & Schaffer, W.A. Resuscitation from out-of-hospital ventricular fibrillation: 4 years follow up. *Circulation 52*, suppl. III, 223–8 (1975)

Cohen, L. Contributions of serum enzymes and isoenzymes to the diagnosis of myocardial injury. I. *Mod. Concepts Cardiovasc. Dis., 36*, 43–7 (1967)

Cohen, L.S., Elliott, W.C., Rolett, E.L. & Gorlin, R. Haemodynamic studies during angina pectoris. *Circulation 31*, 409–16 (1965)

Cohen, S.I., Young, M.W., Lau, S.H., Haft, J.I. & Damato, A.N. Effects of reserpine on cardiac output and A-V conduction at rest and controlled heart rates in patients with essential hypertension. *Circulation 37*, 738–46 (1968)

Cohn, P.F., Gorlin, R., Herman, M.V. *et al.* Relation between contractile reserve and prognosis in patients with coronary artery disease and a depressed ejection fraction. *Circulation 51*, 414–20 (1975)

Cole, J.P. & Ellestad, M.H. Significance of chest pain during treadmill exercise: correlation with coronary events. *Amer. J. Cardiol., 41*, 227–32 (1978)

Cole, D.R., Singian, E.B. & Katz, L.N. Long-term prognosis following myocardial infarction, and some factors which affect it. *Circulation 9*, 321–34 (1954)

Collis, M. *Employee Fitness* (Minister of State for Fitness and Amateur Sport, Ottawa, 1975)

Cooksey, W.B. Letter to the Editor. *J. Amer. Med. Assoc., 113*, 351–2 (1939)

Cooper, J.K. & Willig, S.H. Nonphysicians for coronary care

delivery: Are they legal? *Amer. J. Cardiol., 28*, 363–5 (1971)

Cooper, K.H. *Aerobics* (Evans, New York, 1968)

Cooper, K.H. Guidelines in the management of the exercising patient. *J. Amer. Med. Assoc., 211*, 1663–7 (1970)

Cooper, K.H., Meyer, B.U., Blide, R., Pollock, M. & Gibbons, L. The important role of fitness determination and stress testing in predicting coronary incidence. *Ann. N.Y. Acad. Sci., 301*, 642–52 (1977)

Corliss, R.J. Cardiac catheterization. In: *Heart Disease and Rehabilitation*, ed. M. Pollock & D.H. Schmidt (Houghton Mifflin, Boston, 1979) pp. 140–56

Coronary Drug Project Research Group. Clofibrate and niacin in coronary heart disease. *J. Amer. Med. Assoc., 231*, 360–81 (1975)

Corvisart. *Essai sur les Maladies du Coeur et des Gros Vaisseaux* (Paris, 1806). Cited by L.F. Bishop & P. Reichart, *Psychosomatics 12*, 412–15 (1971)

Council on Rehabilitation. International Society of Cardiology. *Myocardial Infarction. How to Prevent. How to Rehabilitate*. Ed. T. Semple (Brussels, 1973)

Cox, M.H. & Shephard, R.J. Employee fitness, absenteeism, and job satisfaction. *Med. Sci. Sports 11*, 105 (abstr.) (1979)

Crews, J. & Aldinger, E.E. Effect of chronic exercise on myocardial function. *Amer. Heart. J., 74*, 536–42 (1967)

Criterion Committee of New York Heart Association. *Diseases of the Heart and Blood Vessels. Nomenclature and Criteria for Diagnosis* (Little, Brown, Boston, 1964)

Cumming, G.R. & Alexander, W.D. The calibration of bicycle ergometers. *Canad. J. Physiol. Pharm., 46*, 917–19 (1968)

Cumming, G.R., Borysyk, L.M. & Dufresne, C. The maximal exercise ECG in asymptomatic men. *Canad. Med. Assoc. J., 106*, 649–53 (1972)

Cumming, G.R., Dufresne, C., Kich, L. & Samm, J. Exercise electrocardiogram patterns in normal women. *Brit. Heart J., 35*, 1055–61 (1973a)

Cumming, G.R., Dufresne, C. & Samm, J. Exercise ECG changes in normal women. *Canad. Med. Assoc. J., 109*, 108–11 (1973b)

Cumming, G.R. & Edwards, A.H. Indirect measurement of left ventricular function during exercise. *Canad. Med. Assoc., J., 89*, 219–21 (1963)

Cumming, G.R., & Glenn, J. Evaluation of the Canadian Home

Fitness Test in middle-aged men. *Canad. Med. Assoc. J., 117*, 346–9 (1977)

Cunningham, D.A., Ingram, K.J. & Rechnitzer, P.A. The effect of training: physiological responses. *Med. Sci. Sports 11*, 379–81 (1979)

Cunningham, D.A., Ingram, K.J., Rechnitzer, P.A., Jones, N.L., Shephard, R.J., Sangal, S., Andrew, G., Buck, C., Kavanagh, T., Parker, J.O. & Yuhasz, M.S. Effect of a 2-year program of exercise training on cardiovascular fitness and recurrence rates in post-myocardial infarction patients. *Cardiology 62*, 136–7 (1977)

Cunningham, D.A. & Rechnitzer, P.A. Exercise prescription and the post-coronary patient. *Arch. Phys. Med. Rehab., 55*, 296–300 (1974)

Cureton, T.K. Improving the physical fitness of youth. A report of research in the sports-fitness school of the University of Illinois. *Monographs of Society for Research in Child Development 29* (4), 1–221 (1964)

Dagenais, G.R., Pitt, B. & Ross, R.S. Exercise tolerance in patients with angina pectoris. *Amer. J. Cardiol., 28*, 10–16 (1971)

Daoud, A.S., Fritz, K.E., Jarmolych, J., Augustyn, J.M., Lee, K.T. & Thomas, W.A. Regression of complicated atherosclerotic lesions in the abdominal aortas of swine. *Adv. Exp. Med. Biol., 82*, 447–52 (1977)

Davies, C.T.M. Submaximal tests for estimating maximum oxygen intake. Commentary. In: *Proceedings of an International Symposium on Physical Activity and Cardiovascular Health. Canad. Med. Assoc. J., 96*, 743–4 (1967)

Dayton, S., Hashimoto, S.D., Dixon, W.J. & Tomiyasu, W. A controlled clinical trial of a diet high in unsaturated fat in preventing complications of atherosclerosis. *Circulation 40*, Suppl. II, 1–63 (1969)

d'Andrade, B.J.F. & Rose, E.H. Study of the rest e.c.g. of marathon runners. In: *Proceedings of the International Conference on Sports Cardiology*, ed. A. Venerando (A. Gaggi, Bologna, 1979)

Defares, J.G. *A Study of the Carbon Dioxide Time Course during Rebreathing*. Ph.D. Thesis (University of Utrecht, 1956)

Degré, S., Degré-Coustry, C., Hoylaerts, M., Grevisse, M. & Denolin, H. Therapeutic effects of physical training in coronary heart disease. *Cardiology 62*, 206–17 (1977)

Degré, S. & Denolin, H. Bases physiologiques de l'entrainement
musculaire chez les patients atteints d'infarctus du myocarde et
premiers resultats d'un programme de réadaptation physqiue.
Médicine et Hygiene 31, 978–80 (1973)

Degré, S., Messin, R., Vandermoten, P., Bemaret, B., Haissly,
J.C., Salhadin, P.H. & Denolin, H. Aspects physio-
pathologiques de l'entrainement musculaire chez des patients
atteinte d'infarctus du myocarde. *Acta Cardiol.*, *27*, 445–62
(1972)

Delhez, L., Bottin, R., Thonon, A. & Petit, J.M. Influence de
l'entrainment sur la force maximum des muscles repiratoires.
Soc. Med. Belg. Ed. Phys., *20*, 52–63 (1967–8)

Delius, W., Cullhed, I., Björk, L. & Hallen, A. Left ventricular
aneurysmectomy. Clinical, haemodynamic and angiographic
results. In: *Coronary Heart Disease*, ed. M. Kaltenbach, P.
Lichtlen & G.C. Friesinger. (G. Thieme, Stuttgart, 1973) pp.
223–8

de Marées, H. & Barbey, K. Änderung der peripheren
Durchblutung durch Ausdauertraining. *Z. f. Kardiol.*, *62*, 653–
63 (1973)

De Palma, R.G., Bellon, E.M., Klein, L., Koletsky, S. & Insull,
W. Approaches to evaluating regression of experimental
atherosclerosis. *Adv. Exp. Med. Biol.*, *82*, 459–70 (1977)

De Ponti, C., Galli, M.A., Mauri, F., Salvadé, P. & Caru, B.
Effects of association of calcium antagonists with
nitro-derivatives or beta-blocking drugs in effort angina. In:
Coronary Heart Disease, ed. M. Kaltenbach, P. Lichtlen, R.
Balcon & W.D. Bussmann (G. Thieme, Stuttgart, 1978) pp.
316–21

de Soyza, N., Murphy, M.L., Bissett, H.K. *et al.* A comparison of
ventricular arrhythmia in coronary artery disease patients
randomized to surgical and medical therapy. *Clin. Res.*, *24*, 2A
(abstr.) (1976)

Detry, J. & Bruce, R.A. Effects of physical training on exertional
ST segment depression in coronary heart disease. *Circulation 44*,
390–6 (1971)

Detry, J.R., Rousseau, M., Vanden Broucke, G., Kusumi, L.,
Brausseur, A. & Bruce, R.A. Increased arterio-venous oxygen
difference after physical training in coronary heart disease.
Circulation 44, 109–18 (1971)

Devlin, J. The effect of training and acute physical exercise on plasma-insulin like activity. *Irish J. Med. Sci.*, *6*, 423–5 (1963)

de Vries, H.A. Physiological effects of an exercise training regimen upon men aged 52 to 88. *J. Gerontol.*, *25*, 325–36 (1970)

de Wijn, J.F., de Jongste, J.L., Mosterd, W. & Willebrand, D. Haemoglobin, packed cell volume, serum iron-binding capacity of selected athletes during training. *J. Sports Med. Phys. Fitness 11*, 42–51 (1971)

Dimond, G.E. Prognosis of men returning to work after first myocardial infarction. *Circulation 23*, 881–5 (1961)

Doan, A.E., Peterson, D.R., Blackmon, J.R. & Bruce, R.A. Myocardial ischemia after maximal exercise in healthy men. *Amer. Heart. J.*, *69*, 11–21 (1965)

Dobson, M., Tattersfield, A.E., Adler, M.W. and McNicol, M.W. Attitudes and long-term adjustment of patients surviving cardiac arrest. *Brit. Med. J.*, *3*, 207–12 (1971)

Doehrman, S.R. Psycho-social aspects of recovery from coronary heart disease: a review. *Soc. Sci. Med.*, *11*, 199–218 (1977)

Dohm, G.L., Huston, R.L., Askew, H.N. & Weiser, P.C. Effects of exercise on activity of heart and muscle mitochondria. *Amer. J. Physiol.*, *223*, 783–7 (1972)

Doll, E., Keul, J. & Maiwald, C. Oxygen tension and acid-base equilibria in venous blood of working muscle. *Amer. J. Physiol.*, *215*, 23–9 (1968)

Dorossiev, D., Paskova, V. & Zachariev, Z. Psychological problems of cardiac rehabilitation. In: *Psychological Approach to the Rehabilitation of Coronary Patients*, ed. U. Stocksmeier (Springer Verlag, Berlin, 1976) pp. 26–31

Dosch, M., Ozburn, D. & Stephens, M. Motivating the female to exercise. In: *Adult Fitness and Cardiac Rehabilitation*, ed. P.K. Wilson (University Park Press, Baltimore, Md., 1975) pp. 275–9

Dotson, C.O. Analysis of change. *Ex. Sports. Sci. Rev.*, *1*, 393–420 (1973)

Douglas, F.G.V. & Becklake, M.R. Effect of seasonal training on maximal cardiac output. *J. Appl. Physiol.*, *25*, 600–5 (1968)

Doyle, J.T. & Kinch, S.H. The prognosis of an abnormal electrocardiographic stress test. *Circulation 41*, 545–53 (1970)

Draper, H.H. A review of recent nutritional research in the arctic. In: *Circumpolar Health*, ed. R.J. Shephard & S. Itoh (University of Toronto Press, Toronto, 1976) pp. 120–9

Drinkwater, B. & Horvath, S.M. Detraining effects on young women. *Med. Sci. Sports 4*, 91–5 (1972)

Dublin, L.I. Longevity of college athletes. *Harper's Monthly Mag.*, *157*, 229–38 (1928)

Duncan, W.R., Ross, W.D. & Banister, E.W. Heart rate monitoring as a guide to the intensity of an exercise programme. *Brit. Col. Med. J.*, *10* (8), 219–20 (1968)

Dunkman, W.B., Perloff, J.K., Kastor, J.A. *et al.* Medical perspectives in coronary artery surgery — a caveat. *Ann. Intern. Med.*, *81*, 817–37 (1974)

Durnin, J.V.G. & Passmore, R. *Energy, Work and Leisure* (Heinemann, London, 1967)

Durrer, D., Janse, M.J. & Lie, K.I. Electrophysiological mechanisms for sudden coronary death. In: *Sudden Coronary Death*, ed. V. Manninen & P.I. Halonen (Karger, Basel, 1978)

Eckstein, R.W. Effect of exercise and coronary artery narrowing on coronary collateral circulation. *Circ. Res.*, *5*, 230–5 (1957)

Eden, D., Shiron, A., Kellerman, J.J., *et al.* Stress, anxiety, and coronary risk in a supportive society. In: *Stress and Anxiety*, ed. C.D. Spielberger & I.G. Sarason (Hemisphere Publishing, New York, 1977)

Edholm, O.G. The changing pattern of human activity. *Ergonomics 13*, 625–43 (1970)

Edholm, O.G., Humphrey, S., Lourie, J.A., *et al.* Energy expenditure and climatic exposure of Yemenite and Kurdish Jews in Israel. *Philos. Trans. R. Soc. Lond. (Biol. Sci.) 266B*, 127–40 (1973)

Edington, D.W., Cosmas, A.C. & McCaffery, W.B. Exercise and longevity: evidence for a threshold age. *J. Gerontol.*, *27*, 341–3 (1972)

Edler, E.I. The diagnostic use of ultrasound in heart disease. In: *Ultrasonic Energy*, ed. E. Kelly (Univ. of Illinois Press, Urbana, Ill., 1965)

Ekblom, B., Åstrand, P.O., Saltin, B., Stenberg, J. & Wallstrom, B. Effect of training on circulatory response to exercise. *J. Appl. Physiol.*, *24*, 518–28 (1968)

Elder, H.P. The effects of training on middle-aged men. In: *Exercise and Fitness*, ed. D.P. Franks (Athletic Institute, Chicago, 1969)

Elgrishi, I., Ducimetière, P. & Richard, J.L. Reproducibility of analysis of the electrocardiogram in epidemiology using the 'Minnesota Code'. *Brit. J. Prev. Soc. Med.*, *24*, 197–200 (1970)

Eliot, R.S. *Stress and the Heart* (Futura Publishing, Mount Kisko,

N.Y., 1974)

Eliot, R.S. & Miles, R.R. Advising the cardiac patient about sexual intercourse. *Med. Asp. Hum. Sex., 9*, 49–50 (1975)

Ellestad, M.H. *Stress Testing. Principles and Practice* (F.A. Davis, Philadelphia, 1975)

Ellestad, M., Allen, W., Wan, M.K.C. & Kemp, G.L. Maximal treadmill stress testing for cardiovascular evaluation. *Circulation 39*, 517–22 (1969)

Ellestad, M.H. & Wan, M.K.C. Predictive implications of stress testing: follow-up of 2,700 subjects after maximum treadmill stress testing. *Circulation 51*, 363–9 (1975)

Elmfeldt, D., Wilhelmsson, C., Vedin, A., Tibblin, G. & Wilhelmsen, L. Characteristics of representative male survivors of myocardial infarction compared with representative population samples. *Acta Med. Scand., 199*, 387–98 (1976)

Enig, M.G. The problem of trans-fatty acids in modern diet. In: *Topics in Ischaemic Heart Disease — An International Symposium* (Toronto Rehabilitation Centre, Toronto, 1979)

Enos, W.F., Bayer, J.C. & Holmes, R.H. Pathogenesis of coronary disease in American soldiers killed in Korea. *J. Amer. Med. Assoc., 158*, 912–14 (1955)

Enos, W.F., Holmes, R.H. & Bayer, J.C. Coronary artery sclerosis in American soldiers killed during the Korean war. *J. Amer. Med. Assoc., 152*, 1090–3 (1953)

Epstein, F.H. Glucose intolerance and coronary heart disease incidence — recent observations. In: *Lipid Metabolism, Obesity and Diabetes Mellitus: Impact upon Atherosclerosis*, ed. H. Greten, R. Levine, E.F. Pfeiffer & A.E. Renold (G. Thieme, Stuttgart, 1974) pp. 174–9

Epstein, L., Miller, G.J., Stitt, F.W. & Morris, J.N. Vigorous exercise in leisure time, coronary risk factors, and resting electrocardiogram in middle-aged male civil servants. *Brit. Heart J., 38*, 403–9 (1976)

Epstein, S.E., Redwood, D.R., Goldstein, R.E., Beiser, G.D., Rosing, D.R., Glancy, D.L., Reis, R.L. & Stinson, E.B. Angina pectoris — pathophysiology, evaluation and treatment. *Ann. Int. Med., 75*, 263–96 (1971)

Erb, B. *Proceedings, National Conference on Exercise in Prevention, Evaluation, and Treatment of Heart Disease, S. Carol. Med. Assoc. J., 65* suppl. I, 73–85 (1969)

Ericsson, B. Haeger, K. & Lindell, S. Maximal flow capacity before and after training. In: *Coronary Heart Disease and Physical Fitness*, ed. O.A. Lassen & R.O. Malborg (University Park Press, Baltimore, 1971) pp. 155–7

Estes, E.H. Electrocardiography and vectorcardiography. In: *The Heart*, 3rd edn, ed. J.W. Hurst, R.B. Logue, R.C. Schlant & N.K. Wenger (McGraw Hill, New York, 1974) pp. 267–85

Fabian, J., Stolz, I., Janota, M., *et al.* Reproducibility of exercise tests in patients with symptomatic ischaemic heart disease. *Brit. Heart. J., 37*, 785–9 (1975)

Fardy, P.S. Effects of soccer training and detraining upon selected cardiac and metabolic measures. *Res. Quart., 40*, 502–8 (1969)

Fardy, P.S. & Ilmarinen, J. Evaluating the effects and feasibility of an at work stairclimbing intervention program for men. *Med. Sci. Sports 7*, 91–3 (1975)

Fardy, P., Maresh, C.M. & Abbott, R.D. A comparison of myocardial function in former athletes and non-athletes. *Med. Sci. Sports 8*, 26–30 (1976)

Feigenbaum, H. Use of echocardiography to evaluate cardiac performance. In: *Cardiac Mechanics: Physiological, Clinical and Mathematical Considerations*, ed. I. Mirsky, D. Ghista & H. Sandler (Wiley, New York, 1974) pp. 203–31

Feil, H. & Siegel, M.L. Electrocardiographic changes during attacks of angina pectoris. *Amer. J. Med. Sci., 175*, 255–60 (1928)

Feldman, S.A., Ho, K.J., Lewis, L.A., Mikkelson, B. & Taylor, C.B. Lipid and cholesterol metabolism in Alaskan Arctic Eskimos. *Arch. Pathol., 94*, 43–58 (1972)

Ferguson, R.J., Choquette, G., Chanioto, L., Jankowski, L.W. & Huot, E. Role de la marche dans la réadaptation des patients coronariens. *Arch. Mal. Coeur 66* (8), 995–1001 (1973)

Ferguson, R.J., Gauthier, P., Coté, P. & Bourassa, M.G. Coronary hemodynamics during upright exercise in patients with angina pectoris. *Circulation 52*, suppl. II, 115 (abstr.) (1975)

Ferguson, R.J., Petitclerc, R., Choquette, G., *et al.* Effect of physical training on treadmill exercise capacity, collateral circulation and progression of coronary disease. *Amer. J. Cardiol., 34*, 764–9 (1974)

Ferrer, M.I. The sick sinus syndrome. *Circulation 47*, 635–41 (1973)

Finkle, A.L. Sexual potency in aging males. Part I. Frequency of coitus among clinical patients. *J. Amer. Med. Assoc., 170*, 1391–

3 (1959)

Fishbein, M. & Ajzen, J. *Belief, Attitude, Intention and Behavior* (Addison Wesley, Reading, Mass., 1975)

Fisher, F.D. & Tyroler, H.A. Relationship between ventricular premature contractions in routine electrocardiograms and subsequent death from coronary heart disease. *Circulation 47*, 712–19 (1963)

Fisher, S. Impact of physical disability on vocational activity: work status following myocardial infarction. *Scand. J. Rehabil. Med., 3*, 65–70 (1970a)

Fisher, S. International survey on the psychological aspects of cardiac rehabilitation. *Scand. J. Rehab. Med., 2–3*, 71–7 (1970b)

Fitzhugh, G. & Hamilton, B.E. Coronary occlusion and fatal angina pectoris. *J. Amer. Med. Assoc., 100*, 475–80 (1933)

Flaherty, J.T., Ferans, V.J., Pierce, J.E., Carew, T.E. & Fry, D.L. Localizing factors in experimental atherosclerosis. In: *Atherosclerosis and Coronary Heart Disease*, ed. W. Likoff, B.L. Segal & W. Insull (Grune & Stratton, New York, 1972) pp. 40–83

Fleischmann, P. & Kellermann, J.J. Persistent irregular tachycardia in a successful athlete without impairment of performance. *Israeli J. Med. Sci., 5*, 950–2 (1969)

Fletcher, C.M. Chronic bronchitis. Its prevalence, nature and pathogenesis. *Amer. Rev. Resp. Dis., 80*, 483–94 (1959)

Fletcher, G.F. & Cantwell, J.D. *Exercise in the Management of Coronary Heart Disease. A Guide for the Practicing Physician* (C.C. Thomas, Springfield, Ill., 1971)

Fletcher, G.F. & Cantwell, J.D. *Exercise and Coronary Heart Disease. Role in Prevention, Diagnosis, Treatment* (C.C. Thomas, Springfield, Ill., 1974)

Florey, Du V.C., Melia, R.J.W. & Darby, S.C. Changing mortality from ischaemic heart disease in Great Britain 1966–76. *Brit. Med. J., 1*, 635–7 (1978)

Fogelman, M., Abbasi, A.S., Pearce, M.L. & Kattus, A.A. Echocardiographic study of the abnormal motion of the posterior left ventricular wall during angina pectoris. *Circulation 46*, 905–13 (1972)

Ford, A.B. & Hellerstein, H.K. Energy cost of the Master two-step test. *J. Amer. Med. Assoc., 164*, 1868–74 (1957)

Forrester, J.S., Diamond, G.A. & Swan, H.J.C. Correlation classification of clinical and hemodynamic function after acute myocardial infarction. *Amer. J. Cardiol., 39*, 137–45 (1977)

Foster, G.L. & Reeves, T.J. Haemodynamic response to exercise in clinically normal middle-aged men and those with angina pectoris. *J. Clin. Invest., 43*, 1758–68 (1964)

Fox, S.M. Heart disease and rehabilitation: scope of the problem. In: *Heart Disease and Rehabilitation*, ed. M.L. Pollock & D.H. Schmidt. (Houghton Mifflin, Boston, 1979) pp. 3–12

Fox, S.M. & Haskell, W.L. Population studies. *Canad. Med. Assoc. J., 96*, 808–11 (1967)

Fox, S.M. & Haskell, W.L. Physical activity and the prevention of coronary heart disease. *Bull. N.Y. Acad. Sci., 44*, 950–65 (1968a)

Fox, S.M. & Haskell, W.L. The exercise stress test: needs for standardisation. Presented at the Fourth Asian/Pacific Congress of Cardiology, Tel Aviv. Cited by S. Fox, Exercise and stress testing workshop report. National Conference on Exercise in the Prevention, in the Evaluation and in the Treatment of Heart Disease. *J. S. Carol. Med. Assoc., 65*, suppl. 1, 77 (1968b)

Fox, S.M., Naughton, J.P. & Gorman, P.A. Physical activity and cardiovascular health. *Mod. Concepts Cardiovasc. Dis., 41*, 17–30 (1972)

Fox, S.M. Skinner, J.S. Physical activity and cardiovascular health. *Amer. J. Cardiol., 14*, 731–46 (1964)

Framingham Heart Study. *Habits and Coronary Heart Disease*. US National Heart Institute Public Health Service Publication 1515 (US Government Printing Office, Washington, D.C., 1966) pp. 1–13

Franks, B.D. & Cureton, T.K. Effects of training on time components of the left ventricle. *J. Sports. Med. Phys. Fitness 9*, 80–8 (1969)

Fredrickson, D.S. Function and structure of plasma lipoproteins. In: *Lipid Metabolism, Obesity and Diabetes Mellitus: Impact upon Atherosclerosis*, ed. H. Greten, R. Levine, E.F. Pfeiffer & A.E. Renold (G. Thieme, Stuttgart, 1974)

French, A.J. & Dock, W. Fatal coronary arteriosclerosis in young soldiers. *J. Amer. Med. Assoc., 124*, 1233–7 (1944)

French, J.R.P. & Caplan, R.D. *Psychosocial Factors in Coronary Heart Disease* (US National Air & Space Administration, 1970)

Frick, M.H. The response of heart volume and ventricular functions to physical training in coronary heart disease. *Mal. Cardiovasc., 10*, 331–9 (1969)

Frick, M.H., Harjola, P.T. & Valle, M. The prognostic impact of coronary by-pass surgery. In:' *Internal Medicine: 1976 Topics* (Karger, Basel, 1976) pp. 287–92

Frick, M.H., Harjola, P.T. & Valle, M. Influence of coronary bypass surgery on sudden death in chronic artery disease. In: *Sudden Coronary Death*, ed. V. Manninen & P.I. Halonen (Karger, Basel, 1978) pp. 229–31

Frick, M.H. & Katila, M. Hemodynamic consequences of physical training after myocardial infarction. *Circulation 37*, 192–202 (1968)

Frick, M.H., Katila, M. & Sjörgen, A.L. Cardiac function and physical training after myocardial infarction. In: *Coronary Heart Disease and Physical Fitness*, ed. O.A. Larsen & R.O. Malmborg (University Park Press, Baltimore, Md., 1971) pp. 44–7

Frick, M.H., Konttinen, A. & Sarajas, S.H.S. Effects of physical training on circulation at rest and during exercise. *Amer. J. Cardiol., 12*, 142–7 (1963)

Fried, T. & Shephard, R.J. Deterioration and restoration of physical fitness after training. *Canad. Med. Assoc. J., 100*, 831–7 (1969)

Friedberg, C.K. *Diseases of the Heart* (W.B. Saunders, Philadelphia, 1966)

Friedberg, C.K. & Unger, A.H. The natural history of coronary heart disease. In: *Atherosclerotic Vascular Disease*, ed. A.N. Brest & G.H. Moyer (Appleton Century Crofts, New York, 1967) pp. 300–8

Friedman, E.H. Type A or B behavior. *J. Amer. Med. Assoc., 228*, 1369 (1974)

Friedman, E.H. & Hellerstein, H.K. Influence of psychosocial factors on coronary risk and adaptation to a physical fitness evaluation programme. In: *Exercise Testing and Exercise Training in Coronary Heart Disease*, ed. J.P. Naughton & H.K. Hellerstein (Academic Press, New York, 1973)

Friedman, M., Manwaring, J.H., Rosenman, R.H., Donion, G. & Ortega, P. Instantaneous and sudden deaths. *J. Amer. Med. Assoc., 225*, 1319–28 (1973)

Friedman, M. & Rosenman, R.H. Type A behavior and your heart (Fawcett, Greenwich, Conn., 1974)

Friedman, R.J., More, S., Singal., D.P. & Gent, M. Regression of injury-induced atheromatous lesions in rabbits. *Arch. Pathol.*

Lab. Med., 100, 189–95 (1976)

Friend, B., Page, L. & Marston, R. Food consumption patterns in the United States: 1909–13 to 1976. In: *Nutrition, Lipids and Coronary Heart Disease*, ed. R. Levy, B. Rifkind, B. Dennis & N. Ernst (Raven Press, New York, 1979) pp. 489–522

Froehlicher, V.F. Animal studies of the effect of chronic exercise on the heart and atherosclerosis. A review. *Amer. Heart. J., 84*, 496–506 (1972)

Froehlicher, V.F. *The Effect of Chronic Exercise on the Heart and on Coronary Atherosclerotic Heart Disease. A Literature Survey*. US Airforce, Brooks Air Force Base Report SAM-TR-76-69 (1976)

Froehlicher, V.F. & Oberman, A. Analysis of epidemiologic studies of physical inactivity as risk factor for coronary artery disease. *Progr. Cardiovasc. Dis., 15*, 41–65 (1972)

Funderburk, C.F., Hipskind, S.G., Welton, R.C. & Lind, A.R. Development of and recovery from fatigue induced by static effort at various tensions. *J. Appl. Physiol., 37*, 392–6 (1974)

Galbo, H., Hoist, J.J. & Christensen, N.J. Glucagon and plasma catecholamine responses to graded and prolonged exercise in man. *J. Appl. Physiol., 38*, 70–6 (1975)

Ganz, W., Cribier, A., Chew, C., Kanmatsuse, K., Tzivoni, D., Nair, R. & Swan, H.J.C. Effect of nitroglycerin on the acutely ischemic myocardium. In: *Coronary Heart Disease*, ed. M. Kaltenbach, P. Lichtlen, R. Balcon & W.D. Bussmann (G. Thieme, Stuttgart, 1978) pp. 256–61

Gardner, G.W., Danks, D.L. & Scharfstein, L. Use of carotid pulse for heart rate monitoring. *Med. Sci. Sports 11* (1), 111 (abstr.) (1979)

Gauthier, P., Ferguson, R.J., Chaniotis, L., Avon, G. & Choquette, G. Evaluation hémodynamique en position couchée et assise avant et après l'entrainement chez le coronarien. In: *Abstracts from First Canadian Congress of Sport and Physical Activity* (Montreal, 1973) p. 13

Geddes, L.A. & Baker, L.E. The relationship between input impedance and electrode area in recording the ECG. *Med. Biol. Eng., 4*, 439–50 (1966)

Geer, J.C. & McGill, H.C. The evolution of the fatty streak. In: *Atherosclerotic Vascular Disease*, ed. A.N. Brest & J.H. Moyer (Appleton Century Crofts, New York, 1967) pp. 8–22

Geis, W.P., Ardekani, R.G., Rahimtoola, S.H., *et al.* Delineation of improved ventricular wall motion after coronary revascularization. In: *Coronary Artery Surgery*, ed. J.C. Norman. (Appleton Century Crofts, New York, 1975) pp. 846–55

Gelfand, D. Experience at the cardiac work classification unit of the heart association of southeastern Pennsylvania (Philadelphia). In: *Work and the Heart*, ed. F.F. Rosenbaum & E.L. Belknap (P.B. Hoeber, New York, 1959) pp. 322–9

Gentry, W.D. Psychosocial concerns and benefits in cardiac rehabilitation. In: *Heart Disease and Rehabilitation*, ed. M.L. Pollock & D.H. Schmidt (Houghton Mifflin, Boston, 1979)

Georgopoulos, A.J., Proudfit, W.L. & Page, I.H. Effect of exercise on electrocardiograms of patients with low serum potassium. *Circulation 23*, 567–72 (1961)

Gerstenblith, G., Lakatta, E.G. & Weisfeldt, M.L. Age changes in myocardial function and exercise response. *Progr. Cardiovasc. Dis., 19*, 1–21 (1976)

Gertler, M.M. & White, P.D. *Coronary Artery Disease in Young Adults* (Harvard University Printer, Cambridge, Mass., 1954)

Gertler, M.M. & White, P.D. *Coronary Heart Disease. A 25-year Study in Retrospect* (Medical Economics, Oradell, N.J., 1976)

Gettes, L.S. Electrophysiologic basis of arrhythmias and acute myocardial ischemia. In: *Modern trends in Cardiology*, vol. 3, ed. M.F. Olives (Butterworths, London, 1975) pp. 218–46

Gillespie, J.A. Future place of lumbar sympathectomy in obliterative vascular disease of lower limbs. *Brit. Med. J.* (ii), 1640–42 (1960)

Gilson, J.C. & Hugh-Jones, P. *Lung Function in Coalworkers' Pneumoconiosis*. Special Report Series 290 (UK Medical Research Council, 1955) pp. 1–226

Glaser, E.M. *The Physiological Basis of Habituation* (Oxford University Press, London, 1966) pp. 1–102

Glendy, R.E., Levine, S.A. & White, P.D. Coronary disease in youth. Comparison of 100 patients under 40 with 300 persons past 80. *JAMA, 109*, 1775–81 (1937)

Gluckman, M. Sport and conflict. In: *Sport in the Modern World — Chances and Problems*, ed. O. Grupe, D. Kurz & J.M. Teipel (Springer Verlag, New York, 1973) pp. 48–54

Godin, G. & Shephard, R.J. Activity patterns of the Canadian Eskimo. In: *Polar Human Biology*, ed. O.G. Edholm & E.K.E. Gunderson (Heineman, Cambridge, 1973a)

Godin, G. & Shephard, R.J. Body weight and the energy cost of activity. *Arch. Env. Health 27*, 289–93 (1973b)

Goldbarg, A.N. The effects of pharmacological agents on human performance. In: *Exercise Testing and Exercise Training in Coronary Heart Disease*, ed. J.P. Naughton, H.K. Hellerstein & I.C. Mohler (Academic Press, New York, 1973)

Goldbarg, A.N., Ekblom,. B. & Åstrand, P.O. Effects of blocking the autonomic nervous system during exercise. *Circulation 44*, suppl. II, 118 (abstr.) (1971)

Goldberg, D.I. & Shephard, R.J. Stroke volume during recovery from upright bicycle exercise. *J. Appl. Physiol., 48*, 833–7 (1980)

Goldhammer, S. & Schert, D. Elektrokardiographische untersuchungen bei Kranken mit Angina Pectoris ('ambulatorischer' Typus). *Z. f. Klin. Med., 122*, 134–51 (1932)

Goldschlager, N., Cake, D. & Cohn, K. Exercise-induced ventricular arrhythmias in patients with coronary artery disease. Their relation to angiographic findings. *Amer. J. Cardiol., 31*, 434–40 (1973)

Goldstein, R.E. & Epstein, S.E. The use of indirect indices of myocardial oxygen consumption in evaluating angina pectoris. *Chest 63*, 302–6 (1973)

Goldstein, R.E., Rosing, D.R., Redwood, D.R., Beiser, G.D. & Epstein, S.E. Clinical and circulatory effects of isosorbide dinitrate. Comparisons with nitroglycerine. *Circulation 43*, 629–40 (1971)

Goldwater, L.J. & Weiss, N.M. Study of workmen's compensation and heart disease in New York City. *New York J. Med., 51*, 2754–8 (1951)

Gollnick, P. & Hermansen, L. Biochemical adaptations to exercise anaerobic metabolism. *Exercise Sport Sci. Rev., 1*, 1–43 (1973)

Gollnick, P.D. & Ianuzzo, C.D. Hormonal deficiencies and the metabolic adaptations of rats to training. *Amer. J. Physiol., 223*, 278–82 (1972)

Goode, R.C., Firstbrook, J. & Shephard, R.J. Effects of exercise and a cholesterol-free diet on human serum lipids. *Canad. J. Physiol. Pharm., 44*, 575–80 (1966)

Gordon, T., Castelli, W.P., Hjortland, M.C., Kannel, W.B. & Dawber. T.R. High density lipoprotein as a protective factor against coronary heart disease. The Framingham study. *Amer. J. Med., 62*, 707–14 (1977)

Gordon, T., Sorlie, P. & McNamara, P. Physical activity and

coronary vulnerability. The Framingham study. *Cardiol. Digest*
6, 28 (1971)

Gorlin, R. Anginal pain without atherosclerosis. *JAMA, 201* (9),
27–8 (1967)

Gorlin, R. Myocardial blood flow and metabolism in coronary
disease. In: *Coronary Heart Disease and Physical Fitness*, ed.
O.A. Larsen & R.O. Malmborg (University Park Press,
Baltimore, 1971) pp. 97–101

Gorlin, R. *Coronary Artery Disease* (W.B. Saunders, Philadelphia,
1976)

Gottheiner, V. Herzinfarkt und sport. In: *Proceedings of Sports
Medical Symposium of Seventeenth Olympic Games* (Rome,
1960)

Gottheiner, V. Long range strenuous sports training for cardiac
reconditioning and rehabilitation. *Amer. J. Cardiol., 22*, 426–35
(1968)

Gould, K.L. & Lipscomb, K. Effects of coronary stenoses on
coronary flow reserve and resistance. *Amer. J. Cardiol., 34*,
48–55 (1974)

Graievskaia, N.D. & Markov, L.N. Post-mortem anatomical and
histological findings in sudden death in sport. *Brit. J. Sports
Med., 7*, 159–61 (1973)

Granath, A., Johnson, B. & Strandell, T. Circulation in healthy old
men studied by right heart catheterization at rest during exercise
in supine and sitting position. *Acta Med. Scand., 1976*, 425–46
(1964)

Greene, D.G, Klocke, F.J., Schimert, G.L., Bunnell, I.L.,
Wittemberg, S.M. & Lajos, T. Evaluation of venous bypass
grafts from aorta to coronary artery by inert gas desaturation and
direct flowmeter techniques. *J. Clin. Invest., 51*, 191–6 (1972)

Greene, W.A. Psychological factors and reticuloendothelial
disease. *Psychosom. Med., 16*, 220–30 (1954)

Greer, W.E.R. Experience in selective placement and follow-up on
cardiacs. In: *Work and the Heart*, ed. F.F. Rosenbaum & E.L.
Belknap (P.B. Hoeber, New York, 1959) pp. 383–6

Gregg, D.E. & Fisher, L.C. Blood supply to the heart. In:
Handbook of Physiology. Section 2. Circulation, vol. II
(American Physiological Society, Washington, D.C., 1963) pp.
1517–84

Gregg, D.E., Longino, F.H., Green, P.A. & Czerwonka, L.J. A
comparison of coronary flow determined by the nitrous oxide

method and by a direct method using the rotameter. *Circulation* *3*, 89–94 (1951)

Grendahl, H. Early death in acute myocardial infarction. A retrospective study of 302 cases. *Acta Med. Scand., 181*, 655–62 (1967)

Grimby, G., Nilsson, N.J. & Saltin, B. Cardiac output during sub-maximal and maximal exercise in active middle-aged athletes. *J. Appl. Physiol., 21*, 1150–6 (1966)

Groden, B.M. Return to work after myocardial infarction. *Scott. Med. J., 12*, 297–301 (1967)

Groden, B.M. & Brown, R.I.F. Differential psychological effects of early and late mobilization after myocardial infarction. *Scand. J. Rehab. Med., 2–3*, 60–4 (1970)

Grodsky, G.M. & Benoit, F. Effect of massive weight reduction on insulin secretion in obese subjects. *International Diabetes Symposium* (Stockholm, 1967)

Groen, J.J., Tijong, B.K., Willebrandt, A.F. & Kamminga, C.J. Influence of nutrition, individuality and different forms of stress on blood cholesterol. Results of an experiment of 9 months duration in 60 normal volunteers. In: *Proceedings of an International Congress of Dieticians* (1959) p. 19

Grögler, F., Beddermann, C., Frank, G. & Borst, H.G. Myocardial contraction and hemodynamics before, during and after coronary occlusion in the pig. In: *Coronary Heart Disease*, ed. M. Kaltenbach, P. Lichtlen & G.C. Friesinger (G. Thieme, Stuttgart, 1973) pp. 162–6

Grollman, A. The determination of cardiac output of man by the use of acetylene. *Amer. J. Physiol., 88*, 432–45 (1929)

Groom, D. Cardiovascular observations on Tarahumara Indian runners — the modern Spartans. *Amer. Heart J., 81*, 304–14 (1971)

Gueli, D. & Shephard, R.J. Pedal frequency in bicycle ergometry. *Canad. J. Appl. Sports Sci., 1*, 137–42 (1976)

Guinn, G.A. & Mathur, V.S. Surgical versus medical treatment of stable angina pectoris: prospective randomized study with 1- to 4-year follow up. *Ann. Thor. Surg., 22*, 524–7 (1976)

Gwinup, G. Effect of exercise alone on the weight of obese women. *Arch. Int. Med., 135*, 676–80 (1975)

Hacker, R.W. Resection of aneurysms, akinetic areas and infarctions in coronary heart disease. In: *Coronary Heart Disease*, ed. M. Kaltenbach, P. Lichtlen & G.C. Friesinger (G.

Thieme, Stuttgart, 1973) pp. 207–16

Hackett, T.P. & Cassem, N.H. Psychological adaptation to convalescence in myocardial infarction patients. In: *Exercise Testing and Exercise Training in Coronary Heart Disease*, ed. J.P. Naughton & H.K. Hellerstein (Academic Press, New York, 1973) pp. 253–62

Hakkila, J. Studies of the myocardial capillary concentration in cardiac hypertrophy due to training. *Ann. Med. Exp. Biol. Fenn., 33*, suppl. 10, 1–82 (1955)

Halliday, M. & Anderson, T.W. The sex differential in ischaemic heart disease: trends by social class 1931 to 1971. *Epidemiol. & Comm. Health 33*, 74–7 (1979)

Halter, J., Moccetti, T., Gattiker, K. & Lichtlen, P. Left ventricular dynamics before and after aneurysmectomy. In: *Coronary Heart Disease*, ed. M. Kaltenbach, P. Lichtlen & G.C. Friesinger (G. Thieme, Stuttgart, 1973) pp. 228–38

Hames, C. 'Most likely to succeed' as a candidate for a coronary attack. In: *New Horizons in Cardiovascular Practice*, ed. H.I. Russek (University Park Press, Baltimore, Md., 1975)

Hamilton, J.B. The role of testicular secretions as indicated by the effects of castration in men and by studies of pathological conditions and the short life-span associated with maleness. *Recent Prog. in Hormone Res., 3*, 257–322 (1948)

Hamilton, M.J. & Ferguson, J.H. Effects of exercise and cold acclimation on the ventricular and skeletal muscles of white mice (*Mus. musculus*). I. Succinic dehydrogenase activity. *Comp. Biochem. Physiol., A43*, 815–24 (1972)

Hamilton, W.F. Measurement of cardiac output. In: *Handbook of Physiology*. Section 2. *Circulation*, vol. I, ed. W.F. Hamilton (American Physiological Society, Washington, D.C., 1962) pp. 551–84

Hammermeister, K.E., DeRouen, T.A., Murray, J.A., *et al*. Effect of aortocoronary saphenous vein by-pass grafting on death and sudden death: comparison of non-randomized medically and surgically treated cohorts with comparable coronary disease and left ventricular function. *Amer. J. Cardiol., 39*, 925–34 (1977)

Hammermeister, K.E., Kennedy, J.W., Hamilton, G.W., *et al*. Aortocoronary saphenous vein bypass: failure of successful grafting to improve resting left ventricular function in chronic angina. *New Engl. J. Med., 290*, 196–92 (1974)

Hammett, V.B.O. Recognition and management of abnormal

psychological reactions to coronary heart disease. In: *Coronary Heart Disease*, ed. W. Likoff & J.H. Moyer (Grune & Stratton, New York, 1963) pp. 459–63

Hammond, E.C. Smoking in relation to mortality and morbidity. Findings in first thirty-four months of follow-up in a prospective study started in 1959. *J. Nat. Cancer Inst., 32*, 1161–88 (1964)

Hampton, J.R. & Nicholas, C. Randomized trial of a mobile coronary care unit for emergency calls. *Brit. Med. J.* (i), 1118–21 (1978)

Hanne-Paparo, N., Drory, Y., Schoenfeld, Y., Shapira, Y. & Kellermann, J.J. Common ECG changes in athletes. *Cardiology 61*, 267–78 (1976)

Hanson, J.S. & Nedde, W.H. Preliminary observations on physical training for hypertensive males. *Circ. Research 36/37*, suppl. I, 49–53 (1970)

Hanson, J.S., Tabakin, B.S. & Levy, A.M. Comparative exercise cardio-respiratory performance of normal men in the third, fourth and fifth decades of life. *Circulation 37*, 345–60 (1968)

Harken, D.E. Changing concepts in mechanical assistance and surgical excision. In: *Changing Concepts in Cardiovascular Disease*, ed. H.I. Russek & B.L. Zohman (Williams & Wilkins, Baltimore, 1972) pp. 281–7

Harris, D.V. Physical activity history and attitudes of middle-aged men. *Med. Sci. Sports 2*, 203–8 (1970)

Harris, W.S. Systolic time intervals in the non-invasive assessment of left ventricular performance in man. In: *Cardiac Mechanics: Physiological, Clinical and Mathematical Considerations*, ed. I. Mirsky, D. Ghista & H. Sandler (Wiley, New York, 1974) pp. 233–92

Harrison, T.R. & Reeves, T.J. *Principles and Problems of Ischemic Heart Disease* (Year Book Publishers, Chicago, 1968)

Hartley, L.H. Growth hormone and catecholamine response to exercise in relation to physical training. *Med. Sci. Sports 7*, 34–6 (1975)

Hartley, L.H., Grimby, G., Kilbom, A., Nilsson, N.J., Åstrand, I., Bjure, J., Ekblom, B. & Saltin, B. Physical training in sedentary middle-aged and older men. III. Cardiac output and gas exchange at submaximal and maximal exercise. *Scand. J. Clin. Lab. Invest., 24*, 335–44 (1969)

Hartley, L.H., Mason, J.W., Hogan, R.P., Jones, L.G., Kotchen, T.A., Mougey, E.H., Wherry, F.E., Pennington, L.L. &

Ricketts, P.T. Multiple hormone responses to graded exercise in relation to physical training. *J. Appl. Physiol., 33*, 602–6 (1972)

Hartley, L.H. & Saltin, B. Blood gas tensions and pH in brachial artery, femoral vein and brachial vein during maximal exercise. *Med. Sci. Sports 3*, 66–72 (1969)

Hartung, G.H. Physical activity and coronary heart disease risk: a review. *Amer. Corr. Therap. J., 31* (4), 110–15 (1977)

Hartung, G.H., Smith, L.C., Foreyt, J., Gorry, A.G. & Gotto, A.M. Plasma lipid levels in middle-aged runners, joggers, and sedentary men. *International Conference on Sports Cardiology* (Rome, 1978)

Harvey, R.M., Smith, W.M., Parker, J.O. & Ferrer, M.I. The response of the abnormal heart to exercise. *Circulation 26*, 341–62 (1962)

Haskell, W.L. Cardiovascular complications during exercise training of cardiac patients. *Circulation 57*, 920–4 (1978)

Haskell, W.L. Mechanisms by which physical activity may enhance the clinical status of cardiac patients. In: *Heart Disease and Rehabilitation*, ed. M.L. Pollock & D.H. Schmidt (Houghton Mifflin, Boston, Mass., 1979) pp. 276–96

Haskell, W.L. & Fox, S.N. Physical activity in the prevention and therapy of cardiovascular disease. In: *Science and Medicine of Exercise and Sport*, 2nd edn, ed. W.R. Johnson & E.R. Burkirk (Harper & Row, New York, 1974) pp. 455–68

Hatch, T. & Cook, K.M. Partitional respirometry. *AMA Arch. Industr. Health 11*, 142–58 (1955)

Haust, M.D. Injury and repair in the pathogenesis of atherosclerotic lesions. In: *Atherosclerosis*, ed. R.J. Jones (Springer Verlag, Berlin, 1970) pp. 12–20

Heberden, W. Some account of a disorder of the breast. *Med. Trans. Roy. Coll. Phys., 2*, 59 (1772)

Hedley, O.F. Analysis of 5,116 deaths reported as due to coronary occlusion in Philadelphia. *US Weekly Public Health Rep., 54*, 972 (1959)

Hedlund, S. & Porjé, J.B. Cirkulationstörningar hos äldre. Synpunkter på fysiologi och fysisk träning som terapiform. *Svenska Läk-Tidn 61*, 2970–85 (1964)

Heintzen, P.H., Moldenhauer, K. & Lange, P.E. Three dimensional computerized contraction pattern analysis: description of methodology and its validation. *Europ. J. Cardiol., 1*, 229–39 (1974)

Heinzelmann, F. & Baggley, R. Response to physical activity programs and their effects on health behavior. *Publ. Health Rep., 85*, 905–11 (1970)

Helander, S. & Levander, M. Primary mortality and 5-year prognosis of cardiac infarction. Study which considers in particular how prognosis is affected by composition of materials as regards age and sex of patients and severity of infarction. *Acta Med. Scand., 163*, 289–304 (1959)

Helfant, R.H., deVilla, M.A. & Meister, S.G. Effect of sustained isometric handgrip exercise on left ventricular performance. *Circulation 44*, 982–93 (1971)

Heller, E.M. Four year practical experience with a graded exercise program for myocardial infarction patients. Paper presented to Ontario Medical Association Annual Meeting (Toronto, May, 1968)

Heller, E.M. A practical graded exercise program for post-coronary patients — five year review. *Modern Medicine of Canada 27* (7), 529–42 (1972)

Hellerstein, H.K. Active physical reconditioning of coronary patients. *Circulation 32*, suppl. II, 110 (abstr.) (1965)

Hellerstein, H.K. Exercise therapy in coronary disease. *Bull. N.Y. Acad. Med., 44*, 1208–47 (1968)

Hellerstein, H.K. Exercise therapy in coronary heart disease. In: *Ischaemic Heart Disease*, ed. J.H. De Haas *et al.* (Williams & Wilkins, Baltimore, 1970) pp. 406–29

Hellerstein, H.K. A misguided goal or unrealized objective? In: *Critical Evaluation of Cardiac Rehabilitation*, ed. J.J. Kellermann & H. Denolin (Karger, Basel, 1977) pp. 125–35

Hellerstein, H.K. Cardiac rehabilitation: a retrospective view. In: *Heart Disease and Rehabilitation*, ed. M.L. Pollock & D.H. Schmidt (Houghton-Mifflin, Boston, 1979) pp. 509–20

Hellerstein, H.K. & Friedman, E.H. Sexual activity and the post-coronary patient. *Arch. Int. Med., 125*, 987–99 (1970)

Hellerstein, H.K. & Friedman, E.H. Sexual activity and the post-coronary patient. *Med. Aspects Hum. Sex., 3*, 70 (1973)

Hellerstein, H.K., Hornsten, T.R., Goldberg, A., Burlando, A.G., Friedman, E.H., Hirsch, E.Z. & Marik, S. The influence of active conditioning upon subjects with coronary artery disease. Cardio-respiratory changes during training in 67 patients. *Canad. Med. Assoc. J., 96*, 758–9, 901–3 (1967)

Hellerstein, H.K. & Turrell, D.J. The mode of death in coronary artery disease. An electrocardiograophic and clinicopathological correlation. In: *Sudden Cardiac Death*, ed. B. Surawicz & E.E. Pellegrino (Grune & Stratton, New York, 1964)

Herman, M.V., Heinle, R.A., Klein, M.D. & Gorlin, R. Localized disorders in myocardial contraction: asynergy and its role in congestive heart failure. *N. Engl. J. Med.*, *277*, 222–32 (1967)

Hermansen, L. & Ekblom, B. Physical fitness of an arctic and a tropical population. In: *Physical Activity in Health and Disease*, ed. E. Evang & K.L. Andersen (Williams & Wilkins, Baltimore, 1966)

Hermansen, L. & Wachtlová, M. Capillary density of skeletal muscle in well-trained and untrained men. *J. Appl. Physiol.*, *30*, 860–3 (1971)

Herrick, J.B. Clinical features of sudden obstruction of the coronary arteries. *JAMA*, *59*, 2015–20 (1912)

Hettinger, T. *Physiology of Strength* (C.C. Thomas, Springfield, Ill., 1961)

Hickey, N., Mulcahy, R., Bourke, G.J., Graham, I. & Wilson-Davis, K. Study of coronary risk factors related to physical activity in 15,171 men. *Brit. Med. J.* (3), 507–9 (1975)

Higgs, B.E., Clode, M. & Campbell, E.J.M. Changes in ventilation, gas exchange and circulation during exercise after recovery from myocardial infarction. *Lancet* (ii), 793–5 (1968)

Hill, A. Bradford. *Principles of Medical Statistics*, 9th edn. (University Press, New York, 1971)

Hill, J.D., Hampton, J.R. & Mitchell, J.R.A. A randomized trial of home versus hospital management for patients with suspected myocardial infarction. *Lancet* (i), 837–41 (1978)

Hinckle, L.E. An estimate of the effects of 'stress' on the incidence and prevalence of coronary heart disease in a large industrial population in the United States. *Thromb. Diath. Haemorrh.*, *51*, suppl., 15–65 (1972)

Hinckle, L.E., Carver, S.T. & Plakun, A. Slow heart rate and increased risk of cardiac death in middle-aged men. *Arch. Int. Med.*, *129*, 732–48 (1972)

Hinckle, L.E., Carver, S.T. & Stevens, M. The frequency of asymptomatic disturbances of cardiac rhythm and conduction in middle-aged men. *Amer. J. Cardiol.*, *24*, 629–50 (1969)

Hinckle, L.E, Whitney, L.A., Lehman, E.W., Dunn, J. & Benjamin, B. Occupation, education and coronary heart disease. *Science 161*, 238–46 (1968)

Hinckle, L.E. & Wolff, H.G. The role of emotional and environmental factors in essential hypertension. In: *The Pathology of Essential Hypertension*, ed. J.H. Cort, V. Fencl, Z. Hejl & J. Jirka (State Medical Publishing House, Prague, 1962)

Hinohara, S. Psychological aspects in rehabilitation of coronary heart disease. *Scand. J. Rehabil. Med., 2*, 53–9 (1970)

Hirai, M. Muscle blood flow measured by Xe^{133} clearance method and peripheral vascular diseases. Part I. Standard exercise method — with special reference to work load and volume injected. *Jap. Circ. J., 38*, 655–9 (1974)

Hirzel, H.O., Meier, W., Mehmel, H. & Krayenbühl, H.P. Left ventricular dynamics during acute ischemia in the dog. In: *Coronary Heart Disease*, ed. M. Kaltenbach, P. Lichtlen & G.C. Friesinger (G. Thieme, Stuttgart, 1973) pp. 156–61

Hiss, R.G. & Lamb, L.E. Electrocardiographic findings in 122,043 individuals. *Circulation 25*, 947–61 (1962)

Ho, K., Mikkelson, B., Lewis, L.A., Feldman, S.A. & Taylor, C.B. Alaskan Arctic eskimo: responses to a customary high fat diet. *Amer. J. Clin. Nutr., 25*, 737–45 (1972)

Ho, K.J., Taylor, C.B. & Biss, K. Overall control of sterol synthesis in animals and man. In: *Atherosclerosis. Proceedings of Second International Symposium*, ed. R.J. Jones (Springer-Verlag, New York, 1970)

Hoes, M., Binkhorst, R.A., Smeekes-Kuyl, A. & Vissurs, A.C. Measurement of forces exerted on a pedal crank during work on the bicycle ergometer at different loads. *Int. Z. Angew. Physiol., 26*, 33–42 (1968)

Hokanson, J.E. Psychophysiological evaluation of the catharsis hypothesis. In: *The Dynamics of Aggression*, ed. E.I. Megargee & J.E. Hokanson (Harper & Row, New York, 1970)

Holloszy, J.O. The epidemiology of coronary heart disease: national differences and the role of physical activity. *J. Amer. Geriatr. Soc., 11*, 718–25 (1963)

Holloszy, J.O. Biochemical adaptations to exercise: aerobic metabolism. *Ex. Sports Sci. Rev., 1*, 45–71 (1973)

Holloszy, J.O., Oscai, L.B., Molé, P.A., *et al.* Biochemical adaptations to endurance exercise in skeletal muscle. In: *Muscle Metabolism during Exercise*, ed. B. Pernow & B. Saltin (Plenum Press, New York, 1971)

Holmberg, S., Serzysko, W. & Varnauskas, E. Coronary circulation during heavy exercise in control subjects and patients with coronary artery disease. *Acta Med. Scand., 190*, 465–80 (1971)

Holmér, I. & Åstrand, P.O. Swimming training and maximal oxygen uptake. *J. Appl. Physiol., 33*, 510–13 (1972)

Holmes, T.H. & Rahe, R.H. The social readjustment scale. *J. Psychomat. Res., 11*, 213–18 (1967)

Holmgren, A. Cardiorespiratory determinants of cardiovascular fitness. In: *Proceedings of International Symposium on Physical Activity and Cardiovascular Health, Canad. Med. Assoc., J., 96*, 697–702 (1967)

Holmgren, A. & Strandell, J. Relationship between heart volume, total hemoglobin and physical working capacity in former athletes. *Acta Med. Scand., 163*, 149–60 (1959)

Honey, G.E. & Truelove, S.C. Prognostic factors in myocardial infarction — long-term prognosis. *Lancet* (i), 1209–12 (1957)

Horwitz, L.D., Atkins, J.M. & Leshin, S.J. Role of the Frank-Starling mechanism in exercise. *Circ. Res., 57*, 64–70 (1972)

Horwitz, L.D., Herman, M.V. & Gorlin, R. Clinical responses to nitroglycerin as a diagnostic test for coronary artery disease. *Amer. J. Cardiol., 29*, 149–53 (1972)

Howard, A.N. Recent advances in nutrition and atherosclerosis. In: *Atherosclerosis. Proceedings of Second International Symposium*, ed. R.J. Jones (Springer Verlag, Berlin, 1970)

Humphries, J.O., Kuller, L., Ross, R.S., *et al*. Natural history of ischemic heart disease in relation to arteriographic findings: a twelve year study of 224 patients. *Circulation 49*, 489–97 (1974)

Hunyor, S.N., Flynn, J.M. & Cochineas, C. Comparison of performance of various sphygmomanometers with intra-arterial blood pressure readings. *Brit. Med. J., 2*, 159–62 (1978)

Hurry, J.B. *Imhotep* (Oxford University Press, London, 1926)

Ilmarinen, J. & Fardy, P.S. Physical activity intevention for males with high risk of coronary heart disease: a three year follow-up. *Prev. Med., 6*, 416–25 (1977)

Ingraham, H.S. Public health and fitness — the outdoor life and other antidotes to enemies of fitness. In: *Guide to Fitness after Fifty*, ed. R.H. Harris & L.J. Frankel (Plenum Press, New York, 1977) pp. 39–44

Inman, W.H.W. & Vessey, M.P. Investigation of deaths from pulmonary coronary and cerebral thrombosis and embolism in women of child-bearing age. *Brit. Med. J.* (ii), 193–9 (1968)

Innes, J.A., Campbell, I.W., Campbell, C.J., Needle, A.L., &

Munroe, J.F. Long-term follow-up of therapeutic starvation. *Brit. Med. J.* (ii), 357–9 (1974)

Isacsson, S.O. Venous occlusion plethysmography in 55 year old men. *Acta Med. Scand., 537*, suppl., 1–62 (1972)

Ishiko, T. Aerobic capacity and external criteria of performance. *Canad. Med. Assoc. J., 96*, 746–9 (1967)

Izeki, T. Statistical observation on sudden deaths in sport. *Brit. J. Sports Med., 7*, 172–6 (1973)

Jackson, L.K., Simmons, R., Leinbach, R.C., Rosner, S.W., Presto, A.J., Weihrer, A.L. & Caceres, C.A. Noise reduction and representative complex selection in the computer analyzed exercise electrocardiogram. In: *Measurement in Exercise Electrocardiography. The Ernst Simonson Conference*, ed. H. Blackburn (C.C. Thomas, Springfield, Ill., 1969) pp. 73–107

Jacobs, W.F., Nutter, D.O., Siegel, W., Schlant, R.C. & Hurst, J.W. Hemodynamic responses to isometric handgrip in patients with heart disease. *Circulation 42*, suppl. III, 169 (abstr.) (1970)

Jaffé, D. & Manning, M. Coronary arteries in early life. In: *Proceedings of Thirteenth Annual Congress of Pediatrics* (Vienna, 1971)

James, T.N. Angina without coronary disease. *Circulation 42*, 189–91 (1970)

James, T.N. Mysterious sudden death. *Chest 62*, 454–68 (1972)

James, T.N., Froggatt, P. & Marshall, T.K. Sudden death in young athletes. In: *Exercise and Cardiac Death*, ed. E. Jokl & J.T. McClellan (Karger, Basel, 1971)

James, W.E. & Patnoi, C.M. Instrumentation review. In: *Coronary Heart Disease. Prevention, Detection, Rehabilitation with Emphasis on Exercise Testing*, ed. S.M. Fox (International Medical Corporation, Denver, Colorado, 1974) pp. (7-1)–(7-46)

Jamison, P.L. & Zegura, S.L. An anthropometric study of the Eskimos of Wainwright, Alaska. *Arctic Anthropol., 7*, 125–43 (1970)

Jansson, L., Johansson, K., Jonson, B., Olsson, L.G., Werner, O. & Westling, H. Computer assistance in the e.c.g. laboratory — a new look. *Scand. J. Clin. Lab. Invest., 36*, suppl. 145, 1–43 (1976)

Jean, C.F., Streeter, D.D. & Reichenbach, D.D. Fiber orientation in the normal and hypertensive cadaver left ventricle. *Circulation 46*, suppl., 44 (abstr.) (1972)

Jenkins, C.D. Psychologic and social precursors of coronary

disease. II. *New Engl. J. Med., 284*, 307–16 (1971)

Jetté, M., Campbell, J. Mongeon, J. & Routhier, R. The Canadian Home Fitness Test as a prediction of aerobic capacity. *Canad. Med. Assoc. J., 114*, 680–2 (1976)

Jetter, W.W. & White, P.D. Rupture of the heart in patients in mental institutions. *Ann. Intern. Med., 21*, 783–802 (1944)

Jezer, A. & Warshaw, L.J. Detection and evaluation of heart disease in industry. In: *The Heart in Industry*, ed. L.J. Warshaw (P. Hoeber, New York, 1960) p. 163

Johnson, S.A., Robb, R.A., Greenleaf, J.F., Ritman, E.L., Lee, S.L., Herman, G.T., Sturm, R.E. & Wood, E.H. The problem of accurate measurement of left ventricular shape and dimensions from multiplane roentgenographic data. *Europ. J. Cardiol., 1*, 241–58 (1974)

Johnson, W.D. Coronary bypass surgery: its value in the rehabilitation of coronary patients. In: *Heart Disease and Rehabilitation*, ed. M.L. Pollock & D.H. Schmidt (Houghton Mifflin, Boston, 1979) pp. 203–11

Johnson, W.D., Flemma, R.J., Manley, J.C. & Leply, D. Physiologic parameters of ventricular function as affected by direct coronary surgery. *J. Thorac. Cardiovasc. Surg., 60*, 483–90 (1970)

Joint Working Party. Prevention of coronary heart disease. *J. R. Coll. Phys. Surg. (Lond.), 10*, 213–75 (1976)

Jokl, E. *The Clinical Physiology of Physical Fitness and Rehabilitation* (C.C. Thomas, Springfield, Ill., 1958)

Jokl, E., Jokl-Ball, M., Jokl, P. & Frankel, L. Notation of exercise. In: *Medicine and Sport*, vol. 4. *Physical Activity and Aging*, ed. D. Brunner & E. Jokl (Karger, Basel, 1970) pp. 2–18

Jokl, E. & McClellan, J.T. *Exercise and Cardiac Death* (University Park Press, Baltimore, Md., 1971)

Jones, N. & Kane, M. Inter-laboratory standardization of methodology. *Med. Sci. Sports 11*, 368–72 (1979)

Jones, N., McHardy, G.J.R., Naimark, A. & Campbell, E.J.M. Physiological dead space and alveolar-arterial gas pressure differences during exercise. *Clin. Sci., 31*, 19–29 (1966)

Jones, N.L., Campbell, E.J.M., Edwards, R.H.T. & Robertson, D.G. *Clinical Exercise Testing* (W.B. Saunders, Philadelphia, 1975)

Jones, N.L., Campbell, E.J.M., McHardy, G.J.R., Higgs, B. & Clode, M. The estimation of carbon dioxide pressure of mixed venous blood during exercise. *Clin. Sci., 32*, 311–27 (1967)

Jorgensen, C.R. Coronary blood flow and myocardial oxygen consumption in man. In: *Physiology of Fitness and Exercise*, ed. J.F. Alexander, R.C. Serfass & C.M. Tipton (Athletic Institute, Chicago, 1972) pp. 39–50

Jorgensen, C.R., Gobel, F.L., Taylor, H.L. & Wang, Y. Myocardial blood flow and oxygen consumption during exercise. *Ann. N.Y. Acad. Sci., 301*, 213–23 (1977)

Jorgensen, C.R., Kitamura, K., Gobel, F.L., Taylor, H.L. & Wang, Y. Long-term precision of the N_2O method for coronary flow during heavy upright exercise. *J. Appl. Physiol., 30*, 338–44 (1971)

Jorgensen, C.R., Wang, K., Gobel, F.L., *et al.* Effect of propranolol on myocardial oxygen consumption and its hemodynamic correlates during upright exercise. *Circulation 48*, 1173–82 (1973)

Juergens, J.L., Edwards, J.E., Achor, R.W.P. & Burchell, H.B. Prognosis of patients surviving first clinically diagnosed myocardial infarction. *AMA Arch. Int. Med., 105*, 444–50 (1960)

Julian, D.G. The natural history of ischemic heart disease. In: *Advances in Cardiology*, Vol. 8, ed. P. Halönen & A. Louhya (Karger, New York, 1973) pp. 38–48

Julian, D.G., Campbell, R.W.F. & Murray, A. Predicting and preventing ventricular fibrillation in acute myocardial infarction. In: *Sudden Coronary Death*, ed. V. Manninen & P.I. Halonen (Karger, Basel, 1978) pp. 183–90

Julius, S., Amery, A., Whitlock, L.S. & Conway, J. Influence of age on the hemodynamic response to exercise. *Circulation 36*, 222–30 (1967)

Kahler, R.L., Gaffney, T.E & Braunwald, E. Effect of autonomic nervous system inhibition on the circulatory response to exercise. *J. Clin. Invest., 41*, 1981–7 (1962)

Kahn, H. The relationship of reported coronary heart disease mortality to physical activity of work. *Amer. J. Publ. Health 53*, 1058–67 (1963)

Kala, R., Romo, M., Siltanen, P. & Halonen, P.I. Physical activity and sudden cardiac death. In: *Sudden Coronary Death*, ed. R. Kala, M. Romo, P. Siltanen & P.I. Halonen (Karger, Basel, 1978) pp. 27–34

Kallio, V. Results of rehabilitation in coronary patients. In: *Advances in Cardiology*, ed. K. König & H. Denolin (Karger,

Basel, 1978) pp. 153–63

Kannel, W.B. Habitual level of physical activity and risk of coronary heart disease. The Framingham study. *Canad. Med. Ass. J., 96*, 811–12 (1967)

Kannel, W.B. Cardiovascular disease: a multifactorial problem (insights from the Framingham Study). In: *Heart Disease and Rehabilitation*, ed. M.L. Pollock & D.H. Schmidt (Houghton Mifflin, Boston, Mass., 1979) pp. 15–51

Kannel, W.B., Castelli, W.P., Verter, J. & McNamara, P.M. Relative importance of risk factors in the pathogenesis of coronary heart disease. The Framingham Study. In: *Coronary Heart Disease*, ed. H.I. Russek & B.L. Zohman (Lippincott, Philadelphia, 1971a)

Kannel, W.B., McNamara, P.M., Feinleib, M., *et al.* Unrecognized myocardial infarction. *Geratrics 25*, 75–87 (1970)

Kannel, W.B., Sorlie, P. & McNamara, P. The relationship of physical activity to risk of coronary heart disease. The Framingham Study. In: *Coronary Heart Disease and Physical Fitness*, ed. O.A. Larsen & R.O. Malmborg (University Park) Press, Baltimore, Md., 1971b) pp. 256–60

Kaplinsky, E., Hood, W.B., McCarthy, B., McCombs, H.L. & Down, B. Effects of physical training in dogs with coronary artery ligation. *Circulation 37*, 556–65 (1968)

Karlsson, N., Nordesjø, L.O., Jorfeldt, L. & Saltin, B. Muscle lactate, ATP and CP levels during exercise after physical training in man. *J. Appl. Physiol., 33*, 199–203 (1972)

Karvonen, M.J., Klemola, H., Virkajärvi, J. & Kekkonen, A. on heart rate. A 'longitudinal' study. *Ann. Med. Exp. Fenn., 35*, 307–15 (1957)

Karnoven, M.J., Klemola, H., Virkajärvi, J. & Kekkonen, A. Longevity of endurance skiers. *Med. Sci. Sports 6*, 49–51 (1974)

Kasch, F.W. & Boyer, J.L. Changes in maximum work capacity resulting from six months training in patients with ischemic heart disease. *Med. Sci. Sports 1*, 156–9 (1969)

Kasser, I.S. & Bruce, R.A. Comparative effects of aging and coronary heart disease on submaximal and maximal exercise. *Circulation 39*, 759–74 (1969)

Katila, M. & Frick, M.H. A two year circulatory follow-up of physical training after myocardial infarction. *Acta Med. Scand., 187*, 95–100 (1970)

Kato, K. & Watanabe, H. Haemodynamic response to exercise in patients with coronary heart disease. *Jap. Circ. J., 35*, 29–33 (1971)

Kattus, A. Medical versus surgical therapy for ischemic heart disease. *Chest 58*, suppl. 1, 299–304 (1970)

Kattus, A. & Grollman, J. Patterns of coronary collateral circulation in angina pectoris: relation to exercise training. In: *Changing Concepts in Cardiovascular Disease*, ed. H.I. Russek & B.L. Zohman (Williams & Wilkins, Baltimore, 1972)

Kattus, A.A. & McAlpin, R.N. Diagnosis, medical and surgical management of coronary insufficiency. *Ann. Intern. Med., 60*, 115–36 (1968)

Kattus, A.A. & McAlpin, R.N. Role of exercise in discovery, evaluation and management of ischemic heart disease. In: *Cardiovascular Clinics*, vol. 1, No. 2, *Coronary Heart Disease*, ed. A.N. Brest (Davis, Philadelphia, 1969) pp. 225–79

Katz, A.M. Effects of ischemia on the contractile process of heart muscle. *Amer. J. Cardiol., 32*, 456–60 (1973)

Katz, A.M. *Physiology of the Heart* (Raven Press, New York, 1977) pp. 1–433

Katz, A.M. & Katz, P.B. Diseases of the heart, in the works of Hippocrates. *Brit. Heart J., 24*, 257–64 (1962)

Katz, L.J. & Landt, H. The effect of standardized exercise on the four-lead electrocardiogram: its value in study of coronary disease. *Amer. J. Med. Sci., 189*, 346–51 (1935)

Katz, L.N. & Feinberg, H. Relation of cardiac effort to myocardial oxygen consumption and coronary flow. *Circ. Res., 6*, 656–69 (1958)

Kaunitz, H. Causes and consequences of salt consumption. *Nature (Lond.), 178*, 1141–4 (1956)

Kavanagh, T. A cold-weather 'jogging mask' for angina patients. *Canad. Med. Assoc. J., 103*, 1290–1 (1970)

Kavanagh, T. *Heart Attack? Counter Attack!* (Van Nostrand, Toronto, 1976)

Kavanagh, T., Pandit, V. & Shephard, R.J. The application of exercise testing to the elderly amputee. *Canad. Med. Assoc. J., 108*, 314–17 (1973a)

Kavanagh, T. & Shephard, R.J. The immediate antecedents of myocardial infarction in active men. *Canad. Med. Assoc. J., 109*, 19–22 (1973a)

Kavanagh, T. & Shephard, R.J. Importance of physical activity in post-coronary rehabilitation. *Amer. J. Phys. Med., 52*, 304–13

(1973b)

Kavanagh, T. & Shephard, R.J. Conditioning of post-coronary patients. Comparison of continuous and interval training. *Arch. Phys. Med. Rehabil., 56,* 72–6 (1975a)

Kavanagh, T. & Shephard, R.J. Maintenance of hydration in 'post-coronary' marathon runners. *Brit. J. Sports Med., 9,* 130–5 (1975b)

Kavanagh, T. & Shephard, R.J. Maximum exercise tests on 'post-coronary' patients. *J. Appl. Physiol., 40,* 611–18 (1976)

Kavanagh, T. & Shephard, R.J. The effects of continued training on the aging process. *Ann. N.Y. Acad. Sci., 301,* 656–70 (1977a)

Kavanagh, T. & Shephard, R.J. Sexual activity after myocardial infarction. *Canad. Med. Assoc. J., 116,* 1250–3 (1977b)

Kavanagh, T. & Shephard, R.J. Fluid and mineral needs of post-coronary distance runners. In: *Sports Medicine*, ed. F. Landry & W.R. Orban (Symposia Specialists, Miami, Fla., 1978)

Kavanagh, T. & Shephard, R.J. Exercise for post-coronary patients: an assessment of infrequent supervision. *Arch. Phys. Med. Rehab., 61* (3), 114–18 (1980)

Kavanagh, T., Shephard, R.J., Chisholm, A.W., Qureshi, S. & Kennedy, J. Prognostic indexes for patients with ischemic heart disease enrolled in an exercise-centered rehabilitation program. *Amer. J. Cardiol., 44,* 1230–40 (1979)

Kavanagh, T., Shephard, R.J. & Doney, H. Hypnosis and exercise — a possible combined therapy following myocardial infarction. *Amer. J. Clin. Hypnosis 16,* 160–5 (1974a)

Kavanagh, T., Shephard, R.J., Doney, H. & Pandit, V. Intensive exercise in coronary rehabilitation. *Med. Sci. Sports 5,* 34–9 (1973b)

Kavanagh, T., Shephard, R.J. & Kennedy, J. Characteristics of post-coronary marathon runners. *Ann. N.Y. Acad. Sci., 301,* 656–70 (1977a)

Kavanagh, T., Shephard, R.J. & Kennedy, J. Are the benefits of exercise in post-coronary rehabilitation an artefact of patient selection? *Cardiologia 62,* 84–5 (1977c)

Kavanagh, T., Shephard, R.J. & Pandit, V. Marathon running after myocardial infarction. *JAMA, 229,* 1602–5 (1974b)

Kavanagh, T., Shephard, R.J. & Pandit, V. Marathon running after myocardial infarction. In: *Twentieth World Congress of Sports Medicine, Melbourne, Australia*, ed. H. Toyne (Australian Sports Medicine Federation, Melbourne, 1975a)

Kavanagh, T., Shephard, R.J. & Tuck, J.A. Depression after

myocardial infarction. *Canad. Med. Assoc. J., 113*, 23–7 (1975b)

Kavanagh, T., Shephard, R.J., Tuck, J.A. & Qureshi, S. Depression following myocardial infarction: the effects of distance running. *Ann. N.Y. Acad. Sci., 301*, 1029–38 (1977b)

Kay, C. & Shephard, R.J. On muscle strength and the threshold of anaerobic work. *Int. Z. Angew. Physiol., 27*, 311–28 (1969)

Keefer, C.S. & Resnick, W.H. Angina pectoris: a syndrome caused by anoxemia of the myocardium. *Arch. Int. Med., 41*, 769–807 (1928)

Keegan, D.L. The coronary patient: a psychosocial glimpse. *Canad. Fam. Phys., 19*, 66–8 (1973)

Keith, R.A. Personality and coronary heart disease — a review. *J. Chronic Dis., 19*, 1231–43 (1966)

Kellermann, J.J., Ben Ari, E., Chayet, M., Lapidot, C. Drory, Y. & Fisman, E. Cardiocirculatory response to different types of training in patients with angina pectoris. *Cardiology 62*, 218–31 (1977)

Kellerman, J.J. & Kariv, I. *Rehabilitation of Coronary Patients* (Segal Press, Tel Aviv, 1968)

Kellermann, J.J., Modan, B., Feldman, S. & Kariv, I. Evaluation of physical work capacity in coronary patients after myocardial infarction who returned to work with and without a medically directed reconditioning program. In: *Physical Activity and Aging*, ed. D. Brunner & E. Jokl (University Park Press, Baltimore, Md., 1970) pp. 148–55

Kemple, C. Rorschach method and psychosomatic diagnosis: personality traits of patients with rheumatic disease, hypertensive cardiovascular disease, coronary occlusion and fracture. *Psychosom. Med., 7*, 85–9 (1945)

Kemsley, W.F.F. Body weight at different ages and heights. *Ann. Eugen. (Lond.), 16–17*, 316–34 (1951–3)

Kendrick, Z.B., Pollock, M.L., Hickman, T.N. & Miller, H.S. Effects of training and detraining on cardiovascular efficiency. *Amer. Corr. Therap. J., 25*, 79–83 (1971)

Kennedy, C.K., Spiekerman, R.E., Lindsay, M.I., Mankin, H.T., Frye, R.L. & McCallister, B.D. One-year graduated exercise program for men with angina pectoris. Evaluation by physiological studies and coronary arteriography. *Mayo Clin. Proc., 51*, 231–6 (1976)

Kennedy, J.W., Baxley, W.A., Figley, M.M., Dodge, H.T. & Blackburn, J.R. Quantitative angiography. I. The normal left ventricle in man. *Circulation 34*, 272–8 (1966)

Kentala, E. Physical fitness and feasibility of physical rehabilitation after myocardial infarction in men of working age. *Ann. Clin. Res.*, *4*, suppl. 9, 1–84 (1972)

Kentala, E. & Sarna, S. Sudden death and factors related to long term prognosis following acute myocardial infarction. *Scand. J. Rehab. Med.*, *8*, 27–32 (1976)

Kerr, A., Bommer, W.J. & Pilato, S. Coronary artery enlargement in experimental cardiac hypertrophy. *Amer. Heart J.*, *75*, 144 (abstr.) (1968)

Keys, A. Coronary heart disease in seven countries. *Circulation 41*, suppl. 1 (1970)

Keys, A. Coronary heart disease — the global picture. *Atherosclerosis 22*, 149–92 (1975)

Keys, A., Aravanis, C., Blackburn, H., Van Buchem, F.S.P., Buzina, R., Djordjevic, B.S., Fidanza, F., Karvonen, M.J., Menotti, A., Puddu, V. & Taylor, H.L. Coronary heart disease: overweight and obesity. *Ann. Int. Med.*, *77*, 15–27 (1972)

Keys, A. & Parlin, R.W. Serum cholesterol response to changes in dietary lipids. *Amer. J. Clin. Nutr.*, *19*, 175–81 (1966)

Khosla, T. & Lowe, C.R. Indices of obesity derived from body weight and height. *Brit. J. Prev. Soc. Med.*, *21*, 122–8 (1967)

Kiessling, K.H., Pilstrom, L., Karlsson, J. & Piehl, K. Mitochondrial volume in skeletal muscle from young and old physically untrained and trained healthy men and from alcoholics. *Clin. Sci.*, *44*, 547–54 (1973)

Kilböm, Å. Physical training with sub-maximal intensities in women. I. Reaction to exercise and orthostasis. *Scand. J. Clin. Lab. Invest.*, *28*, 141–61 (1971)

Kilböm, Å., Hartley, L.H., Saltin, B., Bjure, J., Grimby, G. & Åstrand, I. Physical training in sedentary middle-aged and older men. I. Medical evaluation. *Scand. J. Clin. Lab. Invest.*, *24*, 315–28 (1969)

Kinderman, W., Keul, J. & Reindell, H. Cardiac function in sports. In: *Basic Book of Sports Medicine*, ed. G. La Cava (International Olympic Committee, Rome, 1978) pp. 47–58

Kinsey, A.C. *Sexual Behaviour in the Human Male* (W.B. Saunders, Philadelphia, 1948)

Kirchheiner, B. & Pedersen-Bjergaard, O. The effect of physical training after myocardial infarction. *Scand. J. Rehabil. Med.*, *5*, 105–10 (1973)

Kitamura, K., Jorgensen, C.R., Gobel, F.L., Taylor, H.L. & Yang, Y. Hemodynamic correlates of myocardial oxygen consumption during upright exercise. *J. Appl. Physiol., 32*, 516–22 (1972)

Kivowitz, C., Marcus, H., Donoso, R., Ganz, W., Swan, H.J.C. & Parmley, W.W. Evaluation of cardiac performance with a handgrip dynamometer in patients with heart disease: 'The grip tests'. *Circulation 42*, suppl. III, 122 (1970); *44*, 994–1002 (1971)

Klarman, H.E. Socio-economic impact of heart disease. In: *The Heart and Circulation. Second National Conference on Cardiovascular Diseases, vol. 2, Community Services and Education*, ed. E.C. Andrus (US Public Health Service, Washington, D.C., 1964)

Klassen, G.A, Woodhouse, S.P., Hathirat, S. & Johnson, A.L. The effect of physical training of post-myocardial infarction patients. A controlled study. *Canad. Med. Assoc. J., 107*, 632 (abstr.) (1972)

Klein, H.P. & Parson, O.A. Self-description of patients with coronary disease. Perceptual and motor skills (Southern Universities Press, Birmingham, Al., 1968)

Klein, R.F., Dean, A., Wilson, M., *et al*. The physician and post-myocardial infarction invalidism. *JAMA, 194*, 143–8 (1965)

Klocke, F.J. & Wittenburg, S.M. Heterogeneity of coronary blood flow in human coronary artery disease and experimental myocardial infarction. *Amer. J. Cardiol., 24*, 782–90 (1969)

Kloster, F., Kremkau, L., Rahimtoola, S., Griswold, H., Ritzmann, L., Neill, W. & Starr, A. Prospective randomized study of coronary by-pass surgery for chronic stable angina. *Circulation 52*, suppl. II, 90, 353 (abstr.) (1975)

Klumbies, G. & Kleinsorge, H. Circulatory dangers and prophylaxis during orgasm. *Int. J. Sexology 10*, 97 (1930)

Kober, G., Kuck, H., Lentz, R.W. & Kaltenbach, M. Angiographic evidence of collateral circulation and its effects on left ventricular function in coronary heart disease. In: *Coronary Heart Disease*, ed. M. Kaltenbach, P. Lichtlen, R. Balcon & W.D. Bussmann (G. Thieme, Stuttgart, 1978) pp. 48–54

Kobernick, S.D., Niawayama, G. & Zuehlewski, A.C. Effect of physical activity on cholesterol atherosclerosis in rabbits. *Proc. Soc. Exp. Biol. Med., N.Y., 96* (3), 623–8 (1957)

Koppes, G., McKiernan, T., Bassan, M., *et al*. Treadmill exercise testing. *Curr. Probl. Cardiol.*, 7 (8), 1–43; 7 (9), 1–45 (1977)

Korsan-Bengtsen, K., Wilhelmsen, L. & Tibblin, G. Blood coagulation and fibrinolysis in relation to degree of physical activity during work and leisure time. *Acta Med. Scand.*, *193*, 73–7 (1973)

Kötter, V., Von Leitner, E. & Schröder, R. Comparison of effects on hemodynamics and myocardial metabolism of phentolamine, sodium nitroprusside and glyceryl trinitrate in acute myocardial infarction. In: *Coronary Heart Disease*, ed. M. Kaltenbach, P. Lichtlen, R. Balcon & W.D. Bussmann (G. Thieme, Stuttgart, 1978) pp 273–8

Krantz, J.C., Lu, G.G., Bell, F.K. & Cascorbi, H.F. Nitrites. XIX. Studies on the mechanism of action of glyceryl trinitrate. *Biochem. Pharmacol.*, *11*, 1095–9 (1962)

Kraus, H. & Kirsten, R. Die Wirkung von körperlichen Training auf die mitochondriale Energieproduktion in Herzmuskel und in der Leber. *Pflügers Archiv.*, *320*, 334–47 (1970)

Kritchevsky, D. Laboratory models for atherosclerosis. In: *Advances in Drug Research*, vol. 9, ed. D. Kritchevsky (Academic Press, London, 1974) pp. 41–53

Kühn, P. Pharmacology of antiarrhythmic therapy. In: *Coronary Heart Disease, Exercise Testing and Cardiac Rehabilitation*, ed. W.E. James and E.A. Amsterdam (Symposia Specialists, Miami, Fla., 1977) pp. 319–24

Kuller, L. Sudden and unexpected non-traumatic deaths in adults. A review of epidemiological and clinical studies. *J. Chron. Dis.*, *19*, 1165–92 (1966)

Kuller, L., Lillienfeld, A. & Fisher, R. An epidemiological study of sudden and unexpected deaths in adults. *Medicine 46*, 341–61 (1967)

Kurita, A., Chaitman, B.R., & Bourassa, M.G. Significance of exercise-induced junctional ST depression in evaluation of coronary artery disease. *Amer. J. Cardiol.*, *40*, 492–7 (1977)

Kushnir, B., Fox, K.M., Tomlinson, I.W. & Aber, C.P. The effect of a pre-discharge consultation on the resumption of work, sexual activity and driving following acute myocardial infarction. *Scand. J. Rehab. Med.*, *8*, 155–9 (1976)

La Due, J.S., Wróblewski, F. & Karmen, A. Serum glutamic oxaloacetic transaminase activity in human acute transmural myocardial infarction. *Science 120*, 497–9 (1954)

Lalonde, M. A new perspective on the health of Canadians

(Information Canada, Ottawa, 1974)

Lamb, L.E. & Hiss, R.G. Influence of exercise on premature contractions. *Amer. J. Cardiol., 10*, 209–16 (1962)

Lamb, L.E., Kelly, R.J., Smith, W.L., LeBlanc, A.D. & Johnson, P.C. Limiting factors in the capacity to achieve maximum cardiac work. *Aerospace Med., 40*, 1291–6 (1969)

Lapiccirella, V., Lapiccirella, R., Abboni, F. & Liotta, S. Enquête clinique, biologie et cardiographique parmi les tribus nomades de le Somalie qui se nourissent seulement de lait. *Bull. WHO 27*, 681–97 (1962)

Largey, L.I. Longevity of college athletes. *Harper's Monthly Mag., 157*, 229–38 (1928)

Larsen, O.A. & Lassen, N.A. Effect of daily muscular exercise in patients with intermittent claudication. *Lancet* (ii), 1093–6 (1968)

Laurenceau, J.L., Turcot, J. & Dumesnil, J.G. Echocardiographic study of Olympic athletes. In: *Proceedings of International Conference on Sports Cardiology*, ed. T. Lubich & A. Venerando (A. Gaggi, Bologna, 1980) p. 705

Laurent, D., Bolene-Williams, C., Williams, F.L., *et al.* Effects of heart rate on coronary flow and cardiac oxygen consumption. *Amer. J. Physiol., 185*, 355–64 (1956)

Lawrie, G.M., Morris, G.C., Hiwell, J.F., *et al.* Results of coronary bypass more than five years after operation in 434 patients. Clinical, treadmill exercise and angiographic correlations. *Amer. J. Cardiol., 40*, 665–72 (1977)

Layman, E.M. Aggression in relation to play and sports. In: *Contemporary Psychology of Sport*, ed. G.S. Kenyon (Athletic Institute, Chicago, Ill., 1970) pp. 25–34

LeBlanc, J. *Man in the Cold* (C.C. Thomas, Springfield, Ill., 1975) pp. 1–195

Lebovits, B., Lichter, E. & Moses, V.K. Personality correlates of coronary heart disease: a re-examination of the MMPI data. *Soc. Sci. Med., 9*, 207–19 (1975)

Lebovits, B.Z., Shekelle, R.B., Ostfeld, A.M. & Paul, O. Prospective and retrospective psychological studies of coronary heart disease. *Psychosom. Med., 29*, 265–72 (1967)

Lee, G., Amsterdam, E.A., de Maria, A.N., Davis, G., LaFave, T. & Mason, D.T. Effect of exercise on hemostatic mechanisms. In: *Exercise in Cardiovascular Health and Disease*, ed. E.A. Amsterdam, J.H. Wilmore & A.N. de Maria (Yorke Medical

Books, New York, 1977) pp. 126–36

Lehtonen, A. & Viikari, J. The effect of vigorous physical activity at work on serum lipids, with special reference to serum high-density lipoprotein cholesterol. *Acta Physiol. Scand., 104*, 117–21 (1978)

Leon, A.S. & Bloor, C.M. Exercise effects on the heart at different ages. *Circulation 41/42*, suppl. III, 50 (1970)

Leon, A., Conrad, J. & Hunninghake, D. Effects of a walking program on body composition, carbohydrate and lipid metabolism of obese young men. *Amer. J. Clin. Nutr., 32*, 1776–87 (1979)

Leon, A.S., Conrad, J., Hunninghake, D., Jacobs, D. & Serfass, R. Exercise effects on body composition, work capacity, and carbohydrate and lipid metabolism of young obese men. *Med. Sci. Sports 9*, 60 (1977)

Lepeschkin, E. Physiological factors influencing the electro-cardiographic response to exercise. In: *Measurements in Exercise Electrocardiography*, ed. H. Blackburn (C.C. Thomas, Springfield, Ill., 1969)

Leppo, J., Yipintsoi, T., Blankstein, R., Bontemps, R., Freeman, L.M., Zohman, L. & Scheuer, J. Thallium-201 myocardial scintigraphy in patients with triple-vessel disease and ischemic exercise stress test. *Circulation 59*, 714–21 (1979)

Leren, P., Askevold, E.M., Foss, O.P., *et al.* The Oslo study. *Acta Med. Scand., 588*, suppl., 1–38 (1975)

Lester, F.M., Sheffield, L.T. & Reeves, J.T. Electrocardiographic changes in clinically normal older men following near maximal and maximal exercise. *Circulation 36*, 5–14 (1967)

Lester, M., Sheffield, L.T., Trammell, P. & Reeves, T.J. The effect of age and athletic training on the maximal heart rate during muscular exercise. *Amer. Heart J., 76*, 370–6 (1968)

Lewes, D. Electrode jelly in electrocardiography. *Brit. Heart J., 27*, 105–15 (1965)

Lewis, B.M., Houssay, H.E.J., Haynes, F.W. & Dexter, L. The dynamics of both right and left ventricles at rest and during exercise in patients with heart failure. *Circ. Res., 1*, 312–20 (1953)

Lichtlen, P., Moccetti, T., Halter, J. & Gattiker, K. Post-operative evaluation of myocardial blood flow in aorta-to-coronary artery vein bypass grafts using the xenon residue detection technique. In: *Coronary Heart Disease*, ed. M. Kaltenbach, P. Lichtlen &

G.C. Friesinger (G. Thieme, Stuttgart, 1973) pp. 286–95

Lie, K.I., Wellens, H.J.J., Downar, E. & Durrer, D. Observations of patients with primary ventricular fibrillation complicating acute myocardial infarction. *Circulation 52*, 755–9 (1975)

Likoff, W. Angina with normally patent coronary arteries. In: *Changing Concepts in Cardiovascular Disease*, ed. H.I. Russek & B.L. Zohman (Williams & Wilkins, Baltimore, 1972) pp. 77–9

Lind, A.R. & McNicol, G.W. Muscular factors which determine the cardiovascular responses to sustained and rhythmic exercise. In: *Proceedings of an International Symposium on Physical Activity and Cardiovascular Health. Canad. Med. Assoc. J., 96*, 706–12 (1967)

Little, J.A., Shanoff, H.M., Roe, R.D., Csima, A. & Yano, R. Studies of male survivors of myocardial infarction. IV. Serum lipids and five year survival. *Circulation 31*, 854–62 (1965)

Littler, W.A., Honour, A.J. & Sleight, P. Direct arterial pressure, heart rate and electrocardiogram during human coitus. *J. Reprod. Fertil., 40*, 321–31 (1974)

Logan, S.E. On the fluid mechanics of human coronary stenosis. *IEEE Trans. Biomed. Eng., BME22*, 327–34 (1975)

Lopez, A., Vial, R., Balart, L. & Arroyave, G. Effect of exercise and physical fitness on serum lipids and lipoproteins. *Atherosclerosis 20*, 1–9 (1974)

Love, W.D. & Burch, G.E. Influence of the rate of coronary plasma flow on the extraction of Rb^{86} from coronary blood. *Circulation Res., 7*, 24–30 (1959)

Lovell, R.R.H. & Verghese, A. Personality traits associated with different chest pains after myocardial infarction. *Brit. Med. J.* (iii), 327–30 (1967)

Lown, B., Kosowsky, B.D. & Whiting, R. Exposure of electrical instability in coronary artery disease by exercise stress. *Circulation 39*, suppl. 3, 136 (abstr.) (1969)

Lundgren, O. & Jodal, M. Regional blood flow. *Ann. Rev. Physiol., 37*, 395–414 (1975)

Mackenzie, G.J., Taylor, S.H., Flenley, D.C., McDonald, A.H., Staunton, H.P. & Donald, K.W. Circulatory and respiratory studies in myocardial infarction and cardiogenic shock. *Lancet* (ii), 825–32 (1964)

Mackintosh, A.F., Crabb, M.E., Grainger, G., Williams, J.H. & Chamberlain, D.A. The Brighton resuscitation ambulances: review of 40 consecutive survivors of out of hospital cardiac arrest. *Brit. Med. J.* (i), 1115–18 (1978)

Maddocks, I. In: *Proceedings of the Sixth International Congress of Nutrition*, ed. C.F. Miles & R. Passmore (Livingstone, Edinburgh, 1964) p. 137

Malleson, A. *The Medical Run-around* (Hart, New York, 1973)

Malmborg, R.O. A clinical and hemodynamic analysis of factors limiting cardiac performance in patients with coronary heart disease. *Acta Med. Scand.*, *117*, suppl. 426, 5–94 (1965)

Malmcrona, R. Cramér, G. & Varnauskas, E. Haemodynamic data during rest and exercise for patients who have or have not been able to retain their occupation after myocardial infarction. *Acta Med. Scand.*, *174*, 557–72 (1963)

Malmcrona, R. & Varnauskas, E. Haemodynamics during rest and during exercise at the end of convalescence from myocardial infarction. *Acta Med. Scand.*, *175*, 19–30 (1964)

Malmros, H. The relation of nutrition to health — a statistical study of the effect of war-time on arteriosclerosis, cardiosclerosis, tuberculosis and diabetes. *Acta Med. Scand.*, *246*, suppl., 137–53 (1950)

Manley, J.C. Hemodynamic performance before and following coronary by-pass surgery. In: *Heart Disease and Rehabilitation*, ed. M.L. Pollock & D.H. Schmidt (Houghton Mifflin, Boston, 1979) pp. 168–82

Manley, J.C. & Johnson, W.D. Effects of surgery on angina (pre- and post-infarction) and myocardial function (failure). *Circulation 46*, 1208–21 (1972)

Mann, G.V. A factor in yogurt which lowers cholesterolemia in man. *Atherosclerosis 26*, 335–40 (1977)

Mann, G.V., Garrett, H.L., Farhi, A., *et al*. Exercise to prevent coronary heart disease. *Amer. J. Med.*, *46*, 12–27 (1969)

Mann, G.V., Schaffer, R.D., Anderson, R.S., *et al*. Cardio-vascular disease in the Masai. *J. Atherosclerosis Res.*, *4*, 289–312 (1965)

Mann, R.H. & Burchell, H.B. Premature ventricular contractions and exercise. *Proc. Staff Mayo Clin.*, *27*, 383–9 (1952)

Manninen, V. & Halonen, P.I. *Sudden Coronary Death* (Karger, Basel, 1978)

Margaria, R., Aghemo, P. & Rovelli, E. Indirect determination of maximal O_2 consumption in man. *J. Appl. Physiol.*, *20*, 1070–3 (1965)

Margolis, J.R. Treadmill stage as a predictor of medical and surgical survival in coronary disease. *Circulation 52*, suppl. II, 109 (abstr.) (1975)

Margolis, J.R., Hirschfield, J.W., McNeer, J.F., *et al.* Sudden death due to coronary artery disease. A clinical, hemodynamic and angiographic profile. *Circulation 52–52*, suppl. III, 180–3 (1975)

Maritz, J.S., Morrison, J.F., Peter, J., Strydom, N.B. & Wyndham, C.H. A practical method of estimating an individual's maximum oxygen intake. *Ergonomics 4*, 97–122 (1961)

Maron, B.J. Cardiac causes of sudden death in athletes and considerations for screening athletic populations. In: *International Congress of Sports Cardiology*, ed. T. Lubich & A. Venerando (A. Gaggi, Bologna, 1980)

Marriott, H.J.L. & Myerburg, R.J. Recognition and treatment of cardiac arrhythmias and conduction disturbances. In: *The Heart*, 3rd edn., ed. J.W. Hurst (McGraw Hill, New York, 1974)

Marshall, R.C., Berger, J.H., Costin, J.C., *et al.* Assessment of cardiac performance with quantitative radionuclide angiography: sequential left ventricular ejection fraction, normalized left ventricular ejection rate and regional wall motion. *Circulation 56*, 820–9 (1977)

Marx, H.J, Rowell, L.B., Conn, R.D., Bruce, R.A. & Kusumi, F. Maintenance of aortic pressure and total peripheral resistance during exercise in heat. *J. Appl. Physiol., 22*, 519–25 (1967)

Marx, J.L. Stress: role in hypertension debated. *Science 198*, 905–7 (1977)

Mason, D.T., Amsterdam, E.A., Miller, R.R., Salel, A.F. & Zelis, R. Physiological basis of antianginal therapy: the nitrites, beta adrenergic receptor blockade, carotid sinus nerve stimulation, and coronary artery-saphenous vein bypass graft. In: *Changing Concepts in Cardiovascular Disease*, ed. H.I. Russek & B.L. Zohman (Williams & Wilkins, Baltimore, 1972) pp. 40–64

Massie, E. Sudden death during coitus: fact or fiction? *Hum. Sex 3*, 22 (1969)

Massie, J., Rode, A., Skrien, T. & Shephard, R.J. A critical review of the 'Aerobics' points system. *Med. Sci. Sports 2*, 1–6 (1970)

Massie, J. & Shephard, R.J. Physiological and psychological effects of training. *Med. Sci. Sports 3*, 110–17 (1971)

Master, A.M. Effect of injury and effort on the normal and the diseased heart. *New York State J. Med.*, *46*, 2634–41 (1946)

Master, A.M. & Jaffe, H.L. Electrocardiographic changes after exercise in angina pectoris. *J. Mt. Sinai Hosp.*, *N.Y.*, *7*, 629–32 (1941)

Master, A.M., Van Liere, E.J., Lindsay, H.A. & Hartroft, W.S. Arterial blood pressure. In: *Biology Data Book*, ed. P.L. Altman & D.S. Dittmer (Federation of American Societies for Experimental Biology, Washington D.C., 1964)

Masuda, M., Shibayama, H. & Ebashi, H. Changes in arterial blood pressure during running and walking determined by a kind of indirect method. *Bull. Phys. Fitness Res. Inst. (Japan), 11*, 1–16 (1967)

Matell, G. Time course of changes in ventilation and arterial gas tensions in man induced by moderate exercise. *Acta Physiol. Scand.*, *58*, suppl. 206, 1–53 (1963)

Mathers, J.A.L., Griffeath, H.I., Levy, R.L. & Nickerson, J.L. Effect of ascending an ordinary flight of stairs on the work of the heart. Observations on normal individuals and on patients with coronary heart disease. *Circulation 3*, 224–9 (1951)

Mathur, V.S. & Guinn, G.A. Prospective randomized study of coronary by-pass surgery in stable angina: the first 100 patients. *Circulation 51/52*, suppl. I, 133–40 (1975)

Mattingly, T.W. The post-exercise electrocardiogram. Its value in the diagnosis and prognosis of coronary arterial disease. *Amer. J. Cardiol.*, *9*, 395–409 (1962)

Mattingly, T.W., Robb, G.P. & Marks, H.H. Stress tests in the detection of coronary disease. *Postgrad. Med.*, *24*, 419–30 (1958)

Mausner, J.S. & Bahn, A.K. *Epidemiology. An Introductory Text* (W.B. Saunders, Philadelphia, 1974)

Maynard, J.E. Coronary heart disease risk factors in relation to urbanization in Eskimo men. In: *Circumpolar Health*, ed. R.J. Shephard & S. Itoh (University of Toronto Press, Toronto, 1976) pp. 294–5

McAllister, F.F., Bertsch, R., Jacobson, J. & D'Allesio, G. The accelerating effect of muscular exercise on experimental atherosclerosis. *Arch. Surg.*, *80*, 54–60 (1959)

McAlpine, V., Milojevic, S. & Monkhouse, F.C. Changes in the electrophoretic patterns of euglobulin fractions following activation of the fibrinolytic system by exercise. *Can. J. Physiol. Pharmacol.*, *49*, 672–7 (1971)

McCrimmon, D.R., Cunningham, D.A., Rechnitzer, P.A. & Griffiths, J. Effect of training on plasma catecholamines in post-myocardial patients. *Med. Sci. Sports 8*, 152–6 (1976)

McDonald, G.A. & Fullerton, H.W. Effect of physical activty on coagulability of blood after ingestion of high-fat meal. *Lancet* (ii), 600–1 (1958)

McDonough, J.R. & Bruce, R.A. Maximal exercise testing in assessing cardiovascular function. In: *Proceedings of National Conference on Exercise in the Prevention, in the Evaluation, and in the Treatment of Heart Disease. J. S. Carol. Med. Ass., 65*, suppl. I, 26–33 (1969)

McDonough, J.R., Danielson, R.A., Wills, R.E. & Vine, P.L. Maximal cardiac output during exercise in patients with coronary artery disease. *Amer. J. Cardiol., 33*, 23–9 (1974)

McDonough, J.R., Haines, C., Stulb, S. & Garrison, G. Coronary heart disease among Negroes and Whites in Evans County, Georgia. *J. Chron. Dis., 18*, 443–68 (1965)

McGee, D. & Gordon, T. *The Framingham Study. An Epidemiological Investigation of Cardiovascular Disease. Section 31. The Results of the Framingham Study Applied to Four Other US Based Epidemiologic Studies of Cardiovascular Disease*, US Department of Health, Education and Welfare Publication, 76–1083 (Washington, D.C., 1976)

McGill, H.C. Comparison of experimentally induced animal atherosclerosis with spontaneous human atherosclerosis. In: *Comparative Atherosclerosis*, ed. J.C. Roberts, R. Strauss & M.S. Cooper (Harper & Row, New York, 1965) pp. 354–9

McGill, H.C. Introduction to the geographic pathology of atherosclerosis. *Lab. Invest., 18*, 465–7 (1968)

McGill, H.C. Abnormalities potentially mediating the effect of cigarette smoking on atherosclerosis. In: *Atherosclerosis IV*, ed. G. Schettler, Y. Goto, Y. Hata & G. Klose (Springer Verlag, Berlin, 1977) pp. 161–5

McHenry, P.L., Fisch, C., Korden, J.W. & Corya, B.R. Cardiac arrhythmias observed during maximal treadmill exercise testing in clinically normal men. *Amer. J. Cardiol., 29*, 331–6 (1972)

McHenry, P.L. & Morris, S.N. Exercise electrocardiography — current state of the art. In: *Advances in Electrocardiography*, vol. 2, ed. R. Schlant & W. Hurst (Grune & Stratton, New York, 1976)

McHenry, P.L., Stowe, D.E. & Lancaster, M.C. Computer

quantitation of the ST segment response during maximal treadmill exercise: clinical correlation. *Circulation 38*, 691–701 (1968)

McIntosh, H.D. & Garcia, J.A. The first decade of aortocoronary bypass grafting 1967–1977. A review. *Circulation 57*, 405–31 (1978)

McNeer, J.F., Starmer, C.F., Bartel, A.G., *et al*. The nature of treatment selection in coronary artery disease. Experience with medical and surgical treatment of a chronic disease. *Circulation 49*, 606–14 (1974)

McPherson, B.D., Paivio, A, & Yuhasz, M.S. Psychological effects of an exercise program for post-infarct and normal adult men. *J. Sports Med., 7*, 95–102 (1967)

Medalie, J.H., Neufeld, H.N., Riss, E., *et al. Physician's Fact Book: Selected Measurements on 10,000 Israeli Males* (Central Printer, Jerusalem, 1968)

Medved, R., Volarić and Pavišić-Medved, V. Sudden death of a top-level football player. *Brit. J. Sports Med., 7*, 164 (1973)

Mellerowicz, H. *Ergometrie* (Von Urban & Schwarzenburg, Munich, 1962)

Messer, J.V., Levine, M.J., Wagman, R.J. & Gorlin, R. Effect of exercise on cardiac performance in human subjects with coronary artery disease. *Circulation 28*, 404–14 (1963)

Metropolitan Life Insurance Company, New York City. Outlook for men disabled by coronary occlusion. *Statist. Bull., 34*, 1–3 (1953)

Meyer, B.M. Methodologic issues and considerations in epidemiologic studies of etiology and prevention of heart disease. In: *Heart Disease and Rehabilitation*, ed. M.L. Pollock & D.H. Schmidt (Houghton Mifflin, Boston, 1979) pp. 57–72

Miettinen, M., Karvonen, M.J., Turpeinen, O., *et al*. Effect of cholesterol-lowering diet on mortality from coronary heart disease and other causes. *Lancet* (ii), 835–9 (1972)

Mikulaj, L., Komadel, L., Vigas, M., Kvetnansky, R., Starka, L. & Vencel, P. Some hormonal changes after different kinds of motor stress in trained and untrained young men. In: *Metabolic Adaptation to Prolonged Physical Exercise*, ed. H. Howald & J.R. Poortmans (Birkhauser Verlag, Basel, 1975) pp. 333–8

Miller, C.K. Psychological correlates of coronary artery disease. *Psychosom. Med., 27*, 257–65 (1965)

Milvy, P. Statistical analysis of deaths from coronary heart disease anticipated in a cohort of marathon runners. *Ann. N.Y. Acad. Sci., 301*, 610–6 (1977)

Mirsky, I. Review of various theories for the evaluation of left ventricular wall stresses. In: *Cardiac Mechanics: Physiological, Clinical and Mathematical Considerations*, ed. I. Mirsky, D. Ghista & H. Sandler (Wiley, New York, 1974) pp. 381–409

Mirsky, I. and Parmlet, W.W. Force-velocity studies in isolated and intact heart muscle. In: *Cardiac Mechanics: Physiological, Clinical and Mathematical Considerations*, ed. I. Mirsky, D. Ghista & H. Sandler (Wiley, New York, 1974) pp. 87–112

Mirwald, R., Bailey, D.A. & Weese, C. Probleme bei der Einschätzung der maximalen aeroben Kraft der Untersuchung des Wachstums in einer Längsschnittstudie. In: *Motorische Entwicklung*, ed. R. Bauss & K. Roth (Institut für Sportswissenschaft, Darmstadt, 1977) pp. 65–75

Mitchell, J.H. & Wildenthal, K. Left ventricular function during exercise. In: *Coronary Heart Disease and Physical Fitness*, ed. O.A. Larsen & R.O. Malmborg (University Park Press, Baltimore, Md., 1971) pp. 93–6

Mitrani, I., Karplus, H. & Brunner, D. Arteriosclerosis of the coronary arteries in cases of traumatic death. *Isr. J. Med. Sci., 3*, 339 (abstr.) (1967)

Mogensen, L. Exercise testing and continuous long-term e.c.g. recording in the detection of arrhythmias and ST-T changes. In: *Coronary Heart Disease, Exercise Testing & Cardiac Rehabilitation*, ed. W.E. James & E.A. Amsterdam (Symposia Specialists, Miami, 1977) pp. 131–41

Moir, T.W. & DeBra, D.W. Effect of left ventricular hypertension, ischemia and vasoactive drugs on the myocardial distribution of coronary flow. *Circ. Res., 21*, 65–74 (1967)

Mojonnier, L., Hall, Y., Berkson, D., *et al.* Experience in changing food habits of hyperlipidaemic men and women. *J. Amer. Diet. Assn.* (1978) Cited by H. Blackburn in: *Heart Disease and Rehabilitation*, ed. M.L. Pollock & D.H. Schmidt (Houghton Mifflin, Boston, Mass., 1979)

Moncur, J. A study of fatalities during sport in Scotland (1969). *Brit. J. Sports Med., 7*, 162–3 (1973)

Monroe, R.G. Myocardial oxygen consumption during ventricular contraction and relaxation. *Circ. Res., 14*, 294–300 (1964)

Monroe, R.G. & French, G.N. Left ventricular pressure-volume relationship and myocardial oxygen consumption in the isolated heart. *Circulation Res., 9*, 362–74 (1961)

Montoye, H.J. Summary of research on the relationship of exercise to heart disease. *J. Sports Med. Fitness 2*, 34–43 (1960)

Montoye, H.J. *Physical Activity and Health. An Epidemiologic Study of an Entire Community* (Prentice Hall, Englewood Cliffs, N.J., 1975)

Montoye, H.J. Epidemiologic studies of exercise and cardiovascular disease. *Physical Educator 34*, 116–21 (1977)

Montoye, H.J., Metzner, H.L., Keller, J.B., *et al.* Habitual physical activity and blood pressure. *Med. Sci. Sports 4*, 175–81 (1972)

Montoye, H.J., Van Huss, W.D., Olson, H., Hudec, A. & Mahoney, E. Study of the longevity and morbidity of college athletes. *JAMA, 162*, 1132–4 (1956)

Montoye, H.J., Van Huss, W.D., Olson, H.W., Pierson, W.R. & Hudec, A.J. *The Longevity and Morbidity of College Athletes* (Phi Epislon Kappa Fraternity, Ann Arbor, 1957)

Montoye, H.J., Willis, P.W., Howard, G.E. & Keller, J.B. Cardiac pre-ejection period: age and sex comparisons. *J. Gerontol., 26*, 208–16 (1971)

Morgan, P., Gildiner, M. & Wright, G.R. Smoking reduction in adults who take up exercise: a survey of a running club for adults. *CAHPER Journal 42*, 39–43 (1976)

Morgan, W.P. Psychologic aspects of heart disease. In: *Heart Disease and Rehabilitation*, ed. M.L. Pollock & D.H. Schmidt (Houghton Mifflin, Boston, 1979) pp. 105–19

Morgan, W.P., Roberts, J.A., Brand, F.R., *et al.* Psychological effect of chronic physical activity. *Med. Sci. Sports 2*, 213–17 (1970)

Morgan, W.P., Roberts, J.A. & Feinerman, A.D. Psychological effect of acute physical activity. *Arch. Phys. Med. Rehab., 52*, 422–6 (1971)

Morgan Jones, A. Heart disease and fitness for work. In: *Work and the Heart*, ed. F.F. Rosenbaum & E.L. Belknap (P.B. Hoeber, New York, 1959) pp. 400–9

Morganroth, J. & Maron, B.J. The athlete's heart syndrome: a new perspective. *Ann. N.Y. Acad. Sci., 301*, 931–9 (1977)

Moritz, A.R. & Zamchek, N. Sudden and unexpected deaths of young soldiers. *Arch. Pathol., 42*, 459–94 (1946)

Moriyama, I.M., Baum, W.S., Haenszel, W.M. & Mattison, B.

Inquiry into diagnostic evidence supporting medical certifications of death. *Amer. J. Publ. Health 48*, 1376–87 (1958)

Morris, J.N. Recent history of coronary disease. *Lancet* (i), 1–7 (1951)

Morris, J.N. The epidemiology of coronary artery disease. In: *International Symposium on Exercise and Coronary Artery Disease*, ed. T. Kavanagh (Toronto Rehabilitation Centre, Toronto, 1975) pp. 76–89

Morris, J.N., Adams, C., Chave, S.P.N., Sirey, C., Epstein, L. & Sheehan, D.J. Vigorous exercise in leisure time and the incidence of coronary heart disease. *Lancet* (i), 333–9 (1973)

Morris, J.N. & Crawford, M.D. Coronary heart disease and physical activity of work. *Brit. Med. J.* (ii), 1485–96 (1958)

Morris, J.N., Heady, J.A. & Raffle, P.A. Physique of London busmen: epidemiology of uniforms. *Lancet* (ii), 569–70 (1956)

Morris, J.N., Heady, J., Raffle, P., Roberts, C. & Parks, J. Coronary heart disease and physical activity of work. *Lancet* (ii), 1053–7, 1111–20 (1953)

Morris, J.N., Kagan, A., Pattison, D.C., Gardner, M.J. & Raffle, P.A.B. Incidence and prediction of ischaemic heart disease in London busmen. *Lancet* (ii), 553–9 (1966)

Morris, J.N. & Raffle, P.A.B. Coronary heart disease in transport workers: progress report. *Brit. J. Industr. Med., 11*, 260–4 (1954)

Most, A.S., Brachfeld, N., Gorlin, R. & Wahren, J. Free fatty acid metabolism of the human heart at rest. *J. Clin. Invest., 48*, 1177–88 (1969)

MRFIT Report of the MRFIT Research Group: contribution of weight reduction to lowering serum cholesterol. *Circulation 56*, suppl. III, 111–13 (1977)

MRFIT Multiple risk factor intervention trial research group: multiple risk factor intervention trial (MRFIT). Smoking cessation procedures and cessation and recidivism patterns for a large cohort of MRFIT participants. In: *Progress in Smoking Cessation*, ed. J.L. Schwartz (American Cancer Society, New York, 1980)

Mulcahy, R., Hickey, N. & Coghlan, N. Rehabilitation of patients with coronary heart disease. *Geriatrics 27*, 120–9 (1972)

Müller, O. & Rørvik. K. Haemodynamic consequences of coronary artery disease with observations during anginal pain and on the effect of nitroglycerine. *Brit. Heart J., 20*, 302–10 (1958)

Mullins, C.B., Leshin, S.J., Mierzwiak, D.S., Matthews, O.A. &

Blomqvist, C.G. Isometric exercise (handgrip) as a stress test for evaluation of left ventricular function. *Circulation 42*, suppl. III, 122 (abstr.) (1970)

Mullins, C.B. & Blomqvist, G. Isometric exercise and the cardiac patient. *Texas Med.*, *69*, 53–8 (1973)

Multicentre Trial. Propranolol in acute myocardial infarction. *Lancet* (ii), 1434–38 (1966)

Munschek, H. Primary illness of the heart and sudden death by physical activity. *Proceedings of International Congress of Sports Cardiology, Rome*, ed. T. Lubich & A. Venerando (A. Gaggi, Bologna, 1980)

Murphy, J. *The Canada Health Survey* (Health & Welfare Canada, Ottawa, 1980)

Murphy, M.L., Hultgren, H.N., Detre, K., Thomsen, J., Takaro, J. and Participants of the Veterans Administration Cooperative Study. Treatment of chronic stable angina: a preliminary report of survival data of the randomized Veterans Administration Cooperative Study. In: *Heart Disease and Rehabilitation*, ed. M.L. Pollock & D.H. Schmidt (Houghton Mifflin, Boston, Mass., 1979) pp. 228–42

Murray, J.A., Kasser, I.S., Rowell, L.B. & Bruce, R.A. Aortic pressure and oxygen transport responses to upright exercise in angina pectoris. *Circulation 37*, suppl. VI, 145 (abstr.) (1968)

Myasnikob, A.L. Influence of some factors on development of experimental cholesterol atherosclerosis. *Circulation 17*, 99–113 (1958)

Myerburg, R.J. & Davis, J.H. The medical ecology of public safety. I. Sudden death due to coronary disease. *Amer. Heart J.*, *68*, 586–95 (1964)

Nager, F., Thomas, M. & Shillingford, J. Changes in cardiac output and stroke volume during first four months after cardiac infarction. *Brit. Heart J.*, *29*, 859–70 (1967)

Nagle, R., Gangola, R. & Picton-Robinson, I. Factors influencing return to work after myocardial infarction. *Lancet 2*, 454–56 (1971)

Najmi, M. & Segal, B.L. Resting and exercise haemodynamics in patients with coronary heart disease with or without previous myocardial infarction. In: *Atherosclerotic Vascular Disease*, ed. A.N. Brest & J.H. Moyer (Appleton Century Crofts, New York, 1967) pp. 321–35

Nakhjavan, F.K., Natarajan, G., Smith, A.M., Drutch, M. &

Goldberg, H. Myocardial lactate metabolism during isometric hand-grip test — comparison with pacing tachycardia. *Brit. Heart J., 37*, 79–84 (1975)

National Diet-Heart Study Research group. The national diet-heart study. Final report. *Circulation 38*, suppl. 1, 428 (1968)

Naughton, J. *The National Exercise and Heart Disease Project. Manual of Operations* (George Washington University, Washington, D.C., 1978)

Naughton, J., Bruhn, J.G. & Lategola, M.T. Effects of physical training on physiological and behavioral characteristics of cardiac patients. *Arch. Phys. Med. Rehab., 49*, 131–7 (1968)

Naughton, J., Shanbour, K., Armstrong, R., McCoy, J. & Lategola, MT.. Cardiovascular response to exercise following myocardial infarction. *Arch. Intern. Med., 117*, 541–5 (1966)

Neill, W.A. Coronary and systemic circulatory adaptations to exercise training and their effects on angina pectoris. In: *Exercise in Cardiovascular Health and Disease*, ed. E.A. Amsterdam, J.H. Wilmore & A.N. DeMaria (Yorke Books, New York, 1977)

Neill, W.A., Duncan, D.A., Kloster, F. & Mahler, D.J. Response of coronary circulation to cutaneous cold. *Amer. J. Med., 56*, 471–6 (1974)

Nelson, R.R., Gobel, F.L., Jorgensen, C.R., Wang, K., Wang, Y & Taylor, H.L. Hemodynamic predictors of myocardial oxygen consumption during static and dynamic exercise. *Circulation 50*, 1179–89 (1974)

Nemec, E.D, Mansfield, L. & Kennedy, J.W. Heart rate and blood pressure responses during sexual activity in normal males. *Amer. Heart J., 92*, 274–7 (1964)

Newman, G. & Nichols, C.R. Sexual activities and attitudes in older persons. *JAMA, 173*, 33–7 (1960)

Niehnes, B., Tauchert, M., Behrenbeck, D.W. & Hilger, H.H. Myocardial oxygen consumption and coronary vascular resistance under the influence of calcium inhibitors. In: *Coronary Heart Disease*, ed. M. Kaltenbach, P. Lichtlen, R. Balcon, & W.P. Bussmann (G. Thieme, Stuttgart, 1978) pp. 279–83

Nielsen, B. Thermoregulation in rest and exercise. *Acta Physiol. Scand., 323*, suppl., 1–74 (1969)

Niinimaa, V., Cole, P., Mintz, S. & Shephard, R.J. Oral augmentation of ventilation. *Respiration Physiol.* (in press,

1980)

Niinimaa, V. & Shephard, R.J. Training and oxygen conductance in the elderly. I. The respiratory system. II. The cardiovascular system. *J. Gerontol., 33*, 354–61 (1978)

Noakes, T., Opie, L. & Beck, W. Coronary heart disease in marathon runners. *Ann. N.Y. Acad. Sci., 301*, 593–619 (1977)

Nolting, D., Mack, R., Luthy, E., Kirsch, M. & Hogancamp, C. Measurement of coronary blood flow and myocardial rubidium uptake with Rb^{86}. *J. Clin. Invest., 37*, 921 (abstr.) (1958)

Norris, R.M., Caughey, D.E. & Scott, P.J. Trial of propranolol in acute myocardial infarction. *Brit. Med. J.* (ii), 398–400 (1968)

Nye, E.R. & Poulsen, W.T. An activity programme for coronary patients: a review of morbidity, mortality and adherence after five years. *New Zealand Med. J., 79*, 1010–13 (1974)

Oberman, A., Jones, W.B., Riley, C.P., *et al*. Natural history of coronary artery disease. *Bull. N.Y. Acad. Med., 48*, 1109–25 (1972)

O'Brien, K.P., Higgs, L.M. & Glancy, D.L. Haemodynamic accompaniments of angina. A comparison during angina induced by exercise and by atrial pacing. *Circulation 39*, 735–43 (1969)

O'Hara, W.J., Allen, C. & Shephard, R.J. Treatment of obesity by exercise in the cold. *Canad. Med. Assoc. J., 117*, 773–9 (1977)

O'Hara, W., Allen, C., Shephard, R.J. & Allen, G. Fat loss in the cold: a controlled study. *J. Appl. Physiol., 46*, 872–7 (1979)

Oldridge, N. What to look for in an exercise class leader. *Phys. Sports Med., 5*, 85–8 (1977)

Oldridge, N.B. Compliance with exercise programs. In: *Heart Disease and Rehabilitation*, ed. M.L. Pollock & D.H. Schmidt (Houghton Mifflin, Boston, 1979a) pp. 619–29

Oldridge, N.B. Compliance of post-myocardial infarction patients to exercise programs. *Med. Sci. Sports 11*, 373–5 (1979b)

Oliver, R.M. Physique and serum lipids of young London busmen in relation to ischaemic heart disease. *Brit. J. Industr. Med., 24*, 181–7 (1967)

Olson, R.E. Vitamin E and its relation to heart disease. *Circulation 48*, 179–84 (1973)

Orban, W.R. *Proceedings of National Conference on Fitness and Health* (Health & Welfare Canada, Ottawa, 1974)

Orlando, J., Aronow, W.S., Cassidy, J., *et al*. Effect of ethanol on angina pectoris. *Ann. Intern. Med., 84*, 652–5 (1976)

Osborn, G.R. *The Incubation Period of Coronary Thrombosis* (Butterworths, London, 1963)

Oscai, L.B., Molé, P.A., Brei, B. & Holloszy, J.O. Cardiac growth and respiratory enzyme levels in male rats subjected to a running program. *Amer. J. Physiol., 220*, 1238–41 (1971)

Oscai, L.B., Molé, P.A. & Holloszy, J.O. Effects of exercise on cardiac weight and mitochondria in male and female rats. *Amer. J. Physiol., 220*, 1944–8 (1971)

Oski, F.A, Miller, L.D., Delicoria-Papadopoulos, M., *et al.* Oxygen affinity in red cells: changes induced *in-vivo* by propranolol. *Science 175*, 1372–3 (1972)

Osler, W. Lectures on angina pectoris and allied states. *N.Y. Med. J., 64*, 177–83 (1896)

Ostfeld, A.M. Lebovits, B.Z., Shekelle, R.B. & Paul, O. A prospective study of the relationship between personality and coronary heart disease. *J. Chron. Dis., 17*, 265–76 (1964)

Ostrander, L.D. & Lamphiear, D.E. Oral contraceptives and physiological variables. *Circulation 58* (4), II-91 (abstr.) (1978)

Otis, A.B. The work of breathing. In: *Handbook of Physiology*, Section 3, *Respiration*, vol. 1, ed. W.O. Fenn & H. Rahn (American Physiological Society, Washington, D.C., 1964)

Paffenbarger, R. Physical activity and fatal heart attack: protection or selection? In: *Exercise in Cardiovascular Health and Disease*, ed. E.A. Amsterdam, J.H. Wilmore & A.N. deMaria (Yorke Medical Books, New York, 1977) pp. 35–49

Paffenbarger, R.S. & Hale, W.E. Work activity and coronary heart mortality. *New Engl. J. Med., 292*, 454–550 (1975)

Paffenbarger, R.S., Hale, W.E., Brand, R.J. & Hyde, R.T. Work-energy level, personal characteristics and fatal heart attack: a birth cohort effect. *Amer. J. Epidemiol., 105*, 200–13 (1977)

Paffenbarger, R.S., Laughlin, M.E., Gima, A.S., *et al.* Work activity of longshoremen as related to death from coronary heart disease and stroke. *New Engl. J. Med., 20*, 1109–14 (1970)

Paffenbarger, R.S., Wing, A.L. & Hyde, R.T. Physical activity as an index of heart attack risk in college alumni. *Amer. J. Epidemiol., 108*, 161–75 (1978)

Palatsi, I. Feasibility of physical training after myocardial infarction and its effect on return to work, morbidity and mortality. *Acta Med. Scand., 599*, suppl., 7–84 (1976)

Pařízková, J. *Body Fat and Physical Fitness* (M. Nijhoff, B.V., The Hague, 1977)

Parker, J.O., DiGiorgi, S. & West, R.O. A hemodynamic study of acute coronary insufficiency precipitated by exercise. With observations on the effects of nitroglycerin. *Amer. J. Cardiol.*, *17*, 470–83 (1966)

Parker, J.O., West, R.O. & diGiorgi, S. The haemodynamic response to exercise in patients with healed myocardial infarction without angina. *Circulation 36*, 734–49 (1967)

Parker, J.O., West, R.O., Ledwich, J.R. & diGiorgi, S. The effect of acute digitalization on the hemodynamic response to exercise in coronary artery disease. *Circulation 40*, 453–62 (1969)

Parkes, C.M., Benjamin, B. & Fitzgerald, R.G. A broken heart. A statistical study of increased mortality among widowers. *Brit. Med. J.* (i), 740–3 (1969)

Parkey, R.W., Bonte, F.J., Meyer, S.L., *et al*. A new method for radionuclide imaging of acute myocardial infarction in humans. *Circulation 50*, 540–6 (1974)

Parr, R.B. & Kerr, J.D. Liability and insurance. In: *Adult Fitness and Cardiac Rehabilitation*, ed. P.K. Wilson (University Park Press, Baltimore, Md., 1975) pp. 219–24

Parran, T.V., Hellerstein, H.K., Cohen, D. & Goldston, E. Results of studies at the work classification clinic of the Cleveland area Heart Society. In: *Work and the Heart*, ed. F.F. Rosenbaum & E.L. Belknap (P.B. Hoeber, New York, 1959) pp. 330–9

Paterson, D.H. *Alterations of Cardiovascular Function with Mild and Intense Physical Training of Post-myocardial Infarction Subjects*. Ph.D. Dissertation (University of Toronto, Toronto, 1977)

Paterson, D.H., Shephard, R.J., Cunningham, D. & Jones, N. Influence of age, angina, and time since infarction upon the cardiovascular response to physical training. *Med. Sci. Sports 12*, 100 (1980)

Paterson, D.H., Shephard, R.H., Cunningham, D., Jones, N.L. & Andrew, G. Effects of physical training upon cardiovascular function following myocardial infarction. *J. Appl. Physiol.*, *47*, 482–9 (1979)

Patton, J.F., Morgan, W.P. & Vogel, J.A. Perceived exertion of absolute work during a military training program. *Europ. J. Appl. Physiol.*, *36*, 107–14 (1977)

Paul, O. Physical activity and coronary heart disease. *Amer. J.*

Cardiol., 23, 303–6 (1969)

Pedersen, A. & Andersen, S.N. Work test with electrocardiogram, analysis by digital computer. In: *Coronary Heart Disease & Physical Fitness*, ed. O.A. Larsen & R.O. Malmborg (University Park Press, Baltimore, Md., 1971) pp. 202–8

Pedersen-Bjergaard, O. The effect of physical training in myocardial infarction. In: *Coronary Heart Disease and Physical Fitness*, ed. O.A. Larsen & R.O. Malmborg (University Park Press, Baltimore, Md., 1971) pp. 115–16

Pedley, F.G. Coronary disease and occupation. *Canad. Med. Assoc. J., 46*, 147–51 (1942)

Pell, S. & D'Alonzo, C.A. Immediate mortality and five year survival of employed men with a first myocardial infarction. *New Engl. J. Med., 270*, 915–22 (1964)

Pelliccia, A. Influenza del lavoro muscolare sul numero e sulle funzioni delle piastrine. *Med. Del. Sport 30*, 275–82 (1978)

Penpargkul, S. & Scheuer, J. The effect of physical training upon the mechanical and metabolic performance of the rat heart. *J. Clin. Invest., 49*, 1859–68 (1970)

Petren, T., Sylven, B. & Sjöstrand, T. Der Einfluss des Trainings auf die Haufigkeit der Capillaren in Herz und Skelettmuskulatur. *Arbeitsphysiol., 9*, 376–86 (1936)

Phibbs, B., Holmes, R.W. & Lowe, C.R. Transient myocardial ischaemia. The significance of dyspnoea. *Amer. J. Med. Sci., 256*, 210–21 (1968)

Phipps, C. Contributory causes of coronary thrombosis. *JAMA, 106*, 761–2 (1936)

Pinto, I.J., Thomas, P., Colaco, F., *et al*. Current developments in India. In: *Atherosclerosis II*, ed. R.J. Jones (Springer Verlag, Berlin, 1970) pp. 328–35

Plas, F. Electrocardiography. In: *Basic Book of Sports Medicine*, ed. G. LaCava (International Olympic Committee, Rome, 1978) pp. 61–5

Polednak, A.P. Longevity and cardiovascular mortality among former college athletes. *Circulation 46*, 649–54 (1972)

Polednak, A.P. & Damon, A. College atheletics, longevity, and cause of death. *Hum. Biol., 42*, 28–46 (1970)

Pollock, M.L. The quantification of endurance training. *Exercise Sport Sci. Rev., 1*, 155–88 (1973)

Pollock, M.L. Physiological characteristics of older champion track athletes. *Res. Quart., 45*, 363–73 (1974)

Pomeroy, W.C. & White, P.D. Coronary heart disease in former football players. *JAMA, 167*, 711–14 (1958)

Poortmans, J.R., Luke, K.H., Zipursky, A. & Bienenstock, J. Fibrinolytic activity and fibrinogen split products in exercise proteinuria. *Clin. Chim. Acta 35*, 449–54 (1971)

Poupa, O., Rakusan, K. & Ostadol, B. The effect of physical activity upon the heart of vertebrates. In: *Physical Activity and Aging*, ed. D. Brunner & E. Jokl (Karger, Basel, 1970) pp. 202–33

Powles, A.C.P., Sutton, J.R., Wicks, J.R., Oldridge, N.B. & Jones, N.L. Reduced heart rate response to exercise in ischemic heart disease: the fallacy of the target heart rate in exercise testing. *Med. Sci. Sports 11*, 227–33 (1979)

President's Council on Fitness. National adult physical fitness survey. *Newsletter*. Special edn, pp. 1–27 (May, 1973)

Price, A.B. Disability due to cardiac impairment under the disability insurance program. In: *Work and the Heart*, ed. F.F. Rosenbaum & E.L. Belknap (P.B. Hoeber, New York, 1959) pp. 499–506

Price, L. Myocardial infarction in garment workers. Characteristics and relationship to time lost from work. In: *Work and the Heart*, ed. F.F. Rosenbaum & E.L. Belknap (P.B. Hoeber, New York, 1959) pp. 387–94

Prior, I.A.M. & Davidson, F. Epidemiology of diabetes in Polynesians and Europeans in New Zealand and the Pacific. *N. Z. Med. J., 65*, 375–83 (1966)

Prior, I.A.M. & Evans, J.G. Current developments in the Pacific. In: *Atherosclerosis II*, ed. R.J. Jones (Springer Verlag, Berlin, 1970) pp. 335–42

Profant, G.R., Early, R.G., Nilson, K.L., Kusumi, F., Hofer, V. & Bruce, R.A. Responses to maximal exercise in healthy middle-aged women. *J. Appl. Physiol., 33*, 595–9 (1972)

Pugh, L.G.C.E. Physiological and medical aspects of the Himalyan Scientific and Mountaineering Expedition 1960–61. *Brit. Med. J.* (ii), 621–7 (1962)

Puska, P. *North Karelia Project. A Programme for Community Control of Cardiovascular Diseases*. University of Kuopio Community Health Series A.1 (1974)

Puska, P., Tuomiletho, J. & Salonen, J. Community control of acute myocardial infarction in Finland. *Pract. Cardiol., 10*, 91–100 (1978)

Pyfer, H. Safety precautions and procedures in cardiac exercise rehabilitation programs. In: *Heart Disease and Rehabilitation*, ed. M.L. Pollock & D.H. Schmidt (Houghton Mifflin, Boston, 1979) pp. 630–9

Pyfer, H.R. & Doane, B.L. Aspects of community exercise programs. A. Economic aspects of cardiac rehabilitation programs. In: *Exercise Testing and Exercise Training in Coronary Heart Disease*, ed. J.P. Naughton, H.K. Hellerstein & I.C. Mohler (Academic Press, New York, 1973) pp. 365–9

Pyfer, H.R., Mead, W.F. & Frederick, R.C. Cardiac arrest during medically supervised exercise training — a report of 13 successful defibrillations, *Med. Sci. Sports* 7, 72 (abstr.) (1975)

Pyörälä, K., Kärävä, R., Punsar, S., *et al*. A controlled study of the effects of 18 months' physical training in sedentary middle-aged men with high indexes of risk relative to coronary heart disease. In: *Coronary Heart Disease and Physical Fitness*, ed. O.A. Larsen & R.O. Malmborg (Munksgaard, Copenhagen, 1971) pp. 261–5

Pyörälä, K., Karvonen, M.J., Taskinen, P., Takkunen, J., Kyrönseppä, H. & Peltokallio, P. Cardiovascular studies on former endurance athletes. *Amer. J. Cardiol., 20*, 191–205 (1967a)

Pyörälä, K., Karvonen, M.J., Taskinen, P., Takkunen, J. & Kyrönseppä, H. Cardiovascular studies on former endurance athletes. In: *Physical Activity and the Heart*, ed. M.J. Karvonen & A.J. Barry (C.C. Thomas, Springfield, Ill., 1967b)

Raab, W. Training, physical activity and the cardiac dynamic cycle. *J. Sports Med. Phys. Fitness* 6, 38–47 (1966)

Rakusan, K., Ost'adal, B. & Wachtlová, M. The influence of muscular work on the capillary density in the heart and skeletal muscle of pigeon. *Canad. J. Physiol. Pharm., 49*, 167–70 (1971)

Rasmussen, R.L., Bell, R.D. & Spencer, G.D. Prepubertal exercise and myocardial collateral circulation. In: *Exercise Physiology*, ed. F. Landry &. W.A.R. Orban (Symposia Specialists, Miami, 1978)

Rautaharju, P.M., Friedrich, H. & Wolf, H. Measurement and interpretation of exercise electrocardiograms. In: *Frontiers of Fitness*, ed. R.J. Shephard (C.C. Thomas, Springfield, Ill., 1971)

Read, R.C., Murphy, M.L., Hultgren, H.N., *et al*. Survival of men treated for chronic stable angina pectoris. A cooperative randomized study. *J. Thoracic. Cardiovasc. Surg., 75*, 1–16 (1978)

Rechnitzer, P.A., Paivio, A., Pickard, H.A. & Yuhasz, M.S. Long-term follow-up study of survival and recurrence rates following myocardial infarction in exercising subjects and matched controls. *Med. Sci. Sport 3*, 502 (C) (abstr.) (1971)

Rechnitzer, P.A., Pickard, H.A., Paivio, A., Yuhasz, M.S. & Cunningham, D.A. Long-term follow-up study of survival and recurrence rates following myocardial infarction in exercising and control subjects. *Circulation 45*, 853–7 (1972)

Rechnitzer, P.A., Sangal, S., Cunningham, D., Andrew, G., Buck, C., Jones, N.L., Kavanagh, T., Parker, J.O., Shephard, R.J. & Yuhasz, M.S. A controlled prospective study of the effect of endurance training on the recurrence rate of myocardial infarction. *Amer. J. Epidemiol., 102*, 358–65 (1975)

Rechnitzer, P.A., Yuhasz, M.S., Paivio, H.A., Pickard, H.A. & Lefcoe, N. Effects of a 24-week exercise programme on normal adults and patients with previous myocardial infarction. *Brit. Med. J.* (i), 734–5 (1967)

Redwood, D.R., Rosing, D.R. & Epstein, S.E. Circulatory and symptomatic effects of physical training in patients with coronary artery disease and angina pectoris. *New Engl. J. Med., 286*, 959–65 (1972)

Rees, G., Bristow, J.D., Kremkau, E.L., Green, G.S., Herr, R.H., Griswold, H.E. & Starr, A. Influence of aortocoronary bypass surgery on left ventricular performance. *New Engl. J. Med., 284*, 1116–20 (1971)

Regestein, Q.R. & Horn, H.R. Coitus in patients with cardiac arrhythmias. *Med. Asp. Hum. Sex., 12*, 108–25 (1978)

Reid, E. *Readiness and Modifying Factors in Exercise Adoption*. Ph.D. Thesis (University of Toronto, 1979)

Reindell, H., Kleipzig, H., Steim, H., Musshoff, K., Roskamm, H. & Schildge, E. *Herz., Kreislaufkrankheiten und Sport* (Johann Ambrosius Barth, Munich, 1960)

Reindell, H., König, K. & Roskamm, H. *Funktionsdiagnostik des Gesunden und Kranken Herzens* (G. Thieme, Stuttgart, 1966)

Remington, R.D. & Schork, M.A. Determination of number of subjects needed for experimental epidemiologic studies of the effect of increased physical activity on incidence of coronary heart disease. Preliminary considerations. In: *Physical Activity and the Heart*, ed. M.J. Karvonen & A.J. Barry (C.C. Thomas, Springfield, Ill., 1967) pp. 311–19

Rennemann, R.S. *Cardiovascular Applications of Ultrasound*

(North Holland Publishing, Amsterdam, 1974)

Renson, R., Beunen, G., Ostyn, M., Simons, J. & Van Gerven, D. Soziale Bedingungen von Körperlicher Fitness. In: *Motorische Entwicklung*, ed. R. Bauss & K. Roth (Institut für Sportwissenschaft, Darmstadt, 1977) pp. 140–50

Rerych, S.K., Scholz, P.M., Newman, G.E., *et al.* Cardiac function at rest and during exercise in normals and in patients with coronary heart disease: evaluation by radionuclide angiography. *Ann. Surg., 187*, 449–64 (1978)

Richards, D.W., Bland, E.F. & White, P.D. Completed 25-year follow-up study of 200 patients with myocardial infarction. *J. Chron. Dis., 4*, 415–22 (1956)

Rigatto, M. Mass spectrometry in the study of the pulmonary circulation. *Bull. Physiol-path. Resp., 3*, 473–86 (1967)

Riley, C.P., Oberman, A., Lampton, T.D. & Hurst, D.C. Submaximal exercise testing in a random sample of an elderly population. *Circulation 42*, 43–51 (1970)

Rinzler, S.H. Primary prevention of coronary heart disease by diet. *Bull. N.Y. Acad. Med., 44*, 936–49 (1968)

Rissanen, V. Occupational physical activity and coronary artery disease. A clinico-pathological appraisal. *Adv. Cardiol., 18*, 113–21 (1976)

Rivard, G., Lavallée, H., Rajic, M., Shephard, R.J., Thibaudeau, P., Davignon, A. & Beaucage, C. Influence of competitive hockey on physical condition and psychological behaviour of children. In: *Frontiers of Activity and Child Health*, ed. H. Lavallée & R.J. Shephard (Editions du Pélican, Quebec City, 1977)

Robb, G.P. & Marks, H.H. Latent coronary artery disease. Determination of its presence and severity by the exercise electrocardiogram. *Amer. J. Cardiol., 13*, 603–18 (1964)

Robb, G.P. & Seltzer, F. Appraisal of the double two-step exercise test. A long-term follow-up study of 3,325 men. *JAMA, 234*, 722–7 (1975)

Robinson, B.F. Relationship of heart rate and systolic blood pressure to the onset of pain in angina pectoris. *Circulation 35*, 1073–83 (1967)

Robinson, B.F. Mode of action of nitroglycerin in angina pectoris. *Brit. Heart J., 30*, 295–301 (1968)

Robinson, J.S., Sloman, G., Mathew, T.H. & Goble, A.J. Survival after resuscitation from cardiac arrest in acute myocardial infarction. *Amer. Heart J., 69*, 740–7 (1965)

Robinson, S. Experimental studies of physical fitness in relation to age. *Arbeitsphysiol., 4*, 251–323 (1938)

Robinson, S., Pearcy, M., Brueckman, F.R., Nicholas, J.R. & Miller, D.I. Effects of atropine on heart rates and oxygen intake in working man. *J. Appl. Physiol., 5*, 508–12 (1953)

Rochelle, R.H., Stumpner, R.L., Robinson, S., Dill, D.B. & Horvath, S.M. Peripheral blood flow response to exercise consequent to physical training. *Med. Sci. Sports 3*, 122–9 (1971)

Rochmis, P. & Blackburn, H. Exercise tests. A survey of procedures, safety and litigation experience in approximately 170,000 tests. *JAMA, 217*, 1061–6 (1971)

Rodbard, S., Williams, F. & Williams, C. The spherical dynamics of the heart (myocardial tension, oxygen consumption, coronary blood flow and efficiency). *Amer. Heart J., 57*, 348–60 (1959)

Rode, A., Ross., R. & Shephard, R.J. Smoking withdrawal program. *AMA Arch. Env. Health 24*, 27–36 (1972)

Rode, A. & Shephard, R.J. Cardio-respiratory fitness of an Arctic community. *J. Appl. Physiol., 31*, 519–26 (1971a)

Rode, A. & Shephard, R.J. The influence of cigarette smoking upon the work of breathing in near maximal exercise. *Med. Sci. Sports 3*, 51–5 (1971b)

Rodstein, M., Wolloch, L. & Gubner, R.S. A mortality study of the significance of extrasystoles in an uninsured population. *Circulation 44*, 617–25 (1971)

Rollett, E.L., Yurchak, P.M., Hood, W.B. & Gorlin, R. Pressure-volume correlates of left ventricular oxygen consumption in the hypervolumic dog. *Circ. Res., 17*, 499–518 (1965)

Romo, M. Factors relating to sudden death in acute ischaemic heart disease. A community study in Helsinki. *Acta Med. Scand., 547*, suppl. (1972)

Rook, A. An investigation into the longevity of Cambridge sportsmen. *Brit. Med. J.* (i), 773–7 (1954)

Rose, C.L. & Cohen, M.L. Relative importance of physical activity for longevity. *Ann. N.Y. Acad. Sci., 301*, 671–97 (1977)

Rose, G. Current developments in Europe. In: *Atherosclerosis II*, ed. R.J. Jones (Springer Verlag, Berlin, 1970) pp. 310–14

Rose, G., Prineas, R.J. & Mitchell, J.R. Myocardial infarction and the intrinsic calibre of coronary arteries. *Brit. Heart J., 29*, 548–52 (1967)

Rosenman, R.H. The influence of different exercise patterns on the incidence of coronary heart disease in the western collaborative group study. In: *Physical Activity and Aging*, ed. D. Brunner & E. Jokl (University Park Press, Baltimore, Md., 1970) pp. 267–73

Rosenman, R.H., Bawol, R.D. & Oscherwitz, M. A 4-year prospective study of the relationship of different habitual vocational physical activity to risk and incidence of ischemic heart disease in volunteer male federal employees. *Ann. N.Y. Acad. Sci., 301*, 627–41 (1977)

Roskamm, H. General circulatory adjustment to exercise in well-trained subjects. In: *Coronary Heart Disease and Physical Fitness*, ed. O.A. Larsen & R.O. Malmborg (University Park Press, Baltimore, Md., 1971) pp. 17–20

Roskamm, H. Limits and age dependency in the adaptation of the heart to physical stress. In: *Sport in the Modern World — Chances and Problems*, ed. O. Grupe, D. Kurz & J.M. Teipel (Springer Verlag, Berlin, 1973a)

Roskamm, H. Myocardial contractility during exercise. In: *Limiting Factors of Physical Performance*, ed. J. Keul (G. Thieme, Stuttgart, 1973b) pp. 225–34

Roskamm, H. & Reindell, H. The heart and circulation of the superior athlete. In: *Training — Scientific Basis and Application*, ed. A.W. Taylor (C.C. Thomas, Springfield, Ill., 1972)

Ross, J. Factors regulating the oxygen consumption of the heart. In: *Changing Concepts in Cardiovascular Disease*, ed. H.I. Russek & B.L. Zohman (Williams & Wilkins, Baltimore, 1972)

Ross, J., Gault, J.H., Mason, D.T., Linhart, J.W. & Braunwald, E. Left ventricular performance during muscular exercise in patients with and without cardiac dysfunction. *Circulation 34*, 597–608 (1966)

Ross, R.S. Ischemic heart disease. An overview. *Amer. J. Cardiol., 36*, 496–505 (1975)

Rothlin, M., Gattiker, K., Huber, R. & Krombach, D. Left ventricular function before and after resection of left ventricular aneurysm. In: *Coronary Heart Disease*, ed. M. Kaltenbach, P. Lichtlen & G.C. Friesinger (G. Thieme, Stuttgart, 1973) pp. 219–22

Rousseau, M., Brasseur, L.A. & Detry, J.M. Haemodynamic determinants of maximal oxygen intake in patients with healed myocardial infarction: influence of physical training. *Circulation 48*, 943–9 (1973)

Rousseau, M., Degré, S., Brasseur, L.A., Denolin, H. & Detry, J.M. Haemodynamic effects of early physical training after acute myocardial infarction, comparison with a control untrained group. *Europ. J. Cardiol., 2*, 29–45 (1974)

Rowe, G.G. The nitrous oxide method for determining coronary blood flow in man. *Amer. Heart J., 58*, 268–81 (1959)

Rowell, L.B. Human cardiovascular adjustments to exercise and thermal stress. *Physiol. Rev., 54*, 75–159 (1974)

Rumball, A. & Acheson, E.D. Latent coronary heart disease detected by electrocardiogram before and after exercise. *Brit. Med. J.* (i), 423–8 (1963)

Ruskin, H.D., Stein, L.L., Shelsky, I.M., *et al*. M.M.P.I. comparison between patients with coronary heart disease and their spouses and other demographic data. *Scand. J. Rehab. Med., 2*, 99–104 (1970)

Russek, H.I. Emotional stress, tobacco smoking and ischemic heart disease. In: *Prevention of Ischemic Heart Disease. Principles and Practice* (C.C. Thomas, Springfield, Ill., 1966) pp. 190–200

Russek, H.I. Propranolol and isosorbide dinitrate synergism in angina pectoris. *Amer. J. Cardiol., 21*, 44–5 (1968)

Russek, H.I. Medical versus surgical therapy in angina pectoris. *Geriatrics 25*, 93–102 (1970)

Russek, H.I. & Russek, L.G. Behavior patterns and emotional stress in the etiology of coronary heart disease: sociological and occupational aspects. In: *Stress and the Heart*, ed. D. Wheatley (Raven Press, New York, 1977)

Russek, H.I. & Zohman, B.L. Relative significance of heredity, diet and occupational stress in coronary heart disease in young adults. *Amer. J. Med. Sci., 235*, 266–75 (1958)

Russek, H.I. & Zohman B.L. The natural history of coronary atherosclerosis. In: *Coronary Heart Disease*, ed. H.I. Russek & B.L. Zohman (Lippincott, Philadelphia, 1971) pp. 167–76

Rutishauser, W., Amende, I., Mehmel, H., Krayenbühl, H.P. & Schönbeck, M. Relaxation of the left ventricle in patients with coronary artery disease. In: *Coronary Heart Disease*, ed. M. Kaltenbach, P. Lichtlen & G.C. Friesinger (G. Thieme, Stuttgart, 1973) pp. 167–72

Ryhming, I. A modified Harvard step test for the evaluation of physical fitness. *Arbeitsphysiol., 15*, 235–50 (1954)

Ryle, J.A. & Russel, W.T. The natural history of coronary disease: clinical and epidemiological study. *Brit. Heart J., 11*, 370–89

(1949)

Sagall, E.L. Legal implications of cardiac rehabilitation programmes. In: *Heart Disease and Rehabilitation*, ed. M.L. Pollock & D.H. Schmidt (Houghton Mifflin, Boston, 1979) pp. 640–9

Saltin, B. Physiological effects of physical conditioning. *Med. Sci. Sports 1*, 50–6 (1969)

Saltin, B. Oxygen transport by the circulatory system during exercise. In: *Limiting Factors of Physical Performance*, ed. J. Keul (G. Thieme, Stuttgart, 1973)

Saltin, B. & Åstrand, P.O. Maximal oxygen uptake in athletes. *J. Appl. Physiol., 23*, 353–8 (1967)

Saltin, B., Blomqvist, G., Mitchell, J.H., Johnson, R.L., Wildenthal, K. & Chapman, C.B. Response to exercise after bed rest and after training. *Amer. Heart Assoc. Monograph 23* (Circulation 37–8, Suppl. 7), 1–68 (1968)

Saltin, B. & Grimby, G. Physiological analysis of middle-aged and old former athletes. Comparison with still active athletes of the same ages. *Circulation 38*, 1104–15 (1968)

Saltin, B. & Karlsson, J. Muscle ATP, CP, and lactate during exercise after physical conditioning. In: *Muscle Metabolism during Exercise*, ed. B. Pernow & B. Saltin (Plenum Press, New York, 1971) pp. 395–9

Saltzman, S.H., Hellerstein, H.K., Radke, J.D., Maistelman, H.W. & Ricklin, R. Quantitative effects of physical conditioning on the exercise electrocardiogram of middle-aged subjects with atherosclerotic heart disease. In: *Measurement in Exercise Electrocardiography*, ed. H. Blackburn (C.C. Thomas, Springfield, Ill., 1969) pp. 388–410

Samson, W.E. & Scher, A.M. Mechanism of S-T segment alteration during acute myocardial injury. *Circ. Res., 8*, 780–7 (1960)

Sanders, T.M., White, F.C. & Bloor, C.M. Myocardial blood flow distribution in the conscious pig during steady state and exhaustive exercise. *Fed. Proc., 34*, 414 (abstr.) (1975)

Sanders, T.M., White, F.C., Peterson, T.M. & Bloor, C.M. Effects of endurance exercise on coronary collateral blood flow in miniature swine. *Amer. J. Physiol., 234*, 614–19 (1978)

Sandler, H. & Dodge, H.T. Angiographic methods for determination of left ventricular geometry and volume. In: *Cardiac Mechanics: Physiological, Clinical and Mathematical*

Considerations, ed. I. Mirsky, D. Ghista & H. Sandler (Wiley, New York, 1974) pp. 141–70

Sanne, H. (in collaboration with D. Elmfeldt, G. Grimby, C. Rydin & L. Wilhelmsen). Exercise tolerance and physical training of non-selected patients after myocardial infarction. *Acta Med. Scand., 551*, suppl., 1–124 (1973)

Sanne, H., Elmfeldt, D. & Wilhelmsen, L. Preventive effect of physical training after a myocardial infarction. In: *Preventive Cardiology*, ed. G. Tibblin, A. Keys & L. Werko (John Wiley, New York, 1972) p. 154

Sanne, H. & Sivertsson, R. The effect of exercise on the development of collateral circulation after experimental occlusion of the femoral artery in the cat. *Acta Physiol. Scand., 73*, 257–63 (1968)

Sannerstedt, R. Hemodynamic response to exercise in patients with arterial hypertension. *Acta Med. Scand., 458*, suppl. (1966)

Sarnoff, S.J., Braunwald, E., Welch, G.H., Case, R.B., Stainsby, W.N. & Macruz, R. Hemodynamic determinants of oxygen consumption of the heart with special reference to the tension time index. *Amer. J. Physiol., 192*, 148–56 (1958)

Sarvotham, S.G. & Berry, J.N. Prevalence of coronary heart disease in an urban population in Northern India. *Circulation 37*, 939–53 (1968)

Sayed, J., Schaefer, O. & Hildes, J.A. Biochemical indices of nutrition of the Iglooligmiut. In: *Circumpolar Health*, ed. R.J. Shephard & S. Itoh (University of Toronto Press, Toronto, 1976) pp. 130–4

Schad, N. Nontraumatic assessment of left ventricular wall motion and regional stroke volume after myocardial infarction. *J. Nucl. Med., 18*, 333–41 (1977)

Schaefer, O. Vigorous exercise and coronary heart disease. *Lancet* (i), 840 (abstr.) (1973)

Scheidt, S., Aschein, R. & Killip, T. Shock after acute myocardial infarction. A clinical and hemodynamic profile. *Amer. J. Cardiol., 26*, 556–64 (1970)

Scheingold, L.D. & Wagner, N.N. *Sound Sex and the Aging Heart* (Human Sciences Press, New York, 1974) pp. 137–41

Schettler, G. Keynote address. In: *Atherosclerosis*, ed. R.J. Jones (Springer Verlag, Berlin, 1970) pp. xxvii–xxxii

Schettler, G. Atherosclerosis, the main problem of the industrialized societies. In: *Atherosclerosis IV*, ed. G. Schettler,

Y. Goto, Y. Hata & G. Klose (Springer Verlag, Berlin, 1977)

Scheuer, J. Physical training and intrinsic cardiac adaptation. *Circulation 47*, 677–80 (1973)

Scheuer, J., Penpargkul, S. & Bhan, A.K. Experimental observations on the effects of physical training upon intrinsic cardiac physiology and biochemistry. *Amer. J. Cardiol., 33*, 744–51 (1974)

Scheuer, J., Penpargkul, S. & Bhan, A.K. Experimental observations on the effects of physical training upon intrinsic cardiac physiology and biochemistry. In: *Exercise in Cardiovascular Health and Disease*, ed. E.A. Amsterdam, J.H. Wilmore & A.N. DeMaria (Yorke Medical Books, New York, 1977) pp. 108–21

Schlant, R.C. Altered cardiovascular physiology of coronary atherosclerotic heart disease. In: *The Heart*, ed. J. Willis Hurst (McGraw Hill, New York, 1974) pp. 1017–37

Schmale, A.H. & Engel, G.L. The giving up-given up complex. *Arch. Gen. Psychiatr., 17*, 135–45 (1967)

Schmid, L. & Hornof, Z. Sudden death in Czechoslovakian sports. *Brit. J. Sports Med., 7*, 156–8 (1973)

Schmidt, D.H., Blau, F.M., Carpenter, J.G. & Hellman, C.K. The clinical and research application of nuclear cardiology. In: *Heart Disease and Rehabilitation*, ed. M.L. Pollock & D.H. Schmidt (Houghton Mifflin, Boston, 1979) pp. 183–202

Schnor, P. Longevity and cause of death in male athletic champions. *Lancet* (ii), 1364–6 (1971)

Schwade, J., Blomqvist, C.G. & Shapiro, W. A comparison of the response to arm and leg work in patients with ischemic heart disease. *Amer. Heart J., 94*, 203–8 (1977)

Scott, R.F., Florentin, R.A., Daoud, A.S., Morrison, E.S., Jones, R.M. & Hutt, M.S.R. Coronary arteries of children and young adults. A comparison of lipids and anatomic features in New Yorkers and East Africans. *Exp. Mol. Pathol., 5*, 12–42 (1966)

Scott, R.F., Likimani, J.C., Morrison, E.S., Thuku, J.J. & Thomas, W.A. Esterified serum fatty acids in subjects eating high and low cholesterol diets. A comparative study of serum lipid metabolism in New Yorkers, indigenous poor East Africans and upper class East Africans. *Amer. J. Clin. Nutr., 13*, 82–91 (1963)

Scrimshaw, N.S. & Guzman, M.A. Diet and atherosclerosis. *Lab. Invest., 18*, 623–8 (1968)

Segers, M.J. & Mertens, C. Psychological and bioclinical CHD risk factors, quantitative differences between obese, normal and thin subjects. *J. Psychosom. Res., 18*, 403–11 (1974)

Selye, H. On the real benefits of eustress. *Psychol. Today 11*, 60–70 (1978)

Semple, T. *Myocardial Infarction. How to Prevent, How to Rehabilitate* (Council on Rehabilitation of International Society of Cardiology, Brussels, 1973)

Semple, T. Acceleration of collaterals by physical activity. In: *Critical Evaluation of Cardiac Rehabilitation*, ed. J.J. Kellermann & H. Denolin (Karger, Basel, 1977) pp. 141–2

Seymour, J. & Conway, N. Value of dual reports on routine electrocardiograms. *Brit. Heart J., 31*, 610–12 (1969)

Shah, V.V., Shah, S.R. & Panse, V.N. Nutritional and physical factors in coronary heart disease. *Geriatrics 23*, 99–103 (1968)

Shaper, A.G. Current developments in atherosclerosis in Africa. In: *Atherosclerosis II*, ed. R.J. Jones (Springer Verlag, Berlin, 1970) pp. 314–20

Shapiro, A.P., Schwartz, G.E., Ferguson, D.C., *et al*. Behavioral methods in the treatment of hypertension. A review of their clinical status. *Ann. Intern. Med., 86*, 626–36 (1977)

Shapiro, S., Weinblatt, E., Frank, C.W. & Sager, R.V. Incidence of coronary heart disease in a population insured for medical care (HIP). *Amer. J. Publ. Health 59*, suppl. 1–101 (1969)

Sharland, D.E. Ability of men to return to work after cardiac infarction. *Brit. Med. J., 2*, 718–20 (1964)

Sharma, B., Goodwin, J.F. & Steiner, R.E. Left ventriculography during angina induced by exercise and atrial pacing. *Amer. J. Cardiol., 37*, 172 (abstr.) (1976)

Sheets, M.F., Eckberg, D.L. & Heisted, D.D. Impairment of autonomic heart rate responses by local sinus node hypoxemia. *Fed. Proc., 34*, 420 (abstr.) (1975)

Sheffield, L.T. The meaning of exercise test findings. In: *Coronary Heart Disease. Prevention, Detection, Rehabilitation, with Emphasis on Exercise Testing*, ed. S.M. Fox (International Medical Corporation, Denver, Col., 1974) pp. (9-1)–(9-35)

Sheffield, L.T. & Roitman, D. Systolic blood pressure, heart rate and treadmill work at anginal threshold. *Chest, 63*, 327–35 (1973)

Sheldon, W.C., Rincon, G., Effler, D.B., *et al*. Surgical treatment of coronary artery disease: pure graft operations, with a study of 741 patients followed 3–7 years. *Progr. Cardiovasc. Dis., 18*,

237–53 (1975)

Sheldon, W.C., Sones, F.M., Shirey, E.K., Fergusson, D.J.G., Favaloro, R.G. & Effler, D.B. Reconstructive coronary artery surgery: post-operative assessment. *Circulation 39*, suppl., 61–6 (1969)

Shephard, R.J. Partitional respirometry in human subjects. *J. Appl. Physiol., 13*, 357–67 (1959)

Shephard, R.J. The development of cardiorespiratory fitness. *Med. Services J., Canada 21*, 533–44 (1965)

Shephard, R.J. The oxygen cost of breathing during vigorous exercise. *Quart. J. Exp. Physiol., 51*, 336–50 (1966)

Shephard, R.J. Normal levels of activity in Canadian city-dwellers. *Canad. Med. Assoc. J., 97*, 313–18 (1967a)

Shephard, R.J. The prediction of 'maximal' oxygen consumption using a new progressive step test. *Ergonomics 10*, 1–15 (1967b)

Shephard, R.J. Intensity, duration and frequency of exercise as determinants of the response to a training regime. *Int. Z. Angew. Physiol., 26*, 272–8 (1968a)

Shephard, R.J. Oscillations of acid-base equilibrium during maximum exercise. *Int. Z. Angew. Physiol., 26*, 258–71 (1968b)

Shephard, R.J. A nomogram to calculate the oxygen cost of running at slow speeds. *J. Sports Med. Phys. Fitness 9*, 10–16 (1968c)

Shephard, R.J. Learning, habituation and training. *Int. Z. Angew. Physiol., 26*, 272–8 (1969)

Shephard, R.J. Standard tests of aerobic power. In: *Frontiers of Fitness*, ed. R.J. Shephard (C.C. Thomas, Springfield, Ill., 1971) pp. 233–64

Shephard, R.J. The influences of race and environment on ischemic heart disease. *Canad. Med. Ass. J., 111*, 1336–40 (1974a)

Shephard, R.J. Sudden death — a significant hazard of exercise? *Brit. J. Sports Med., 8*, 101–10 (1974b)

Shephard, R.J. Exercise test methodology. In: *Coronary Disease. Exercise Testing, Rehabilitation Therapy*, ed. S.M. Fox (International Medical Corporation, Denver, Col., 1974c)

Shephard, R.J. *Men at Work: Applications of Ergonomics to Performance and Design* (C.C. Thomas, Springfield, Ill., 1974d)

Shephard, R.J. Future research on the quantifying of endurance training. *J. Human Ergol., 3*, 163–81 (1975)

Shephard, R.J. Coronary artery disease — the magnitude of the problem. In: *Proceedings of International Symposium on*

Exercise and Coronary Artery Disease, ed. T. Kavanagh
(Toronto Rehabilitation Centre, Toronto, 1976)

Shephard, R.J. *Endurance Fitness*, 2nd edn (University of Toronto
Press, Toronto, 1977a)

Shephard, R.J. Exercise-induced bronchospasm — a review. *Med.
Sci. Sports 9*, 1–10 (1977b)

Shephard, R.J. *Human Physiological Work Capacity* (Cambridge
University Press, London, 1978a)

Shephard, R.J. *Physical Activity and Aging* (Croom Helm,
London, 1978b)

Shephard, R.J. *The Fit Athlete* (Oxford University Press, London,
1978c)

Shephard, R.J. Recurrence of myocardial infarction in an
exercising population. *Brit. Heart J., 42*, 133–8 (1979a)

Shephard, R.J. Cardiac rehabilitation in prospect. In: *Heart
Disease and Rehabilitation*, ed. M.L. Pollock and D.H. Schmidt
(Houghton Mifflin, Boston, 1979b) pp. 521–47

Shephard, R.J. Current status and prospects for post-coronary
exercise multicentre studies. *Med. Sci. Sports 11*, 383–5 (1979c)

Shephard, R.J. Current status of the Canadian Home Fitness Test.
S. Afr. J. Sports Sci., 2, 19–35 (1980a)

Shephard, R.J. Recurrence of myocardial infarction. Observations
on patients participating in the Ontario Multi-Centre Exercise-
heart Trial. *Europ. J. Cardiol., 11*, 147–57 (1980b)

Shephard, R.J. *Textbook of Exercise Physiology and Biochemistry*
(Prager, Philadelphia, 1980c)

Shephard, R.J. Evaluation of earlier studies — Canadian study. In:
*N.I.H. Conference on Exercise and Cardiac Rehabilitation, May
1979*, ed. N. Epstein (Bethesda, Md., 1980d)

Shephard, R.J. A critique: coronary disease and exercise stress
tests. *Canad. Fam. Physician 26*, 555–9 (1980e)

Shephard, R.J. The sick sinus syndrome. *Med. Sci. Sports* (in press,
1980f)

Shephard, R.J., Allen, C., Benade, A.J.S., Davies, C.T.M.,
diPrampero, P.E., Hedman, R., Merriman, J.E., Myhre, K. &
Simmons, R. The maximum oxygen intake — an international
reference standard of cardio-respiratory fitness. *Bull. WHO, 38*,
757–64 (1968a)

Shephard, R.J., Allen, C., Benade, A.J.S., Davies, C.T.M.,
diPrampero, P.E., Hedman, R., Merriman, J.E., Myhre, K. &
Simmons, R. Standardization of sub-maximal exercise tests.

Bull. WHO, 38, 765–76 (1968b)

Shephard, R.J., Corey, P. & Kavanagh, T. Exercise compliance and the prevention of a recurrence of myocardial infarction. *Can. J. Appl. Sports Sci., 4*, 236 (1979a)

Shephard, R.J. & Cox, M. Some characteristics of participants in an industrial fitness programme. *Canad. J. Appl. Sports Sci., 5*, 69–76 (1980)

Shephard, R.J., Cox, M. and Simper, K. *An Analysis of 'Par-Q' Responses in an Office Population* (Fitness & Amateur Sport Branch, Department of National Health & Welfare, 1979b)

Shephard, R.J., Hatcher, J. & Rode, A. On the body composition of the Eskimo. *Europ. J. Appl. Physiol., 30*, 1–13 (1973)

Shephard, R.J., Jones, C. & Brown, J.R. Some observations on the fitness of a Canadian population. *Canad. Med. Assoc. J., 98*, 977–84 (1968c)

Shephard, R.J. & Kavanagh, T. Biochemical changes with marathon running — observations on 'post-coronary' patients. In: *Metabolic Adaptations to prolonged Exercise*, ed. J.R. Poortmans & H. Howald (Karger, Basel, 1975)

Shephard, R.J. & Kavanagh, T. Predicting the exercise catastrophe in the post-coronary patient. *Canad. Fam. Phys., 24*, 614–18 (1978a)

Shephard, R.J. & Kavanagh, T. Does 'post-coronary' rehabilitation increase longevity? In: *Proceedings of International Conference on Sports Cardiology*, ed. A. Venerando (Fondazione Giovanni Lorenzi, Rome, 1978b)

Shephard, R.J. & Kavanagh, T. On the stage duration for a progressive exercise test protocol. In: *Physical Fitness Assessment*, ed. R.J. Shephard & H. Lavallée (C.C. Thomas, Springfield, Ill., 1978c) pp. 335–44

Shephard, R.J. & Kavanagh, T. Patient reactions to a regular conditioning programme following myocardial infarction. *J. Sports Med. Phys. Fitness 18*, 373–8 (1978d)

Shephard, R.J., Kavanagh, T. & Moore, R. Fluid and mineral balance of post-coronary distance runners. Studies on the 1975 Boston marathon. In: *Nutrition, Dietetics and Sport*, ed. G. Ricci & A. Venerando (Ed. Minerva Medica, Torino, 1978a) pp. 217–28

Shephard, R.J., Killinger, D. & Fried, T. Responses to sustained use of anabolic steroid. *Brit. J. Sports Med., 11*, 170–3 (1977a)

Shephard, R.J. & Lavallée, H. Probleme der Längsschnittuntersuchung motorischer Entwicklung. In: *Motorische Entwicklung. Probleme und Ergebnisse von Längsschnittuntersuchungen*, ed. R. Bauss & K. Roth (Institüt für Sportwissenschaft, Darmstadt, 1977)

Shephard, R.J., Lavallée, H., Jéquier, J.C., LaBarre, R., Rajic, M. & Beaucage, C. Seasonal differences in aerobic power. In: *Physical Fitness Assessment: Principles, Practice and Application*, ed. R.J. Shephard & H. Lavallée (C.C. Thomas, Springfield, Ill., 1978b) pp. 194–210

Shephard, R.J., Lavallée, H., Jéquier, J.C., Rajic, M. & Beaucage, C. Un programme complémentaire d'éducation physique. Etude préliminaire de l'expérience pratiquée dans le district de Trois Rivières. In: *Facteurs Limitant l'Endurance Humaine*, ed. J.R. LaCour (Université de St. Etienne, St Etienne, France, 1977b)

Shephard, R.J., Morgan, P., Finucane, R. & Schimmelfing, L. Factors influencing participation in an employee fitness programme. *J. Occup. Med., 22*, 389–98 (1980a)

Shephard, R.J., Rode, A. & Ross, R. Reinforcement of a smoking withdrawal program: the role of the physiologist and the psychologist. *Canad. J. Publ. Health 64*, S41–S51 (1972)

Shephard, R.J. & Sidney, K.H. Effects of physical exercise on plasma growth hormone and cortisol levels in human subjects. *Ex. Sport Sci. Rev., 3*, 1–30 (1975)

Shephard, R.J., Youldon, P.E., Cox, M. & West, C. Effects of a 6-month industrial fitness programme on serum lipid concentrations. *Atherosclerosis 35*, 277–85 (1980b)

Sherman, M. *Diet, Lipid Metabolism and Atherosclerosis* (US Department of Health, Education and Welfare, Bethesda, Md., 1964)

Sidney, K.H. & Shephard, R.J. Physiological characteristics and performance of the whitewater paddler. *Int. Z. Angew. Physiol., 32*, 55–70 (1973)

Sidney, K.H. & Shephard, R.J. Attitudes towards health and physical activity in the elderly. Effects of a physical training programme. *Med. Sci. Sports 8*, 246–52 (1977a)

Sidney, K.H. & Shephard, R.J. Training and e.c.g. abnormalities in the elderly. *Brit. Heart J., 39*, 1114–20 (1977b)

Sidney, K.H. & Shephard, R.J. Maximum and sub-maximum exercise tests in men and women in the seventh, eighth and ninth decades of life. *J. Appl. Physiol., 43*, 280–7 (1977c)

Sidney, K.H. & Shephard, R.J. Frequency and intensity of exercise as determinants of the response to training in elderly subjects. *Med. Sci. Sports 10*, 125–31 (1978)

Sidney, K.H., Shephard, R.J. & Harrison. J. Endurance training and body composition of the elderly. *Amer. J. Clin. Nutr., 30*, 326–33 (1977)

Siegel, G.H. The law and cardiac rehabilitation. A. Legal aspects of informed consent. In: *Exercise Testing and Exercise Training in Coronary Heart Disease*, ed. J. Naughton, H.K. Hellerstein & I.C. Mohler (Academic Press, New York, 1973) pp. 387–413

Siegel, W. Exercise-induced indicators of coronary atherosclerotic heart disease. In: *Coronary Heart Disease. Prevention, Detection, Rehabilitation, with Emphasis on Exercise Testing*, ed. S.M. Fox (International Medical Corporation, Denver, Colorado, 1974) pp. (3-1)–(3-21)

Siegel, W., Blomqvist, G. & Mitchell, J.H. Effects of a quantitated physical training program on middle-aged sedentary men. *Circulation 41*, 19–29 (1970)

Sigwart, U., Schmidt, H., Bonzel, T., *et al.* Biplane cineangiographic evaluation of left ventricular contraction in ischemic heart disease at rest and during bicycle exercise. *Circulation 51/52*, suppl. II, 37 (141) (abstr.) (1975)

Siltanen, P. Mobile coronary care unit and sudden coronary death. In: *Sudden Coronary Death*, ed. V. Manninen & P.I. Halonen (Karger, Basel, 1978) pp. 193–5

Siltanen, P., Lauroma, M., Mirkko, O., *et al.* Psychological characteristics related to coronary heart disease. *J. Psychosom. Res., 19*, 183–95 (1975)

Sim, D.N. & Neill, W.A. Investigation of the physiological basis for increased exercise threshold for angina pectoris after physical conditioning. *J. Clin. Invest., 54*, 763–70 (1974)

Simmons, R. & Shephard, R.J. Effects of physical conditioning upon the central and peripheral circulatory responses to arm work. *Int. Z. Angew. Physiol., 30*, 73–84 (1971a)

Simmons, R. & Shephard, R.J. Measurement of cardiac output in maximum exercise. Application of an acetylene rebreathing method to arm and leg exercise. *Int. Z. Angew. Physiol., 29*, 159–72 (1971b)

Simonson, E. & Berman, R. Myocardial infarction in young people — experience in USSR. *Amer. Heart J., 84*, 814–22 (1972)

Simoons, M.L. *Computer Assisted Interpretation of Exercise*

Electrocardiograms (Bronder-Offset B.V., Rotterdam, 1976)

Simoons, M.L. Computer processing of exercise electro-cardiograms: In: *Coronary Heart Disease, Exercise Testing and Cardiac Rehabilitation*, ed. W.E. James & E.A. Amsterdam (Symposia Specialists, Miami, Fla., 1977) pp. 154–64

Simpson, F.O. Beta-adrenergic receptor blocking drugs in hypertension. *Drugs 7*, 85–105 (1974)

Singer, A. & Rob, C. The fate of the claudicator. *Brit. Med. J.* (ii), 633–6 (1960)

Skelton, M. & Dominian, J. Psychological stress in wives of patients with myocardial infarction. *Brit. Med. J.* (ii), 101–3 (1973)

Skinner, J.S. Sexual relations and the cardiac patient. In: *Heart Disease and Rehabilitation*, ed. M.L. Pollock & D.H. Schmidt (Houghton Mifflin, Boston, 1979) pp. 587–99

Smith, C., Sauls, H.C. & Ballew, J. Coronary occlusion: a clinical study of 100 patients. *Ann. Int. Med., 17*, 681–92 (1942)

Smith, E.B., Evans, P.H. & Downham, M.D. Lipid in the aortic intima: the correlation of morphological and chemical characteristics. *J. Atheroscler. Res., 7*, 171–86 (1967)

Smith, E.E., Guyton, A.C., Manning, R.D. & White, R.J. Integrated mechanisms of cardiovascular response and control during exercise in the normal human. *Progr. Cardiovasc. Dis., 18*, 421–43 (1976)

Smith, E.P. Lipoproteins — steady state aspects. In: *Atherosclerosis IV*, ed. G. Schettler, Y. Goto, Y. Hata & G. Klose (Springer Verlag, Berlin, 1977)

Smoking and Health. Report of the Advisory Committee to the Surgeon General of the Public Health Service. Public Health Service Publication 1103 (US Government Printing Office, Washington, D.C., 1964) pp. 1–387

Smoking in Canada. Health and Welfare, Canada, Bulletin 5 (1973) pp. 101–6

Snow, J. *On the Mode of Communication of Cholera*, 2nd edn (Churchill, London, 1855)

Society of Actuaries. *Build and Blood Pressure Study* (Society of Actuaries, Chicago, 1959)

Sodhi, H.S., Kudchodkar, B.J., Mason, D.T. & Borhani, N. Relationships between metabolism of cholesterol and the turnover of plasma lipoproteins. In: *Atherosclerosis IV*, ed. G. Schettler, Y. Goto, Y. Hata & G. Klose (Springer Verlag, Berlin, 1977) pp. 298–301

Sohar, E. & Sneh, E. Follow-up of obese patients: 14 years after a successful reducing diet. *Amer. J. Clin. Nutr., 26*, 845–8 (1973)

Sonnenblick, E.H. Oxygen consumption of the heart. In: *Coronary Heart Disease and Physical Fitness*, ed. O.A. Larsen & R.O. Malmborg (University Park Press, Baltimore, Md., 1971) pp. 89–92

Sonnenblick, E.H., Ross, J., Covell, J.W., Kaiser, G.A. & Braunwald, E. Velocity of contraction as a determinant of myocardial oxygen consumption. *Amer. J. Physiol., 209*, 919–27 (1965)

Spain, D.M. & Bradess, V.A. The relationship of coronary thrombosis to coronary atherosclerosis and ischaemic heart disease. *Amer. J. Med. Sci., 240*, 701–10 (1960a)

Spain, D.M. & Bradess, V.A. Occupational physical activity and the degree of coronary atherosclerosis in 'normal' men. A postmortem study. *Circulation 22*, 239–42 (1960b)

Stamler, J. Acute myocardial infarction — progress in primary prevention. *Brit. Heart J., 33*, suppl., 145–64 (1971)

Stamler, J. (With Coronary Drug Project Research Group). Clofibrate and niacin in coronary heart disease. *JAMA, 231*, 360–81 (1975)

Stamler, J. Improving life styles to control the coronary epidemic. In: *Nutrition, Dietetics and Sport*, ed. G. Ricci & A. Venerando (Ed. Minerva Medica, Torino, 1978) pp. 5–48

Stamler, J., Berkson, D.M., Lindberg, H.A., *et al*. Socio-economic factors in the epidemiology of hypertensive disease. In: *The Epidemiology of Hypertension*, ed. J. Stamler, R. Stamler & T.N. Pullman (Grune & Stratton, New York, 1967) pp. 289–313

Stamler, J., Lindbergh, H.A., Berkson, D.M., Shaffer, A., Miller, W. & Poindexter, A. Prevalence and incidence of coronary heart disease in strata of the labour force of a Chicago industrial corporation. *J. Chron. Dis., 11*, 405–20 (1960)

Stary, H.C., Eggen, D.A. & Strong, J.P. The mechanism of atherosclerosis regression. In: *Atherosclerosis IV*, ed. G. Schettler, Y. Goto, Y. Hata & G. Klose (Springer Verlag, Berlin, 1977) pp. 394–404

Steele, P., Battock, D., Pappas, G., *et al*. Effect of patent coronary arterial occlusion on left ventricular function after aortocoronary by-pass surgery. *Amer. J. Cardiol., 39*, 39–42 (1977)

Stein, R.A. The effect of exercise training on heart rate during coitus in the post-myocardial infarction patient. *Circulation 55*,

738–40 (1977)

Steinhaus, A. Chronic effects of exercise. *Physiol. Rev., 13*, 103–47 (1933)

Stensaasen, S. The sport role socialization process in four industrialized countries: comments from a Norwegian perspective. In: *Sociology of Sport*, ed. F. Landry & W.A.R. Orban (Symposia Specialists, Miami, Fla., 1978) pp. 61–5

Sternby, N.H. Atherosclerosis and risk factors. In: *Atherosclerosis IV*, ed. G. Schettler, Y. Goto, Y. Hata & G. Klose (Springer Verlag, Berlin, 1977) pp. 102–4

Stevenson, J.A.F. Exercise, food intake, and health in experimental animals. *Canad. Med. Assoc. J., 96*, 862–6 (1967)

Stiles, M.H. Motivation for sports participation in the community. In: *Proceedings of International Symposium on Physical Activity and Cardiovascular Health*, ed. R.J. Shephard. *Canad. Med. Assoc. J., 96*, 889–92 (1967)

Stokes, W.R. Sexual functioning in the aging male. *Geriatrics 6*, 304–8 (1951)

Strauer, B.E. Studies concerning the effect of nitroglycerin on the contractile and relaxing properties of the isolated human ventricular myocardium. In: *Coronary Heart Disease*, ed. M. Kaltenbach, P. Lichtlen & G.C. Friesinger (G. Thieme, Stuttgart, 1973) pp. 20–4

Streeter, D.D., Spotnitz, H.M., Patel, D.P. & Sonnenblick, E.H. Fiber orientation in the canine left ventricle during systole and diastole. *Circ. Res., 24*, 339–47 (1969)

Strong, J.P. An introduction to the epidemiology of atherosclerosis. In: *Atherosclerosis IV*, ed. G. Schettler, Y. Goto, Y. Hata & G. Klose (Springer-Verlag, Berlin, 1977)

Stroud, M.W. & Feil, H.S. The terminal electrocardiogram: twenty three case reports of a review of the literature. *Amer. Heart J., 35*, 910–23 (1948)

Surawicz, B. The input of cellular electrophysiology into the practice of clinical electrocardiography. *Mod. Concepts Cardiovasc. Dis., 44*, 41–6 (1975)

Tabakin, B.S., Hanson, J.S. & Levy, A.M. Effects of physical training on the cardiovascular and respiratory response to graded upright exercise in distance runners. *Brit. Heart J., 27*, 205–10 (1965)

Takaro, T., Hultgren, H.N., Lipton, M.J., *et al*. The VA cooperative randomized study of surgery for coronary arterial occlusive disease. II. Subgroup with significant left main lesions. *Circulation 54*, suppl. III, 107–17 (1976)

Tauchart, M., Kochsiek, K., Heiss, H.W., Strauer, B.E., Kettler, D., Reploh, H.D., Rau, G. & Bretschneider, H.J. Measurement of coronary blood flow in man by the argon method. In: *Myocardial Blood Flow in Man. Methods and Significance in Coronary Disease*, ed. A. Maseri (Ed. Minerva Medica, Torino, 1972) pp. 139–44

Taylor, A.W. The effects of exercise and training on the activities of human glycogen cycle enzymes. In: *Metabolic Adaptation to Prolonged Physical Exercise*, ed. H. Howald & J.R. Poortmans (Birkhauser Verlag, Basel, 1975)

Taylor, C.B., Farquhar, J.W., Nelson, E., *et al*. Relaxation therapy and high blood pressure. *Arch. Gen. Psychiatry 34*, 339–42 (1977)

Taylor, H.L., Henschel, A., Brozek, J. & Keys, A. The effect of bed controlled trials of the prevention of coronary heart disease. *Fed. Proc., 32*, 1623–7 (1973)

Taylor, H.L., Henscel, A., Brozek, J. & Keys, A. The effect of bed rest on cardiovascular function and work performance. *J. Appl. Physiol., 2*, 223–39 (1949)

Taylor, H.L., Klepetar, E., Keys, A., *et al*. Death rates among physically active and sedentary employees of the railroad industry. *Amer. J. Publ. Health 52*, 1697–1707 (1962)

Taylor, H.L., Parlin, R.W., Blackburn, H. & Keys, A. Problems in the analysis of the relationship of coronary heart disease to physical activity or its lack, with special reference to sample size and occupational withdrawal. In: *Physical Activity in Health and Disease*, ed. K. Evang & K.L. Andersen (Williams & Wilkins, Baltimore, 1966)

Tepperman, J. & Pearlman, D. Effects of exercise and anemia on coronary arteries of small animals as revealed by the corrosion cast technique. *Circ. Res., 9*, 576–84 (1961)

Teräslinna, P., Partanen, T., Oja, P. & Koskela, A. Some social characteristics and living habits associated with willingness to participate in a physical activity intervention study. *J. Sports Med. Phys. Fitness 10*, 138–44 (1970)

Teräslinna, P., Partanen, T., Pyörälä, K., *et al*. Feasibility study on physical activity intervention. Report on recruiting design, training program, and three months' experience. *Work Environ. Health 6*, 24–31 (1969)

Terjung, R.L. & Tipton, C.M. Plasma thyroxine and thyroid-stimulation hormone levels during submaximal exercise in humans. *Amer. J. Physiol., 220,* 1840–5 (1971)

Terjung, R.L. & Winder, W.W. Exercise and thyroid function. *Med. Sci. Sports 7,* 20–6 (1975)

Texon, M. Causal relationships in heart disease in workmen's compensation cases. In: *Work and the Heart,* ed. F.F. Rosenbaum & E.L. Belknap (P.B. Hoeber, New York, 1959) pp. 426–31

Texon, M. Mechanical factors involved in atherosclerosis. In: *Atherosclerotic Vascular Disease,* ed. A.N. Brest & J.H. Moyer (Appleton Century Crofts, New York, 1967) pp. 23–42

Texon, M. The role of vascular dynamics (mechanical factors) in the development of atherosclerosis. In: *Coronary Heart Disease,* ed. H.I. Russek & B.L. Zohman (Lippincott, Philadelphia, 1971) pp. 121–36

Thompson, P.L. & Lown, B. Exercise and coronary occlusion: experimental studies. In: *Proceedings of Twentieth World Congress of Sports and Medicine,* ed. H. Toyne (Australian Sports Medicine Federation, Melbourne, 1975) p. 278

Tibblin, G., Wilhelmsen, L. & Werkö, L. Risk factors for myocardial infarction and death due to ischemic disease and other causes. *Amer. J. Cardiol., 35,* 514–22 (1975)

Tilkian, A.G., Pfeifer, J.F., Barry, W.H., *et al.* The effect of coronary bypass surgery on exercise-induced ventricular arrhythmias. *Amer. Heart J., 92,* 707–14 (1976)

Tomanek, R.J. Effects of age and exercise on the extent on the myocardial capillary bed. *Anat. Rec., 167,* 55–62 (1970)

Tominaga, S. & Blackburn, H. Prognostic importance of premature beats following myocardial infarction. *JAMA, 223,* 1116–23 (1973)

Trautwein, W., Gottstein, U. & Dudel, J. Der Aktionstrom der Myokardfaser im Sauerstoffmangel. *Pflüg. Archiv., 260,* 40–60 (1954)

Tregear, R.T. Interpretation of skin impedance measurements. *Nature 205,* 600–1 (1965)

Treumann, F. & Schroeder, W. Trainingseinfluss auf Muskeldurchblutung und Herzfrequenz. *Z. f. Kreislauff., 57,* 1024–33 (1968)

Triebwasser, J.H., Johnson, R.L., Burop, R.P., Campbell, J.C., Reardon, W.C. & Blomqvist, C.G. Non-invasive determination of cardiac output by a modified acetylene rebreathing procedure utilizing mass spectrometric measurements. *Aviat. Space Env. Med., 48*, 203–5 (1977)

Truett, J., Cornfield, J. & Kannel, W. A multivariate analysis of the risk of coronary heart disease in Framingham. *J. Chronic Dis., 20*, 511–24 (1967)

Turell, D.J. & Hellerstein, H.K. Six-year average follow-up of 460 consecutive cardiac patients. *Circulation 18*, 790 (abstr.) (1958)

Turpeinen, O., Miettinen, M., Karvonen, M.J., Roine, P., Pekkarinen, M., Lehtosuo, E.J. & Alivirtam, P. Dietary prevention of coronary heart disease: long-term experiment. I. Observation on male subjects. *Amer. J. Clin. Nutr., 21*, 255–76 (1968)

Tuttle, W.B., Cook, W.L. & Fitch, E. Sexual behavior in post-myocardial infarction patients. *Amer. J. Cardiol., 13*, 140–53 (1964)

Ueno, M. The so-called coition death. *Jap. J. Leg. Med., 17*, 33–40 (1963)

Ungerleider, H.E. & Gubner, R.S. Magnitude of the problem of the cardiac-in-industry. In: *Work and the Heart*, ed. F.F. Rosenbaum & E.L. Belknap (P.B. Hoeber, New York, 1959) pp. 417–25

Valentine, P.A., Fluck, D.C., Mounsey, J.P.D., Reid, D., Shillingford, J.P. & Steiner, R.E. Blood-gas changes after acute myocardial infarction. *Lancet* (ii), 837–41 (1966)

Van der Hoeven, G.M.A., Clerens, P.J.A., Donders, J.J.H., Beneken, J.E.W. & Vonk, J.T.C. A study of systolic time intervals during uninterrupted exercise. *Brit. Heart J., 39*, 242–54 (1977)

Van Tassel, R.A. & Edwards, J.E. Rupture of heart complicating myocardial infarction; analysis of 40 cases, including nine examples of left ventricular false aneurysm. *Chest, 61*, 104–16 (1972)

Varnauskas, E. The circulatory adjustment to training in patients with coronary disease. In: *Physical Activity in Health and Disease*, ed. K. Evang & K.L. Andersen (Williams & Wilkins, Baltimore, Md., 1966) pp. 135–45

Varnauskas, E., Bergman, H., Houk, P. & Björntorp, P. Hemodynamic effects of physical training in coronary patients. *Lancet* (ii), 8–12 (1966)

Varnauskas, E. & Holmberg, S. Myocardial blood flow during

exercise in patients with coronary heart disease. Comments on training effects. In: *Coronary Heart Disease and Physical Fitness*, ed. O.A. Lassen & R.O. Malmborg (University Park Press, Baltimore, Md., 1971) pp. 102–4

Vatner, S.F., Higgins, C.B., Franklin, D. & Braunwald, E. Role of tachycardia in mediating the coronary hemodynamic response to severe exercise. *J. Appl. Physiol., 32*, 380—5 (1972)

Vedin, J.A., Wilhelmsson, C.E., Wilhelmsen, L., Bjure, J. & Ekström, J.B. Relation of resting and exercise-induced ectopic beats to other ischemic manifestations and to coronary risk factors. *Amer. J. Cardiol., 30*, 25–31 (1972)

Vedin, J.A., Wilhelmsson,. C., Elmfeldt, D., Säve-Söderbergh, J., Tibblin, G. & Wilhelmsen, L. Deaths and non-fatal reinfarctions during two years' follow up after myocardial infarction. *Acta Med. Scand., 198*, 353–64 (1975)

Venco, A., Saviotte, M., Barzizza, F., Bianchi, C., Tramarin, R. & Zolezzi, F. Electrocardiographic and echocardiographic findings in well-trained athletes. In: *Proceedings of International Conference on Sports Cardiology*, ed. T. Lubich & A. Venerando (A. Gaggi, Bologna, 1980) pp. 717–22

Venerando, A. Electrocardiography in sports medicine. *J. Sports Med. Phys. Fitness 19*, 107–28 (1979)

Verwoerdt, A. & Dovenmuehle, R.H. Heart disease and depression. *Geriatrics 19*, 856–64 (1964)

Vesselinovitch, D., Wissler, R.W., Fisher-Dzoga, K., Hughes, R. & Dubien, L. Regression of atherosclerosis in rabbits. *Atherosclerosis 19*, 259–75 (1974)

Virchow, R. Aus dem pathologisch-anatomischen Curse. *Wien. med. Wschr., 6*, 809 (1856). Cited by D.E. Bowyer & G.A. Gresham. In: *Atherosclerosis*, ed. R.J. Jones (Springer Verlag, Berlin, 1970)

Von der Groeben, J., Toole, J.G., Weaver, C.S. & Fitzgerald, J.W. Noise reduction in exercise electrocardiograms by digital filter techniques. In: *Measurement in Exercise Electrocardiography. The Ernst Simonson Conference*, ed. H. Blackburn (C.C. Thomas, Springfield, Ill., 1969) pp. 41–60

Von Euler, U.S. Sympatho-adrenal activity in physical exercise. *Med. Sci. Sports 6*, 165–73 (1973)

Vuori, I. Studies in the feasibility of long-distance (20–90 km) ski-hikes as a mass sport. In: *Proceedings of Twentieth World Congress of Sports Medicine*, ed. H. Toyne (Australian Sports

Medicine Federation, Melbourne, Australia, 1975)

Wakefield, M.C. A study of mortality amongst the men who have played in the Indiana high school state final basketball tournament. *Res. Quart., 15*, 3–11 (1944)

Wald, A. *Sequential Analysis* (Wiley, New York, 1947)

Wald, N., Howard, S., Smith, P.G. & Kjeldsen, K. Association between atherosclerotic diseases and carboxyhaemoglobin levels in smokers. *Brit. Med. J.* (i), 761–5 (1973)

Walker, J.A, Friedberg, H.D., Flemma, R.J. & Johnson, W.D. Determinants of angiographic patency of aortocoronary vein by-pass grafts. In: *Cardiovascular Surgery 1971*. American Heart Association Monograph 35 (1971)

Walker, W.J. Changing United States life-style and declining vascular mortality: cause or coincidence? *New Engl. J. Med., 297*, 163–5 (1977)

Wang, Y. Reaction to coronary blood flow during exercise. In: *Fitness and Exercise*, ed. J.F. Alexander, R.C. Serfass & C.M. Tipton (Athletic Institute, Chicago, 1972) pp. 51–4

Warnock, N.H., Clarkson, T.B. & Stevenson, R. Effect of exercise on blood coagulation time and atherosclerosis of cholesterol-fed cockerels. *Circ. Res., 5*, 478–80 (1957)

Wassermill, M. & Toor, M. The effects of graded work exercise in 100 patients with ischemic heart disease. In: *Prevention of Ischaemic Heart Disease*, ed. W. Raab (C.C. Thomas, Springfield, Ill., 1966) pp. 348–50

Watanabe, Y. & Dreifus, L.S. Mechanisms of cardiac arrhythmias. In: *Changing Concepts in Cardiovascular Disease*, ed. H.I. Russek & B.L. Zohman (Williams & Wilkins, Baltimore, Md., 1972) pp. 171–82

Weaver, N.K. The selective placement of cardiacs in industry. In: *Work and the Heart*, ed. F.F. Rosenbaum & E L. Belknap (P.B. Hoeber, New York, 1959) pp. 368–74

Weber, G. Regression of arterial lesions: facts and problems. In: *International Conference on Atherosclerosis*, ed. L.A. Carlson, R.A. Paoletti, C.R. Sirtori & G. Weber (Raven Press, New York, 1978) pp. 1–13

Weber, G., Fabbrini, P., Capaccioli, E. & Resi, L. Repair of early cholesterol-induced aortic lesions in rabbits after withdrawal from short-term atherogenic diet. *Atherosclerosis 22*, 565–72 (1975)

Weinblatt, E., Shapiro, S. & Frank, C.W. Prognosis of women with newly diagnosed coronary heart disease — a comparison with course of disease among men. *Amer. J. Publ. Health 63*, 577–93 (1973)

Weinblatt, E., Shapiro, R., Frank, C.W., *et al*. Return to work and work status following first myocardial infarction. *Amer. J. Publ. Health 56*, 169–85 (1966)

Weinblatt, E., Shapiro, S., Frank, C.W. & Singer, R. Prognosis of men after first myocardial infarction: mortality and first recurrence in relation to selected parameters. *Amer. J. Publ. Health 58*, 1329–47 (1968)

Weisman, A.D. & Hackett, T.P. Predilection to death: death and dying as a psychiatric problem. *Psychosom. Med., 23*, 232–57 (1961)

Weiss, E. & English, O.S. *Psychosomatic Medicine* (W.B. Saunders, Philadelphia, 1957)

Wen, C.P. & Gershoff, S.N. Changes in serum cholesterol and coronary heart disease mortality associated with changes in the postwar Japanese diet. *Amer. J. Clin. Nutr., 26*, 616–19 (1973)

Wenger, N.K. Early ambulation after myocardial infarction: Grady Memorial Hospital — Emory University, School of Medicine. In: *Exercise Testing and Exercise Training in Coronary Heart Disease*, ed. J.P. Naughton, H.K. Hellerstein and I.C. Mohler (Academic Press, New York, 1973) pp. 324–8

Wenger, N.K. Does exercise training enhance collateral circulation? In: *Critical Evaluation of Cardiac Rehabilitation*, ed. J. Kellermann & H. Denolin (Karger, Basel, 1977) pp. 143–5

Wenger, N.K., Hellerstein, H.K., Blackburn, H., *et al*. Uncomplicated myocardial infarction: current physician practice in patient management. *JAMA, 224*, 511–14 (1973)

Westling, H. Comnments on mechanism of angina pectoris and effects of drugs. In: *Coronary Heart Disease and Physical Fitness*, ed. O.A. Larsen & R.O. Malmborg (University Park Press, Baltimore, Md., 1971) pp. 119–21

Wexler, B.C. & Greenberg, B.P. Effect of exercise on myocardial infarction in young vs old male rats: electocardiographic changes. *Amer. Heart J., 88*, 343–50 (1974)

Whipp, B.J., Torres, F., Davis, J.A., Wasserman, K. & Casaburi, R. A test to determine the parameters of aerobic function during exercise. *Fed. Proc., 36*, 449 (abstr.) (1977)

White, J.R. EKG changes using carotid artery for heart rate

monitoring. *Med. Sci. Sports 9*, 88–94 (1977)

White, K.L. & Ibrahim, M.A. The distribution of cardiovascular disease in the community. *Ann. Int. Med., 58*, 627–36 (1963)

Widdicombe, J.G. *MTP International Reviews of Science Physiology*, Series 1, *Respiratory Physiology* (Butterworths, London, 1974)

Widmer, L.K., Hartmann, G., Duchosal, F. & Plechl, S.Ch. Risikofaktoren und Gliedmassenarterienverschluss. *Dtsch. med. Wschr., 94*, 1107–10 (1969)

Wiener, L., Dwyer, E.M. & Cos, J.W. Left ventricular haemodynamics in exercise-induced angina patients. *Circulation 38*, 240–9 (1968)

Wikland, B. Medically unattended fatal cases of ischaemic heart disease in a defined population. *Acta Med. Scand., 524*, suppl. (1971)

Wildenthal, K., Morgan, H.E., Opie, L.H. & Srere, P.A. Regulation of cardiac metabolism (symposium). *Circ. Res., 38* (5), suppl., 1, 1–160 (1976)

Wiley, J.F. Effects of 10 weeks of endurance training on left ventricular intervals. *J. Sports Med. Phys. Fitness 11*, 104–11 (1971)

Wilhelmsen, L., Ljungberg, S., Wedel, H., *et al.* A comparison between participants and non-participants in a primary preventive trial. *J. Chronic Dis., 29*, 331–9 (1976)

Wilhelmsen, L., Sanne, H., Elmfelt, D., Grimby, G., Tibblin, G. & Wedel, H. A controlled trial of physical training after myocardial infarction. *Prev. Medicine 4*, 491–508 (1975)

Wilhelmsen, L. & Tibblin, G. Physical inactivity and risk of myocardial infarction — the men born in 1913 study. In: *Coronary Heart Disease and Physical Fitness*, ed. O.A. Larsen & R.O. Malmborg (Munksgaard, Copenhagen, 1971)

Wilhelmsen, L., Tibblin, G. & Werkö, L. A primary preventive study in Göteburg, Sweden. *Prev. Medicine 1*, 153–60 (1972)

Williams, M.H. & Edwards, R.L. Effects of variant training regimens upon submaximal and maximal cardiovascular performance. *Amer. Corr. Therapy J., 25*, 11–15 (1971)

Williamson, J.S., Bauman, D.J. & Tsargaris, T.J. A comparison of hemodynamic and angiographic indices of left ventricular performance in patients with coronary artery disease. *Cardiology 63*, 220–36 (1978)

Wilmore, J.H. & Norton, A.C. *The Heart and Lungs at Work. A*

Primer of Exercise Physiology. (Beckman Instruments, Schiller Park, Ill., 1974)

Wilmore, J.H., Royce, J., Girandola, R.N., Katch, F.I. & Katch, V.L. Physiological alterations resulting from a ten week program of jogging. *Med. Sci. Sports 2*, 7–14 (1970)

Wilson, F.N. The precordial electrocardiogram. *Amer. Heart J., 27*, 19–85 (1944)

Winter, D.A. Noise measurement and quality control techniques in recording and processing of electrocardiograms. In: *Measurement in Exercise Electrocardiography. The Ernst Simonson Conference*, ed. H. Blackburn (C.C. Thomas, Springfield, Ill., 1971) pp. 159–68

Winter, D.A. & Trenholm, B.G. Reliable triggering for exercise electrocardiograms. *IEEE Trans. on Biomed. Eng., 16*, 75–9 (1969)

Wishnie, H.A., Hackett, T.P. & Cassem, N.H. Psychological hazards of convalescence following a myocardial infarction. *JAMA, 215*, 1292–6 (1971)

Wissler, R.W. & Vesselinovitch, D. Animal models of regression. In: *Atherosclerosis IV*, ed. G. Schettler, Y. Goto, Y. Hata & G. Klose (Springer Verlag, Berlin, 1977) pp. 377–85

Wohl, A.J., Lewis, M.R. & Campbell, M.R. Cardiovascular function during early recovery from myocardial infarction. *Circulation 56*, 931–7 (1977)

Wolferth, C.C. & Wood, F.C. Electrocardiographic diagnosis of coronary occlusion by use of chest leads. *Amer. J. Med. Sci., 183*, 30–5 (1932)

Wong, H.O., Kasser, I.S. & Bruce, R.A. Impaired maximal exercise performance with hypertensive cardiovascular disease. *Circulation 39*, 633–8 (1969)

Wood, J.E. The cardiovascular effects of oral contraceptives. *Mod. Concepts Cardiovasc. Dis., 41*, 37–40 (1972)

Wood, P.D. Effect of exercise on plasma lipids and high density lipoprotein levels. In: *Topics in Ischaemic Heart Disease. An International Symposium* (Toronto Rehabilitation Centre, Toronto, 1979)

Wood, P.D., Haskell, W., Klein, H., Lewis, S., Stern, M.P. & Farquhar, J. The distribution of plasma lipoproteins in middle-aged runners. *Metabolism 25*, 1249–57 (1976)

Wood, P.D., McGregor, M., Magidson, O. & Whittaker, W. The effort test in angina pectoris. *Brit. Heart J., 12*, 363–71 (1950)

Woods, J.D. Relative ischemia in the hypertrophied heart. *Lancet* (i), 696–8 (1961)

World Health Organization. *Classification of Atherosclerotic Lesions*, WHO Tech. Rept. 143 (Geneva, 1958)

World Health Organization. *International Classification of Diseases and Causes of Death* (WHO, Geneva, 1968)

World Health Organization. Myocardial infarction community registers. In: *Public Health in Europe 5* (World Health Organization, Geneva, 1976)

World Health Organization. *The Prevention of Coronary Heart Diseases*, WHO Report ICP/CVD 002 (10) (Copenhagen, 1977)

Wright, G.R. & Shephard, R.J. Carbon monoxide, nicotine, and the 'safer' cigarette. *Respiration 35*, 40–52 (1978)

Wright, G.R. & Shephard, R.J. Physiological effects of carbon monoxide. *International Review of Physiology. Environmental Physiology III*, *20*, 311–68 (1979)

Wyatt, H.L. & Mitchell, J.H. Influences of physical training on the heart of dogs. *Circulation Res.*, *35*, 883–9 (1974)

Wyman, M.G. & Hammersmith, L. Comprehensive treatment plan for the prevention of primary ventricular fibrillation in acute myocardial infarction. *Amer. J. Cardiol.*, *33*, 661–7 (1974)

Wynder, E.L., Lemon, F.L. & Bross, I.J. Cancer and coronary artery diseases among seventh-day adventists. *Cancer 12*, 1016–28 (1959)

Wyndham, C.H. & Strydom, N.B. Körperliche Arbeit bei hoher Temperatur. In: *Zentrale Themen der Sportmedizin*, ed. W. Hollmann (Springer Verlag, New York, 1972)

Yamaji, K. & Shephard, R.J. Longevity and causes of death of athletes: a review of the literature. *J. Human Ergol.*, *6*, 13–25 (1977)

Yater, W.M., Welsh, P.P., Stapleton, J.F. & Clark, M.L. Comparison of clinical and pathological aspects of coronary artery disease in men of various age groups: a study of 950 autopsied cases from the Armed Forces Institute of Pathology. *Ann. Int. Med.*, *34*, 353–92 (1971)

Young, M. & Willmot, P. *The Symmetrical Family* (Routledge & Kegan Paul, London, 1973)

Zakopoulos, K.S. Sudden death in football in Greece. *Brit. J. Sports Med.*, *7*, 165 (1973)

Zaret, B.L. Strauss, H.W., Martin, N.D., Wells, H.P. & Flamm, M.D. Non-invasive evaluation of myocardial perfusion with potassium 43. Study of patients at rest, exercise, and during angina pectoris. *New Engl. J. Med., 288*, 809–12 (1973)

Zebe, H., Mehmel, H.C., Leinberger, H., Mäurer, W., Tillmanns, H. & Kübler, W. Phentolamine: short and long-term effects in the treatment of congestive heart failure. In: *Coronary Heart Disease*, ed. M. Kaltenbach, P. Lichtlen, R. Balcon & W.D. Bussmann (G. Thieme, Stuttgart, 1978) pp. 262–5

Zetterquist, S. Effect of training in intermittent claudication. Redistribution of blood flow due to training. In: *Coronary Heart Disease and Physical Fitness*, ed. O.A. Larsen & R.O. Malmborg (University Park Press, Baltimore, Md., 1971) pp. 158–62

Zir, L.M., Miller, S.W., Dinsmore, R.E., *et al*. Interobserver variability in coronary angiography. *Circulation 27*, suppl. II, 51–52 (1975)

Zohman, L.R. Early ambulation of post-myocardial infarction patients: Montefiore Hospital. In: *Exercise Testing and Exercise Training in Coronary Heart Disease*, ed. J.P. Naughton, H.K. Hellerstein & I.C. Mohler (Academic Press, New York, 1973)

Zohman, L.R. & Tobis, J.S. The effect of exercise training on patients with angina pectoris. *Phys. Med., 48*, 525–32 (1967)

Zohman, L.R. & Tobis, J.S. *Cardiac Rehabilitation* (Grune & Stratton, New York, 1970)

Zonereich, S., Rhee, J.J., Zoneraich, O., Jordan, D. & Appel, J. Assessment of cardiac function in marathon runners by graphic non-invasive techniques. *Ann. N.Y. Acad. Sci., 301*, 900–17 (1977)

Zukel, W.J., Lewis, R.H., Enterline, P.E., Painter, R.C., Ralston, L.S., Fawcett, R.M., Meredith, A.P. & Peterson, B. A short-term community study of the epidemiology of coronary heart disease. A preliminary report on the North Dakota study. *Amer. J. Publ. Health 49*, 1630–9 (1959)

Zwillinger, L. Die Digitalis Entwirkung auf das Arbeits Elektrokardiogramm. *Med. Klin., 31*, 977–9 (1935)

INDEX

419